Prevention Practice and Health Promotion

A Health Care Professional's Guide to Health, Fitness, and Wellness

Second Edition

Prevention Practice and Health Promotion

A Health Care Professional's Guide to Health, Fitness, and Wellness

Second Edition

Catherine Rush Thompson, PT, PhD, MS
Associate Professor of Physical Therapy
Department of Physical Therapy Education
Rockhurst University
Kansas City, Missouri

Routledge
Taylor & Francis Group
NEW YORK AND LONDON

Prevention Practice and Health Promotion: A Health Care Professional's Guide to Health, Fitness, and Wellness includes ancillary materials specifically available for faculty use. Included are PowerPoint slides. Please visit www.routledge.com/9781032957975 to obtain access.

First published in hardback 2024

First published 2015 by SLACK Incorporated

Published 2024 by Routledge
605 Third Avenue, New York, NY 10158

and by Routledge
4 Park Square, Milton Park, Abingdon, Oxon OX14 4RN

Routledge is an imprint of the Taylor & Francis Group, an informa business

Publisher's Note
The publisher has gone to great lengths to ensure the quality of this reprint but points out that some imperfections in the original copies may be apparent.

Library of Congress Cataloging-in-Publication Data
Prevention practice (Thompson)
Prevention practice and health promotion : a health care professional's guide to health, fitness, and wellness / edited by Catherine Rush Thompson. -- Second edition.
p. ; cm.
Preceded by: Prevention practice : a physical therapist's guide to health, fitness, and wellness / edited by Catherine Rush Thompson. 2007.
Includes bibliographical references and index.
I. Thompson, Catherine Rush, 1954- editor. II. Title.
[DNLM: 1. Health Promotion--methods. 2. Primary Prevention--methods. WA 108]
RM700
613.7--dc23

ISBN: 978-1-03-295797-5 (hbk)
ISBN: 978-1-61711-084-9 (pbk)
ISBN: 978-1-00-352588-2 (ebk)

DOI: 10.4324/9781003525882

DEDICATION

"Man is a knot into which relationships are tied."—Antoine de Saint-Exupéry, *Flight to Arras* (1942), translated from French by Lewis Galantière

This book is dedicated those who are my "knot": my family, both nuclear and extended. May my two sons, Richard and Eric, live long and healthy lives, and may Jerry Thompson (1951-2003) be remembered for his humor, grace, and dignity.

CONTENTS

Acknowledgments

"We are what we repeatedly do. Excellence, then, is not an act, but a habit."—Aristotle

I would like to personally thank my professional colleagues who have supported this effort and provided valuable insight regarding the growing role of preventive care in health care. More specifically, I would like to thank those who contributed their time and effort to this book through sharing their expertise and reviewing the book's content for accuracy and relevance. I am also indebted to my family members, friends, colleagues, students, and patients, who provided both the incentive and the inspiration for expanding my book promoting health, fitness, and wellness. I am very grateful for lessons learned in life through friendship, love, loss, and hope.

About the Author

Catherine Rush Thompson, PT, PhD, MS, was born in Kansas City and attended the University of Colorado Medical Center, graduating with distinction with a BS in physical therapy. With support from the Hillman Medical Student Fellowship, she attended and graduated with distinction from the University of Kansas Medical Center with an MS in special education with an emphasis on children with illness and other health impairments. With support from the Arthur Mag Fellowship and the UMKC Community Scholars Fellowship at the University of Missouri at Kansas City, she completed her interdisciplinary PhD, incorporating studies in physiology, psychology, biochemistry, neuroscience, exercise science, and education. Although her primary clinical practice focuses on individuals with developmental disabilities across the lifespan, she has worked in practice settings in acute care, outpatient care, long-term care, school-based therapy, home health, and private practice. Currently she is an associate professor in the Department of Physical Therapy Education at Rockhurst University.

Dr. Thompson's travel to more than 50 countries gives her insight into global health care disparities and the need for multicultural education and advocacy for populations at risk for health problems. Her research interests focus on growth and development across the lifespan, motor learning, and prevention practice. She hopes this book will encourage health care professionals to advocate for healthy lifestyles and collaboratively work toward a healthier world.

Contributing Authors

Shawn T. Blakeley, PT, CWI, CEES, MBA (Chapter 20)
Area Vice President
Aegis Therapies
Chicago, Illinois

Ann Marie Decker, PT, MSA, GCS, CEEAA (Chapter 9)
Clinical Assistant Professor of Physical Therapy and Academic Coordinator of Clinical Education
Department of Physical Therapy Education
Rockhurst University
Kansas City, Missouri

Shannon DeSalvo, PT (Chapter 8)
Physical Therapist Specialist in Pelvic Rehabilitation
Foundational Concepts, PA
Kansas City, Missouri

Amy Foley, DPT, PT (Chapters 13, 14, 16)
Associate Professor of Physical Therapy
Department of Physical Therapy Education
Rockhurst University
Kansas City, Missouri

Martha Highfield, PhD, RN (Chapter 10)
Professor of Nursing
California State University
Northridge, California

Steven G. Lesh, PhD, PT, SCS, ATC (Chapter 19)
Chair, Physical Therapy Department
Professor of Physical Therapy
Southwest Baptist University
Bolivar, Missouri

Gail Regan, PhD, MS, PT (Chapters 9, 13, 14)
Associate Professor
Physical Education Department
Castleton State College
Castleton, Vermont

Mike Studer, PT, MHS, NCS, CEEAA, CWT (Chapter 15)
President
Northwest Rehabilitation Associates
Salem, Oregon

Preface

"Prevention is better than cure."—Desiderius Erasmus

This is the second edition of *Prevention Practice: A Guide for Health, Fitness, and Wellness*, expanded to offer evidence-based resources to all health care professionals incorporating health promotion and preventive care in their practice settings. Whereas health promotion encourages others to improve their health, my definition of *prevention practice* is the conscious habit of caring for one's health, fitness, and wellness mentally, physically, spiritually, psychosocially, and environmentally. As with any type of practice, prevention practice relies on mindfulness and consistency to become a lifestyle habit. As health care professionals, we need to support and advocate for prevention practice for ourselves, our patients, our communities, and society at large.

The intent of this book is to provide health information contributing to "a society in which all people live long, healthy lives" (Healthy People 2020) and supporting health care professionals in their efforts to "improve equity in health, reduce health risks, promote healthy lifestyles and settings, and respond to the underlying determinants of health" (World Health Organization). The authors of *Prevention Practice and Health Promotion: A Health Care Professional's Guide to Health, Fitness, and Wellness* compiled information relevant to health, wellness, and fitness as a ready resource for those promoting holistic health care in diverse practice settings. Written for students and clinicians, this book introduces key concepts of health, fitness, and wellness and offers detailed information for screening individuals across the lifespan, identifying key risk factors for specific populations, educating clients and their families about healthy lifestyle behaviors, and developing effective interventions to promote health, fitness, and wellness. Additionally, this book provides a theoretical framework for program development, including marketing and management strategies to address both individual and community needs. Recognizing the cost-effectiveness of preventive care, health care professionals must work collaboratively in their expanded roles in health promotion and wellness, complementing evidence-based management of medical conditions. Finally, the publisher offers accompanying PowerPoint presentations to facilitate educating others about prevention practice and health promotion.

Through the process of writing and editing this book, I discovered a wealth of resources that can be readily accessed through technology and current literature. My hope is that fellow health care providers and those seeking healthy lifestyles will further explore needed resources to holistically counsel others in preventing illness and injury and in mindfully managing health conditions, ultimately improving their quality of life.

"The cure of the part should not be attempted without the cure of the whole."—Plato

Catherine Rush Thompson, PT, PhD, MS

FOREWORD

"An ounce of prevention is worth a pound of cure."—Benjamin Franklin

The importance of quality of life and a healthy lifestyle has been recognized for decades, with the World Health Organization (WHO) promoting the importance of a healthy state of being since the late 1940s. Although slow to evolve, virtually every health care organization and professional association today speaks clearly to the need for promotion of health and well-being, through policy and position statements on the importance of prevention, health, fitness, and wellness. Although still present, the dichotomy between prevention and wellness on one hand and disease management and treatment on the other is beginning to be addressed. Since the inception of the Healthy People initiative in 2000, when the first set of national strategies for improving the health of Americans by the end of the 21st century was released by the Department of Health and Human Services, there has been a very gradual paradigm shift from an emphasis on illness to an emphasis on health and well-being. In keeping with this vision toward a commitment to health, *Prevention Practice and Health Promotion: A Health Care Professional's Guide to Health, Fitness, and Wellness*, offers the health care professional an evidence-based approach to preventive care and health promotion across a variety of practice settings and age groups. Addressing the broad compendium of a holistic approach to health, wellness, and fitness, this comprehensive book emphasizes the action of primary care vs the treatment of tertiary care and serves as an important resource for health care professionals. This notable book is a testament to Dr. Thompson's long-standing and dedicated career and her commitment to the health and well-being of others.

Ellen F. Spake, PhD
Assistant to the President
Office of Mission and Ministry
Rockhurst University
Kansas City, Missouri

1

Prevention Practice
A Holistic Perspective for Health Care

Catherine Rush Thompson, PT, PhD, MS

"The Doctor of the future will give no medicine, but will interest his patient in the care of the human frame, in diet, and in the cause and prevention of disease."—Thomas Edison, *The Newark Advocate*, January 2, 1903

Health

The word *health* is derived from the Old English term *hal*, meaning sound or whole. Health is essentially the purpose of medicine, the promotion and restoration of wholeness. Although *health* is broadly defined as "the condition of being sound in mind, body, and spirit,"[1] the World Health Organization defines *health* as "a state of complete physical, mental, and social well-being, and not merely the absence of disease or infirmity."[2] Health is a more dynamic process, "a quality of life involving dynamic interaction and independence among an individual's physical well-being, his [her] mental and emotional reactions, and the social complex in which he [she] exists."[3] Finally, "spiritual health" or "the passion one has to fulfill a need" or personal goal is yet another aspect of health that should be recognized by health professionals. In all of these definitions of health, there are physical, mental, social, and spiritual components: key factors for the comprehensive health examination.

Health care professionals are shifting their paradigm perspective from one emphasizing illness to one stressing health, function, quality of life, and well-being. This shift in health care has resulted in a surge in preventive strategies designed to reduce disease by helping individuals modify their lifestyle behaviors to optimize health. *Optimal health* is defined as the conscious pursuit of the highest qualities of the physical, environmental, mental, emotional, spiritual, and social aspects of the human experience.[4] Lifestyle changes promoting optimal health can be facilitated through a combination of efforts that (1) enhance self-awareness and knowledge of healthy habits, (2) change behaviors that interfere with good health, and (3) create environments that support good health practices. The importance of supportive environments for producing lasting change cannot be overemphasized.

Thompson CR.
Prevention Practice and Health Promotion: A Health Care Professional's Guide to Health, Fitness, and Wellness, Second Edition (pp 1-17).

Poor health may include physical ailments causing acute or chronic disabilities, as well as mental health issues that limit independent functioning. Poor health has a significant effect on the individual, the family, the community, and society at large. Depending on the severity of illness, the individual may lose functional independence and the opportunity to fulfill a role in the home and community. Family members also lose the support of those who are ill and often must adjust their roles and goals to meet the needs of someone who is disabled. Society also suffers from injury and disease that may be preventable. One example of a preventable health condition leading to acute or chronic disabilities is obesity. According to the Centers for Disease Control and Prevention, "obesity-related conditions include heart disease, stroke, type 2 diabetes and certain types of cancer, some of the leading causes of preventable death."[5] Obesity is also a contributing factor to physically disabling conditions, such as osteoarthritis, infertility, and sleep apnea. The cost of this health condition has had a major effect on American society; it is estimated that the medical care costs of obesity total more than $147 billion.[5]

A rising trend in poor health reported in the United States indicates an immediate need for preventive care to reduce medical conditions that lead to disability. According to the Behavioral Risk Factor Surveillance System,[6] 3.9% of Americans reported poor health in 2010 (up from 3.5% reporting poor health in 1993), whereas only 20.2% reported excellent health in 2010 (down from 25.3% in 1993). Only 28.4% of adults exercise at the level of moderate intensity for more than 300 minutes/week or vigorous intensity for more than 150 minutes/week, as recommended by the Surgeon General. Nationwide, more than half of the adult population is overweight (36.2%) or obese (27.2%), and only 23.5% consume the recommended 5 fruits or vegetables daily. These data indicate the growing need for preventive care (Table 1-1).[6]

Poor health affects personal satisfaction and the ability to meet family needs, personal responsibilities, and the demands of the workplace. Poor health is not only financially costly, but it also takes a toll on the emotional, psychological, and social well-being of all affected. According to the National Center for Chronic Disease Prevention and Health Promotion,[7] "certain behaviors—often begun while young—put people at high risk for premature death, disability, or chronic diseases. The following are the most common of such behaviors:

- Smoking and other forms of tobacco use
- Eating high-fat and low-fiber foods
- Not engaging in enough physical activity
- Abusing alcohol or other drugs
- Not availing oneself of proven medical methods for preventing disease or diagnosing disease early (eg, flu shots and evidenced-based screening procedures)
- Engaging in violent behavior or behavior that may cause unintentional injuries (eg, driving while intoxicated)"

A study conducted by the Centers for Disease Control and Prevention[8] determined that depression, anxiety, and other emotional problems were a leading cause of limited activity, as measured in a quality-of-life profile. Mental health issues were followed by cancer, diabetes mellitus, stroke, high blood pressure, back and neck problems, heart problems, walking problems, and joint problems. All of these conditions can be positively affected by health promotion activities and a healthy lifestyle.

Wellness

Wellness is often used synonymously with health; however, wellness is a more comprehensive construct. According to the National Wellness Institute, "wellness is an active process of becoming aware of and making choices toward a more successful existence."[9] In other words, wellness is an

Table 1-1. 2009 Behavioral Risk Survey Results of Adults Aged 18 to 75+ Years (N=422,199)				
VARIABLE	**CATEGORY**	**NO. OF RESPONDENTS**	**PERCENT**	**95% CONFIDENCE INTERVAL***
Race/ethnicity	White non-Hispanic	336,768	13.4	13.2 to 13.7
	Black non-Hispanic	32,687	20.8	19.9 to 21.7
	Asian	6974	9.2	7.9 to 10.4
	Pacific Islander	689	18.7	12.2 to 25.1
	American Indian/ Alaskan Native	5900	24.3	21.9 to 26.6
	Other non-Hispanic	9170	20.7	18.9 to 22.5
	Hispanic	25,420	24.7	23.6 to 25.8
Educational level	<High school	38,788	37.0	35.8 to 38.1
	High school graduate	126,094	20.0	19.5 to 20.5
	Some college	113,360	14.4	13.9 to 14.8
	College graduate	142,517	7.1	6.8 to 7.4
Annual household income level	<$15,000	40,578	39.6	38.5 to 40.8
	$15,000 to $24,999	64,396	27.3	26.5 to 28.1
	$25,000 to $34,999	44,409	20.2	19.3 to 21.0
	$35,000 to $49,999	56,660	13.4	12.8 to 14.0
	$50,000 or more	159,624	6.2	5.9 to 6.5
	Unknown/ refused	56,532	18.6	17.8 to 19.4
Employment status	Employed	175,980	8.6	8.3 to 8.9
	Self-employed	35,747	9.5	8.7 to 10.2
	Out of work 1 year or more	9862	26.1	24.3 to 27.9
	Homemaker	31,482	16.8	15.9 to 17.7
	Student	6520	6.5	5.5 to 7.6

(continued)

Table 1-1 (continued). 2009 Behavioral Risk Survey Results of Adults Aged 18 to 75+ Years (N = 422,199)

VARIABLE	CATEGORY	NO. OF RESPONDENTS	PERCENT	95% CONFIDENCE INTERVAL*
	Retired	118,064	24.6	24.1 to 25.0
	Unable to work	28,272	66.7	65.4 to 68.0
Body mass index category	Underweight	6411	21.2	19.1 to 23.3
	Normal weight	135,384	10.9	10.5 to 11.3
	Overweight	147,537	13.5	13.1 to 13.9
	Obese	113,658	24.0	23.5 to 24.6
Cigarette smoking status	Current smoker, every day	50,476	23.6	22.8 to 24.4
	Current smoker, some days	18,101	20.6	19.2 to 22.0
	Former smoker	127,400	18.8	18.4 to 19.3
	Never smoked	223,536	12.4	12.0 to 12.7
Binge drinking	Yes	43,893	10.4	9.7 to 11.1
	No	365,836	16.8	16.5 to 17.1
Leisure time physical activity	Yes	307,156	11.3	11.0 to 11.5
	No	114,516	30.2	29.6 to 30.8
Self-rated health	Good-excellent	341,245	0.0	0.0 to 0.0
	Fair-poor	80,954	100.0	100.0 to 100.0
Diabetes mellitus	Yes	50,749	45.0	44.1 to 46.0
	No	371,058	13.0	12.7 to 13.3
High blood pressure	Yes	163,836	29.0	28.5 to 29.5
	No	257,484	10.5	10.2 to 10.8

*A confidence interval describes the level of variability in a sample estimate and specifies the range in which the true value of the population that the sample represents is likely to fall.

Source: Health, United States, 2012: with special feature on emergency care. Hyattsville, MD: National Center for Health Statistics (US); May 2013.

active, lifelong process of becoming aware of choices and making decisions toward a more balanced and fulfilling life. Wellness involves choices about one's life and the priorities that determine one's lifestyle. Wellness integrates mental, social, occupational, emotional, spiritual, and physical dimensions of one's life and reflects how one feels about life, as well as one's ability to function effectively.

Dimensions of Wellness

According to the systems theory of wellness, the multiple dimensions of wellness are essential subelements of a larger system, yet these dimensions function independently as their own subelements.[10] When one dimension of wellness is disrupted, such as when an individual gets injured in an accident, other dimensions of wellness reciprocally interrelated to that dimension are also disrupted, requiring adaptation of the whole individual. When an individual has emotional problems, these problems affect the mental, social, occupational, spiritual, and physical dimensions of that person.

Corbin et al,[11] prominent educators in the field of exercise and health promotion, outline the 6 dimensions of wellness described by the National Wellness Institute. These descriptions include examples of physical wellness, spiritual wellness, social wellness, psychological wellness, emotional wellness, and intellectual wellness.

1. *Physical wellness* is the positive perception and expectation of health. Physical wellness includes the ability to effectively meet daily demands at work and to use free time. A person with a positive perception and expectation of health may be more likely to embrace healthy lifestyle behaviors that prevent injury and illness.
2. *Spiritual wellness* is the belief in a unifying force between the mind and body. Spiritual wellness includes a person's ability to establish values and act on a system of beliefs as well as to establish and carry out meaningful and constructive lifetime goals. Those individuals with a strong belief system may be more likely to carry out goals that keep both the mind and body healthy.
3. *Social wellness* is the perception of having support available from family or friends in times of need and the perception of being a valued support provider. Social wellness includes a person's ability to successfully interact with others and to establish meaningful relationships that enhance the quality of life for all people involved in the interaction, including oneself. Social support is a valuable asset for health and wellness, as well as recovery from illness and injury.
4. *Psychological wellness* is a general perception that one will experience positive outcomes to the events and circumstances in life. This perception suggests a positive attitude or outlook about life. The intangible qualities of optimism, determination, and hope are vital in preventive practice and positively dealing with life problems.
5. *Emotional wellness* is the progression of a secure self-identity and a positive sense of self-regard, both of which are facets of self-esteem. Emotional wellness includes the ability to cope with daily circumstances and to deal with personal feelings in a positive, optimistic, and constructive manner. A person who dwells on negative emotions and who has negative self-esteem does not reap the benefits of a positive self-attitude. It is important for health care professionals to consider that ill or injured individuals are at risk for lower self-esteem as they lose functional abilities and, potentially, their significant roles in life.
6. *Intellectual wellness* is the perception of being internally energized by an optimal amount of intellectually stimulating activity. This type of intellectual stimulation must be sufficient to challenge intellectual abilities but not so overwhelming that there is no time for mental repose. Both intellectual overload and intellectual underload can adversely affect health. Intellectual wellness includes a person's ability to learn and to use information to enhance the quality of daily living and optimal functioning.

Theologian Howard Clinebell[12] offers an even more comprehensive perspective of wellness with his 7 dimensions of wellness. His dimensions are more encompassing of the environment and a world perspective. The definitions of his 7 dimensions of wellness include spiritual well-being, mental well-being, physical well-being, relationship well-being, work well-being, play well-being, and the well-being of our world.

1. The *Spiritual Well-Being Dimension* incorporates healthy religious beliefs, practices, values, and institutions that energize and enrich all aspects of our lives. This dimension of well-being addresses an individual's need for purpose, guidance, meaning, and values. The ill person who

has healthy religious or spiritual beliefs and values has a sense of personal value and spiritual security.

2. The *Mental Well-Being Dimension* represents the profound interdependence of the mind and body that manifests itself in our mental and physical health. Mental well-being incorporates problem solving, creativity, clarity in thinking, service, and productivity. Those who are given the opportunity to creatively problem solve and provide services to others are believed to have an improved mental well-being.
3. The *Physical Well-Being Dimension* reflects the body's health. Physical well-being is evidenced by the ability to experience sensations without pain, to effectively function with adequate energy, to be responsible for self-care, and to nurture others. Many pathologies and injuries significantly affect this dimension, particularly those presenting with pain.
4. The *Relationship Well-Being Dimension* represents the most important factor for our healing and general wellness. This dimension incorporates the need for nurturing and love, for giving and receiving, for empowering others, and for creating interpersonal bonds. On a larger scale, this well-being relates to peaceful coexistence with others.
5. The *Work Well-Being Dimension* satisfies the thirst for purpose. This dimension of wellness addresses the need for fulfilling a purpose in one's vocation. Self-worth, satisfaction, and personal fulfillment are all related to the individual's ability to serve the community in a meaningful way.
6. The *Play Well-Being Dimension* acknowledges that play provides the individual with laughter, cheer, energy, and balance. It is the ability to successfully play that provides the needed healing and revitalization to meet the demands of the other dimensions. Allowing time for this important dimension is a high priority for overall well-being, as noted in the following quote by Kahil Gibran[13]: "In the sweetness of friendship let there be laughter, and sharing of pleasures. For in the dew of little things, the heart finds its morning and is refreshed."
7. The *Well-Being of Our World Dimension* reflects an individual's perspective on living in a healthy environment and protecting natural resources. This final dimension incorporates a broad overview of the world. Wellness in this dimension includes responsibility, justice, an earth-caring lifestyle, a desire of well-being for all, adequate health care, dependence on others in the community, political participation, and the recognition of institutions as potential resources for meeting needs beyond the self.

These 7 dimensions are more holistic and provide a framework for exploring various aspects of health and wellness, including cultural perspectives of the world. Although the health care provider is often trained to provide education focusing on the physical dimensions of wellness, a more comprehensive or holistic perspective enables these professionals to make appropriate referrals to address other dimensions of well-being. Those in poor health benefit from additional resources, such as educational materials, support groups, and referrals to professionals with expert knowledge.

Models of Wellness

Various theorists have developed models and simplified descriptions of the multidimensional aspects of wellness. In addition to providing a framework for identifying clients' needs, these models of wellness offer insight into the management of illness and prevention practice. As early as 1972, Travis and Ryan[14] developed a continuum of wellness illustrating the effect of wellness on health and premature death (Figure 1-1). The Illness-Wellness Continuum illustrates the spectrum from good health—characterized by awareness, education, and growth—to poor health leading to premature death, experienced as signs and symptoms of disease and disability.

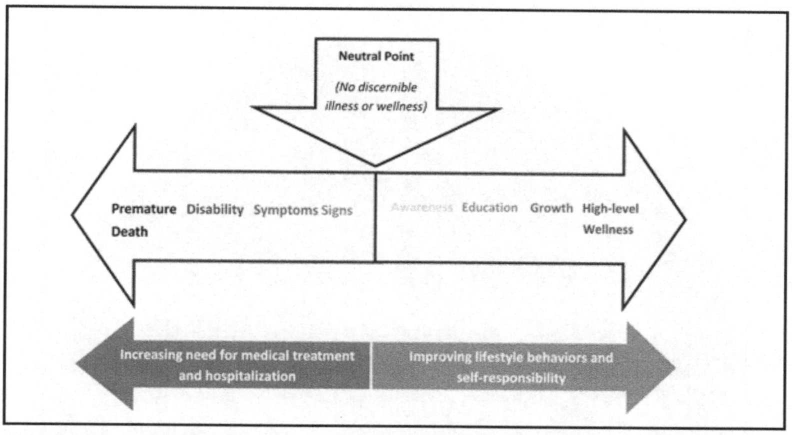

Figure 1-1. Travis and Ryan's Illness-Wellness Continuum. (Adapted from Travis J, Ryan R. *Wellness Workbook: How to Achieve Enduring Health and Vitality.* 3rd ed. Berkeley, CA: Ten Speed Press; 2003.)

Signs of pathology, such as abnormal blood counts and hypertension, may not be perceived by the individual but can generally be detected by medical testing, such as blood tests, vital signs, and imaging studies (ie, physiological and anatomical markers of pathology or illness). Symptoms of pathology are generally more subjective and often include an individual's report of pain, discomfort, fatigue, or feeling "ill." The individual often experiences symptoms of pathology or the awareness of illness after pathophysiological changes have taken place at the subcellular and cellular level. *Disability* is the inability to engage in gainful activity or work and commonly ensues when the individual feels very ill. Disability often results from illness and has a significant effect on all aspects of an individual's well-being.[15] According to the Social Security Administration, disability is "an inability to engage in any substantial gainful work activity because of a medically determinable physical or mental impairment that is expected to last for 12 continuous months or result in death."[16]

Both *acute disability* and *chronic disability* can significantly affect multiple dimensions of wellness, including mental well-being, physical well-being, work well-being, and relationship well-being. Travis and Ryan's[14] model illustrates the point where prevention practices (eg, awareness of and engagement in healthy lifestyle practices) most positively affect health and wellness. Prevention practice should be initiated when the individual is healthy and free of clinical manifestations of illness. Although medical intervention often initiates when an individual presents with signs or symptoms of pathology, earlier intervention (emphasizing awareness and avoidance of risk factors for illness, education about healthy lifestyle behaviors, and access to up-to-date and accurate knowledge) can provide a level of wisdom that buffers individuals from pathology and premature death. For example, if an individual knows that a sedentary lifestyle and high-fat diet can increase the risks of heart disease, engaging in regular, moderate-intensity exercise and eating healthy, nutritional meals could postpone illness. If an individual who is predisposed to illness has routine screenings, then these tests can often detect signs of pathology earlier in the course of disease and allow more immediate and effective interventions.

A wellness perspective invites the health care professional to provide interventions across the spectrum of health and wellness, offering healthy individuals the awareness and knowledge to develop appropriate lifestyle behaviors. Even when an individual presents with signs and symptoms of pathology, education of secondary complications prevents further signs and symptoms leading to disability. In 1977, Donald B. Ardell[17] introduced a new model of wellness that placed self-responsibility at the center his wellness paradigm (Figure 1-2). In this model, *self-responsibility* is surrounded by nutritional awareness and physical fitness, emotional intelligence, meaning and purpose, and relationship dynamics. According to Ardell,[17] "Wellness is first and foremost a

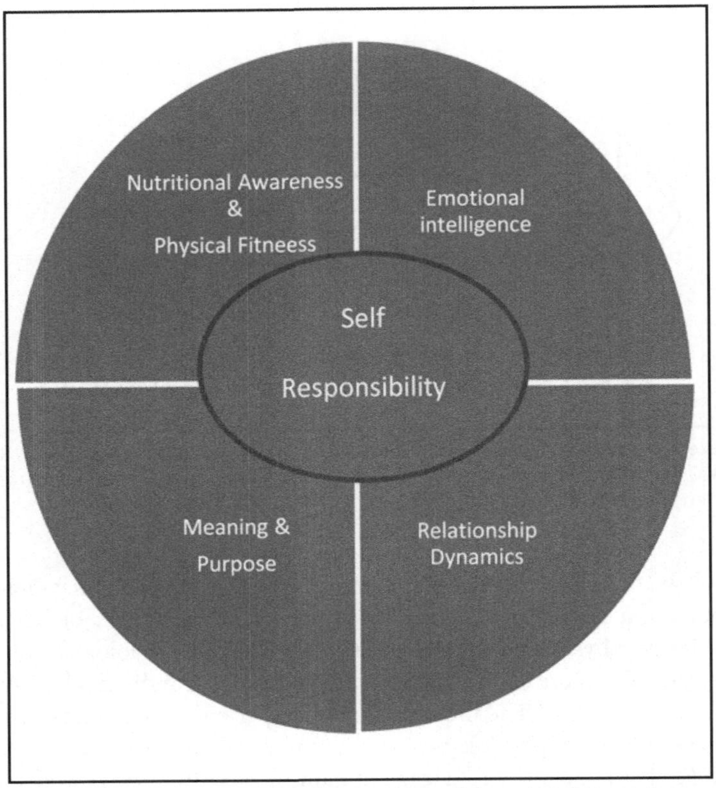

Figure 1-2. Ardell's model of wellness. (Adapted from Ardell D. *14 Days to Wellness: The Easy, Effective, and Fun Way to Optimum Health.* New York, NY: New World Library; 1999.)

choice to assume responsibility for the quality of your life. It begins with a conscious decision to shape a healthy lifestyle. Wellness is a mind-set, a predisposition to adopt a series of key principles in varied life areas that lead to high levels of well-being and life satisfaction." Self-responsibility in assuming wellness behaviors is recognized as one, if not the most, significant factor determining health status.[17] This model emphasizing self-responsibility suggests that health professionals need to provide not only educational programs that promote health and wellness, but also relationship skills and the importance of nurturing one's well-being.

Ardell[17] acknowledged the personal values that motivate individuals—meaning and purpose as well as interpersonal relationships—and developed the domains of wellness to include the physical domain, the mental domain, and the meaning and purpose domain, with 14 skill areas across these 3 domains. Exercise, nutrition, appearance, adaptation and challenges, and lifestyle habits are included in the physical domain. Emotional intelligence, effective decisions, stress management, factual knowledge, and mental health are listed in the mental domain. Finally, meaning/purpose, relationships, humor, and play are incorporated in the meaning and purpose domain, emphasizing the role of self-responsibility in controlling personal health and wellness.

Although health care professionals might focus on the physical domain (particularly addressing exercise, nutrition, knowledge of potential impairments, functional limitations, and lifestyle behaviors influencing health), effective strategies to manage stress, receive social support, and achieve personal goals are also key components of intervention. This model suggests that humor, play, mentally engaging activities, and physically challenging activities should be incorporated into comprehensive wellness programs.

Quality of Life

Quality of life is defined in various ways, ranging from the ability to lead a normal life to the fulfillment of personal goals and self-actualization. According to the World Health Organization (WHO), quality of life is "the individuals' perceptions of their positions in life, in the context of the cultural and value systems in which they live, and in relation to their goals, expectations, standards, and concerns. It is a broad-ranging concept affected in a complex way by each individual's physical health, psychological state, level of independence, social relationships, personal beliefs and their relationship to salient features of their environment."[18] The WHO Quality of Life Measure[18] includes the following domains, with unique facets included in each domain:

- Physical health (energy and fatigue, pain and discomfort, and sleep and rest)
- Psychological health (bodily image and appearance, negative feelings, positive feelings, self-esteem, thinking, learning, memory and concentration)
- Level of independence (mobility, activities of daily living, dependence on medicinal substances and medical aids, and work capacity)
- Social relationships (personal relationships, social support, sexual activity)
- Environment (financial resources, freedom, physical safety and security, accessibility and quality of health and social care, home environment, opportunities for acquiring new information and skill, and participation in and opportunities for recreation/leisure, physical environment, including pollution/noise/traffic/climate and transportation)
- Spirituality/religion/personal beliefs

A quality-of life-measure commonly used across health care settings is the most recent version of the Short Form (SF)-36.[19] The SF-36 is a measure that relies on a consumer's report of his or her health status. It is practical, cost-effective, and easy to use. The survey assesses the following 8 health areas of health:

1. Limitations in physical activities because of health problems
2. Limitations in social activities because of physical or emotional problems
3. Limitations in usual role activities because of physical health problems
4. Limitations in bodily pain
5. General mental health (psychological distress and well-being)
6. Limitations in usual role activities because of emotional problems
7. Vitality (energy and fatigue)
8. General health perceptions

Other types of measures focus on health indices that determine the *quality adjusted life years* (QALY) or a year of life adjusted for its "quality" or its "value."[20] A year in perfect health is considered equal to 1.0 QALY. For this measure, the QALY would be discounted by each year in ill health. For example, a year during which the individual was bedridden for 6 months might have a value equal to 0.5 QALY.[20] While considering objective quality-of-life measures, the health care professional must keep in mind that multiple personal, social, and environmental factors can affect an individual's quality of life on any given day.

Holistic Health

The philosophy of holistic health care is compatible with medicine designed to restore health and wellness. The clinician's comprehensive role in health care requires a holistic perspective of the individual seeking care. This holistic perspective looks beyond the physical functioning of the individual and recognizes the importance of multiple factors contributing to good health and optimal wellness, emphasizing the unity of mind, spirit, and body. According to the American Holistic Health Association,[21] this expanded perspective of holistic health care considers the whole person and the whole situation. Although there are many definitions of holistic health care, the characteristics of holistic medicine that apply to a wellness practice incorporate recognizing the interdependent parts of the whole being, including the physical, mental, emotional, and spiritual aspects of the individual. This recognition of the multiple factors influencing health and wellness leads to the following:

- Identifying and managing the root causes of disease processes
- Empowering the individual to manage these pathological processes
- Providing a comprehensive perspective of the individual in multiple social roles[22]

According to this holistic perspective, disease or illness manifests when the individual's state of being ("ideally the balanced state of mind, body, and spirit"[21]) is not in equilibrium. Holistic health recognizes the multiple dimensions of wellness and the importance of balancing these dimensions for optimal health. Health care professionals can choose to use a more holistic approach for client management as compared with a more traditional approach; however, evidence-based practice is essential. Additional research is needed in the areas of alternative medicine to determine whether less traditional approaches are cost-effective and are the most appropriate. The holistic approach tends to be more health-oriented and teaches the patient to be responsible for his or her own health. Table 1-2 illustrates the differences between traditional or conventional medicine, and holistic medicine, as well as the strengths and weaknesses of these 2 approaches.[21]

According to the American Holistic Medicine Association,[21] the holistic medical practice involves the following principles of care:

- Optimal health is the primary goal of holistic medical practice. It is the conscious pursuit of the highest level of functioning and balance of the physical, environmental, mental, emotional, social, and spiritual aspects of human experience, resulting in a dynamic state of being fully alive. This creates a condition of well-being regardless of the presence or absence of disease.
- Love has healing power. Holistic health care practitioners strive to meet the patient with grace, kindness, acceptance, and spirit without condition because love is life's most powerful healer.
- Holistic medicine addresses the whole person. Holistic health care practitioners view people as the unity of body, mind, spirit, and the systems in which they live.
- Treatment emphasizes prevention. Holistic health care practitioners promote health, prevent illness, and help raise awareness of "dis-ease" in our lives rather than merely managing symptoms. A holistic approach relieves symptoms, modifies contributing factors, and enhances the patient's life system to optimize future well-being.
- Holistic care relies on innate healing power. All people have innate powers of healing in their bodies, minds, and spirits. Holistic health care practitioners evoke and help patients use these powers to affect the healing process.
- Holistic medicine integrates healing systems. Holistic health care practitioners embrace a lifetime of learning about all safe and effective options in diagnosis and treatment. These options come from a variety of traditions and are selected to best meet the unique needs of the patient. The realm of choices may include lifestyle modification and complementary approaches, as well as conventional drugs and surgery.
- Holistic medicine offers relationship-centered care. The ideal practitioner-patient relationship is a partnership that encourages patient autonomy and values the needs and insights of both parties. The quality of this relationship is an essential contributor to the healing process.

Table 1-2. Comparing Holistic Medicine and Conventional Medicine

	HOLISTIC MEDICINE	CONVENTIONAL MEDICINE
Philosophy	Based on allopathic, osteopathic, naturopathic, energy, and ethno-medicine	Based on allopathic medicine
Primary objective of care	Designed to promote optimal health and to prevent and treat disease	Designed to cure or reduce pathology
Diagnosis	Includes a medical history, physical examination, laboratory data, holistic health care sheet	Includes a medical history, physical examination, laboratory data
Primary method of care	Empowers patients to heal themselves through health promotion and lifestyle changes	Eliminates signs and symptoms
Primary care treatment options	Emphasizes diet, exercise, environmental measures, attitudinal and behavioral modifications, relationship and spiritual counseling	Emphasizes medications and surgery
Secondary care treatment options	Offers options of botanical (herbal) medicine, homeopathy, acupuncture, manual medicine, biomolecular therapies, physical therapy, medications, and surgery	Offers options of diet, exercise, physical therapy, and stress management
Weaknesses	Shortage of holistic physicians and training programs; time intensive, requiring a commitment to a healing process, not a quick fix	Ineffective in preventing and curing chronic disease; expensive
Strengths	Teaches patients to take responsibility for their own health, and is cost-effective in treating both acute and chronic illness, therapeutic in preventing and treating chronic disease, essential in creating optimal health	Highly therapeutic in treating both acute and life-threatening illness and injuries

Adapted from Ivker RS. Comparing holistic and conventional medicine. *Holistic Medicine: The Journal of the American Holistic Medical Association.* Winter 1999.

- Individuality is emphasized in holistic care. Holistic health care practitioners focus patient care on the unique needs and nature of the person who has an illness, rather than the illness that has the person.
- Holistic practitioners teach by example. Holistic health care practitioners continually work toward the personal incorporation of the principles of holistic health, which then profoundly influence the quality of the healing relationship.
- Holistic care incorporates a lifetime of learning opportunities. All life experiences, including birth, joy, suffering, and the dying process, are profound learning opportunities for clients and those who care for them.

Prevention Practice

Prevention practice encompasses health care designed to promote health, fitness, and wellness through education and appropriate guidance designed to prevent or delay the progression of pathology. Preventive care not only focuses on the promotion of general health in susceptible or potentially susceptible populations but also aims to minimize the impairments and functional limitations arising from pathological conditions, potentially affecting an individual's quality of life. According to the *Guide to Physical Therapist Practice*,[22] health care professionals are involved in 3 types of preventive practice: primary prevention, secondary prevention, and tertiary prevention.

1. *Primary prevention* is "preventing a target condition in a susceptible or potentially susceptible population through specific measures, such as general health promotion efforts."[22]
2. *Secondary prevention* is "decreasing the duration of illness, severity of disease, and number of sequelae (abnormalities following or resulting from disease, injury, or treatment) through early diagnosis and prompt intervention."[22]
3. *Tertiary prevention* involves "limiting the degree of disability and promoting rehabilitation and restoration of function in patients with chronic or reversible disease."[22]

Examples of preventive care performed by health care providers include screening for potential health problems and providing education or activities to promote health, fitness, and wellness. Screening activities may include identification of children with possible developmental delays, detection of ergonomic risk factors in the workplace, and recognition of factors increasing the risk of falls by older adults. Examples of prevention activities designed to promote general health include prepartum and postpartum exercise classes to improve women's health, exercise classes for well elders to enhance balance and flexibility, and cardiovascular conditioning activities for individuals who are at risk for obesity.

Preventive care also includes instruction to minimize or eliminate injurious forces throughout daily life. This instruction includes recommendations to optimize conditions for performance, whether the performance is related to simple activities of daily living, work activities, leisure activities, or activities related to competitive sports. With back pain affecting 80% of people at some point during their lives,[23] programs to prevent back problems through proper exercise and body mechanics are essential. Finally, individuals with chronic or progressive pathology can benefit from programs that reduce the intensity, duration, and frequency of complications arising from their conditions while improving their health and wellness. Customized exercises for individuals with musculoskeletal, neurological, cardiopulmonary, and integumentary pathologies may forestall secondary complications arising from their conditions, as well as improve their overall health.

Risk Reduction

Identification of populations at risk for developing physical and mental health problems help curtail the number of people whose quality of life is diminished by preventable pathology. Although many pathological conditions are genetic, some conditions are preventable. Knowing the populations at risk for a particular disease allows health care providers to target health promotion education and screening programs to populations at the greatest risk for illness. The website for Healthy People 2020, described in Chapter 2, provides more information about specific populations at the greatest risk for particular types of pathology.

One key to achieving wellness is developing an awareness of how to achieve a balance among the various dimensions affecting health and well-being. Populations that are susceptible to illness or injury are in particular need of this awareness, accomplished through appropriate education and guidance. Risk factors that may predispose an individual to diminished well-being and health problems include physical risk factors (poor nutrition, physical inactivity, a poor physical environment, and substance abuse); psychological, spiritual, and social risk factors (low self-esteem and lacking values and a direction in one's life plan); and environmental risk factors (persons, things, or conditions that negatively influence other dimensions). By identifying and addressing these risk factors, the health professional can reduce the incidence of injury and illness.

Key Players in Promoting Health and Wellness

According to recent statistics from the National Center for Chronic Disease Prevention and Health Promotion, nearly 6% of Americans spend 14 or more days per year limited in their activity.[7] Disability not only affects an individual's independent functioning, but it also places a burden on others who must either care for the individual or assume the individual's roles. Health promotion is essential for the well-being of society. All health care providers can play a role as prevention practitioners to improve the general health of our country. Although many have traditionally been involved in the management of physical impairments and functional limitations associated with medical problems, current roles encompass identifying risk factors and developing health promotion strategies that significantly influence health, fitness, and wellness.

A key element of health care management is directing clients' energies toward improving capabilities for functional independence, maintaining optimal health, and fulfilling important roles in their lives. Health care professionals need to determine an individual's functional capabilities by examining the requisite motor skills and behaviors needed to perform tasks relevant to that individual's role in society. Functional capabilities comprise not only the physical capabilities of the individual, but also the psychosocial environment and well-being of the individual. Social support can contribute significantly to individual well-being. This well-being, in turn, leads to the individual's ability to develop a personal sense of meaningful living.

Physicians and Physician Assistants

Physicians and physician assistants play an essential role in promoting healthier lifestyles and preventing disease through the provision of medical care and early identification of pathological conditions. Both participate in public health activities and direct patient care by providing health education, preventing fragmentation of services, and cooperating and participating with health departments.[24] Health promotion and risk reduction are accomplished through regular risk assessment, counseling, immunizations, education, and research.

Physical Therapists and Physical Therapy Assistants

Physical therapists are experts in examining and evaluating sensorimotor function, gross and skilled movement, physical capabilities, and activity limitations of those with musculoskeletal, neurological, cardiopulmonary, integumentary, and other body system impairments. Under the supervision of physical therapists, physical therapy assistants can ensure exercise adherence and provide health education.

According to the *Guide to Physical Therapist Practice*,[22] physical therapists "restore, maintain, and promote not only optimal physical function, but optimal wellness and fitness and optimal quality of life as it relates to movement and health." The practice of physical therapy encompasses the full spectrum of health and wellness that includes preventing disease and illness and optimizing health. Physical therapy plays a key role in providing education, guidance, consultation, and direct interventions to enable individuals to maintain physical activity for self-care, mobility, leisure skills, work, and play.

Occupational Therapists and Occupational Therapy Assistants

Occupational therapists and occupational therapy assistants aim to help people achieve independence, meaning, and satisfaction in all aspects of their lives by enabling people to engage in activities of daily living that have personal meaning and value.[25] Their role is to "develop, improve, sustain, or restore independence to any person who has an injury, illness, disability, or psychological dysfunction; consult with the person and the family or caregivers and, through evaluation and treatment, promote the client's capacity to participate in satisfying daily activities, and address by intervention the person's capacity to perform, the activity being performed, or the environment in which it is performed. The occupational therapist's goal is to provide the client with skills for the job of living—those necessary to function in the community or in the client's chosen environment."[25]

Clinical Exercise Physiologists

Clinical exercise physiologists work in primarily supervised environments that provide services directed by a licensed physician.[26] Clinical exercise physiologists are trained to work with patients with chronic diseases where exercise training has been shown to be of therapeutic benefit, including, but not limited to, cardiovascular disease, pulmonary disease, and metabolic disorders.[26]

Nurses

Nurses play an integral role in promoting public health with a focus on disease prevention and changing health behaviors. Public health nurses are involved in working with communities and populations on primary prevention and health promotion. They serve as advocates, collaborators, educators, partners, policy makers, and researchers in the area of community health promotion and prevention, with a greater emphasis on community participatory and ethnographic approaches.[27] Nurse practitioners provide advanced practice that enables them to serve as a patient's primary health care provider and to see patients of all ages, depending on their specialty (eg, family, pediatrics, geriatrics). Their scope of practice includes examining for a diagnosis and providing management of acute and uncomplicated chronic illness and disease, such as high blood pressure.[28]

Physical Educators

Physical educators introduce children and adolescents to psychomotor learning and physical activity through play, leisure activities, and competitive sports during primary and secondary education. Physical educators also incorporate nutrition and health behaviors in their classes, along with technologies that encourage play, such as Kinect (Microsoft) and Wii Fit (Nintendo).[29] Adaptive physical education (APE) is federally mandated for students with disabilities. Typically, APE is provided by a certified educator who adapts or modifies physical activities that enable this population to engage in activities that promote psychomotor development and play skills.[30] Because physical educators work with children and adolescents, they provide foundational concepts for health promotion.

Dieticians and Nutritionists

Both dieticians and nutritionists advise people about healthy food and nutrition. Although "every registered dietitian is a nutritionist…not every nutritionist is a registered dietitian."[31] Nutritionists are not considered legal experts because training varies between individuals. Registered dietitians (RDs) or registered dietician nutritionists (RDNs) are legally considered experts because they have specialized professional training that expands their knowledge for practicing in a broad array of settings, ranging from hospital settings to corporate wellness.[31] Some RDs have advanced certifications to provide specialized nutritional consultation for sports, community health, pediatrics, renal conditions, oncological disorders, food allergies, and gerontology.

Certified Athletic Trainers and Personal Trainers

According to the National Athletic Training Association,[32] certified athletic trainers "provide prevention, emergency care, clinical diagnosis, therapeutic intervention and rehabilitation of injuries and medical conditions" under the supervision of physicians. Athletic trainers typically work with individuals for fitness training that emphasizes strength, cardiorespiratory fitness, and performance enhancement. Personal trainers prescribe exercises and provide nutritional advice to promote health and fitness. Although various agencies certify personal trainers, those holding certifications from the American College of Sports Medicine (ACSM), the International Sports Sciences Association (ISSA), or the National Strength and Conditioning Association (NSCA) are considered the most knowledgeable.[33]

Health Psychologists

Health psychologists use a biopsychosocial approach to promote health and wellness in the community. In addition to considering biological processes affecting health, fitness, and wellness, health psychologists also consider psychological factors (eg, stressors, health beliefs, and personal health behaviors) and social processes (eg, socioeconomic status, culture, and ethnicity).[34] Health psychologists advise individuals, other health professionals, and community programs to promote general well-being and to develop public policies that promote healthy psychosocial environments.

Recreation Therapists

Recreation therapists work closely with other health care professionals in a variety of settings, providing primarily structured activities emphasizing leisure skills. Recreation therapists are required to have a bachelor's degree to be certified to provide treatment services and recreation activities to individuals with disabilities or illness.[35]

Community Resources

Professionals need to work collaboratively to integrate resources for health and wellness into their communities. Opportunities to advocate for health and wellness exist in day care centers, schools, fitness centers, community settings, and geriatric care facilities, as well as business and corporate settings. For example, in many communities the YMCA provides programming for children and adults with special needs. In addition, many schools, community centers, and clinics provide programs designed to promote community health. Prevention practice (ie, practicing healthy lifestyle habits that prevent injury and illness) involves a societal commitment to a culture of wellness. Each health care professional can provide a unique perspective on how to improve health and wellness.

Summary

Prevention practice is the holistic practice of medicine encompassing care of the individual in the context of that person's home, work, and community. The effect of prevention practice influences not only the individual, but also society. As a member of the health care team, each professional can play a key role in identifying risk factors for poor health and promoting wellness through various strategies, including screening, health education to encourage self-responsibility and awareness of risk factors, and promoting healthy lifestyle behaviors. The following chapters outline "healthy people" goals for our nation with key concepts for fitness training, stress management, and healthy nutrition. In addition, screening tools and evidence-based interventions are included for at-risk individuals as well as individuals with common conditions. Finally, suggestions for developing and promoting a health promotion business are provided.

References

1. "health." Miriam-Webster.com. http://www.merriam-webster.com/dictionary/health. Accessed June 5, 2012.
2. Definition of health. World Health Organization. https://www.who.int/about/definition/en/print.html. Accessed May 19, 2014.
3. Aspen Health and Administration Development Group. *Community Health Education and Promotion Manual.* New York, NY: Wolters Kluwer Law & Business; 1996.
4. Kidd P. Towards optimal health: managing the multiple factors that cause disease. *Total Health Magazine.* July/August 2001.
5. Work-related musculoskeletal disorders (WMSDs) prevention. Centers for Disease Control and Prevention. http://www.cdc.gov/workplacehealthpromotion/evaluation/topics/disorders.html. Accessed June 5, 2012.
6. Behavioral risk factor surveillance system. Centers for Disease Control and Prevention. http://www.cdc.gov/brfss/. Accessed June 1, 2013.
7. Chronic disease overview. Centers for Disease Control and Prevention. http://www.cdc.gov/nccdphp. Accessed June 1, 2013.
8. Health-related quality of life (HRQOL) key findings. Centers for Disease Control and Prevention. http://www.cdc.gov/hrqol/key_findings.htm. Accessed July 11, 2012.
9. Definition of wellness. National Wellness Institute. http://www.nationalwellness.org/. Accessed June 1, 2013.
10. Dacher E. A systems theory approach to an expanded medical mode: a change for biomedicine. *Altern Ther Health Med.* 1996;1:2.
11. Corbin C, Corbin W, Lindsey R, Welk G. *Concepts of Fitness.* 11th ed. New York, NY: McGraw-Hill; 2003.
12. Clinebell H. *Anchoring Your Well-being: Christian Wholeness in a Fractured World.* Nashville, TN: McMillan Publishing Co; 1997.
13. Quotation #31761 from Classic Quotes: Kahil Gibran. The Quotations Page. http://www.quotationspage.com/quote/31761.html. Accessed June 1, 2013.
14. Travis J, Ryan R. *Wellness Workbook: How to Achieve Enduring Health and Vitality.* 3rd ed. Berkley, CA: Ten Speed Press; 2003.
15. Disabilities. World Health Organization. http://www.who.int/topics/disabilities/en/. Accessed May 19, 2014.
16. What we mean by disability. Social Security Administration. http://www.ssa.gov/dibplan/dqualify4.htm. Accessed June 1, 2013.
17. Ardell D. *14 Days to Wellness: The Easy, Effective, and Fun Way to Optimum Health.* New York, NY: New World Library; 1999.
18. Quality of life and wellbeing: measuring the benefits of culture and sport: literature review and thinkpiece. Scottish Executive. www.scotland.gov.uk/Resource/Doc/89281/0021350.pdf. Accessed June 1, 2013.
19. Brazier JE, Harper R, Jones NM, et al. Validating the SF-36 health survey questionnaire: new outcome measure for primary care. *BMJ.* 1992;305(6846):160-164.
20. Measuring healthy days: population assessment of health-related quality of life. Centers for Disease Control and Prevention. http://www.cdc.gov/hrqol/pdfs/mhd.pdf. Accessed May 19, 2014.
21. The principles of holistic medical practice. American Holistic Medical Association. http://www.holisticmedicine.org/about/about_principles.shtml. Accessed December 10, 2004.
22. Guide to Physical Therapist Practice. American Physical Therapy Association. http://guidetoptpractice.apta.org/. Accessed May 19, 2014.
23. Hoy DG, Bain C, Williams G, et al. A systematic review of the global prevalence of low back pain. *Arthritis Rheum.* 2012;64(6):2028-2037.
24. Competencies for the physician assistant profession. American Academy of Physician Assistants. http://www.nccpa.net/App/PDFs/Definition%20of%20PA%20Competencies%203.5%20for%20Publication.pdf. Accessed May 19, 2014.
25. A definition of occupational therapy. NYU Steinhardt School of Culture, Education, and Human Development. http://www.steinhardt.nyu.edu/ot/definition. Accessed May 25, 2013.
26. What is a clinical exercise physiologist? Clinical Exercise Physiology Association. http://www.acsm-cepa.org/i4a/pages/index.cfm?pageid=3304. Accessed May 25, 2013.
27. Gott M, O'Brien M. The role of the nurse in health promotion. *Health Promot Int.* 1990;5(2):137-143.

28. Horrocks S, Anderson E, Salisbury C. Systematic review of whether nurse practitioners working in primary care can provide equivalent care to doctors. *BMJ*. 2002;324:819-823.
29. Who we are. American Alliance for Health, Physical Education, Recreation and Dance. http://www.aahperd.org/about/. Accessed May 25, 2013.
30. What is adapted physical education? Adapted Physical Education National Standards. http://www.apens.org/whatisape.html. Accessed September 5, 2013.
31. RDs=nutrition experts. Academy of Nutrition and Dietetics. http://www.eatright.org/HealthProfessionals/content.aspx?id=6856. Accessed September 5, 2013.
32. Terminology. National Athletic Trainers Association. http://www.nata.org/athletic-training/terminology. Accessed September 5, 2013.
33. Malek MH, Nalbone DP, Berger DE, Coburn JW. Importance of health science education for personal fitness trainers. *J Strength Cond Res*. 2002;16(1):19-24.
34. Health Psychology Center Presents: What is Health Psychology? http://healthpsychology.org/what-is-health-psychology/. Accessed May 19, 2014.
35. "recreation therapist." *Mosby's Dictionary of Medicine, Nursing and Health Professions*. 8th ed. St. Louis, MO: Mosby; 2009.

2

Healthy People 2020

Catherine Rush Thompson, PT, PhD, MS

"The greatest wealth is health."—Virgil, *The Aeneid*

Healthy People 2020 is a federal health promotion and disease prevention agenda developed to improve the health of Americans.[1] The developers of this government initiative include the Healthy People Consortium, an alliance of more than 350 national organizations and 250 public health, mental health, substance abuse, and environmental agencies and teams of experts from a variety of federal agencies under the direction of Health and Human Services and working in conjunction with the Office of Disease Prevention and Health Promotion. The Healthy People 2020 document was developed through a broad consultation process, including focus groups and representatives from varied populations, built on a foundation of scientific evidence, and designed to measure progress over time.[1]

According to its developers, the vision of Healthy People 2020 is to promote "a society in which all people live long, healthy lives."[1] As stated on its website, Healthy People 2020[1] strives to do the following:

- Identify nationwide health improvement priorities
- Increase public awareness and understanding of the determinants of health, disease, and disability and the opportunities for progress
- Provide measurable objectives and goals that are applicable at the national, state, and local levels
- Engage multiple sectors to take actions to strengthen policies and improve practices that are driven by the best available evidence and knowledge
- Identify critical research, evaluation, and data collection needs

The overarching goals that Healthy People 2020[1] hopes to achieve by 2020 are the following:

- Attain high-quality, longer lives free of preventable disease, disability, injury, and premature death

Thompson CR.
Prevention Practice and Health Promotion: A Health Care Professional's Guide to Health, Fitness, and Wellness, Second Edition (pp 19–36).

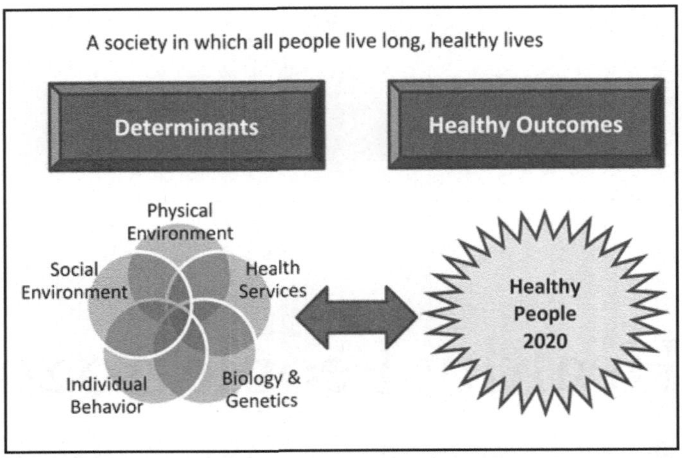

Figure 2-1. Healthy People 2020. (Adapted from Healthypeople.gov. http://www.healthypeople.gov/2020/about/default.aspx. Accessed May 20, 2014.)

This space left blank on purpose.
Please see print edition for figure.

Figure 2-2. International Classification of Functioning, Health and Disability. (Reproduced with permission from the World Health Organization. Towards a Common Language for Functioning, Disability and Health: ICF. http://www.who.int/classifications/icf/icfbeginnersguide.pdf?ua=1. Accessed May 20, 2014.)

- Achieve health equity, eliminate disparities, and improve the health of all groups
- Create social and physical environments that promote good health for all
- Promote quality of life, healthy development, and healthy behaviors across all life stages

The framework for Healthy People 2020, illustrated in Figure 2-1, acknowledges the multiple determinants that affect societal health outcomes, including the physical environment, the social environment, available health services, and individual behavior as it affects biological and genetic risk factors. These determinants involve assessment at many levels, as reflected in the World Health Organization's (WHO's) model of disability, the International Classification of Functioning, Disability and Health[2] (ICF), illustrated in Figure 2-2.

The ICF model enables health care providers to use standardized language and common framework for describing health and health-related states.[3] The ICF model similarly identifies individual factors and contextual factors affecting an individual's health status. This classification helps health care providers to "describe changes in body function and structure, what a person with a health condition can do in a standard environment (their level of capacity), as well as what they actually do in their usual environment (their level of performance)."[4] The definitions of domains within the ICF model are listed in Table 2-1.

Both Healthy People 2020 and the WHO ICF model provide frames of reference that enable health care providers to see the bigger picture—a framework that includes both the individual and the context of each individual's life in a community. This larger framework encourages health care providers to look beyond the individual for factors affecting a person's health, including the physical environment, the psychosocial environment, and the environment created by policies for a given community. Health care providers can use the ICF model and the resources from the Healthy People 2020 website (www.healthypeople.gov) to locate resources for positively influencing the health status of individuals and their communities.

Leading Health Indicators

Health indicators are factors that provide information about the health and well-being of a population.[1] National health indicators are used to help public policy makers and health professionals to measure the general health and wellness of the United States. These indicators are not used individually, but rather as an overview of key national health concerns that need attention. The top leading health indicators of our nation are addressed by at least one objective from Healthy People 2020 and are monitored regularly to determine the effectiveness of health and wellness programs established to improve national health.

Various communities have increased risk due to geographic, economic, and other factors. The Healthy People 2020 website lists leading health indicators that reflect the high-priority health issues across the nation and offers suggested actions that can be taken to address each indicator. The leading health indicators identified for the next decade include the following[1]:

- *Access to health services.* As recently as 2010, almost 1 in 4 Americans did not have a primary care provider or health center where they could receive regular medical services.
- *Clinical preventive services.* Routine screenings and scheduled immunizations reduce illness and disability, yet many do not take advantage of services offered through Medicare, Medicaid, and the Affordable Care Act. For example, in the United States only 25% of adults aged 50 to 64 and fewer than 40% of adults aged 65 and older are up to date on colorectal cancer screening and other recommended clinical preventive services.[3]
- *Environmental quality.* "Safe air, land, and water are fundamental to a healthy community environment. An environment free of hazards, such as secondhand smoke, carbon monoxide, allergens, lead, and toxic chemicals, helps prevent disease and other health problems. Implementing and enforcing environmental standards and regulations, monitoring pollution levels and human exposures, building environments that support healthy lifestyles, and considering the risks of pollution in decision making can improve health and quality of life for all Americans."[3]
- *Injury and violence.* This leading health indicator includes both unintentional and intention injuries, such as motor vehicle accidents, homicide, domestic and school violence, child abuse and neglect, suicide, and unintentional drug overdoses. "Injuries are the leading cause of death for Americans age 1 to 44, and a leading cause of disability for all ages, regardless of sex, race and ethnicity, or socioeconomic status."[5] Consequences of injury and violence, which are both preventable, range from minor concussions to premature death and have a significant emotional and financial effect on the individual and his or her family, as well as the community.
- *Maternal, infant, and child health.* The health of mothers and their offspring is critical for the future of our nation. More than 80% of women in the United States will become pregnant,

Table 2-1. Definitions for the International Classification of Functioning, Health and Disability Model

TERM AND DEFINITION	EXAMPLES
Body functions are physiological functions of body systems (including psychological functions). **Body structures** are anatomical parts of the body such as organs, limbs, and their components. **Impairments** are problems in body function or structure such as a significant deviation or loss.	Mental functions Sensory functions and pain Voice and speech functions Functions of the cardiovascular, hematological, immunological, and respiratory systems Functions of the digestive, metabolic, and endocrine systems Genitourinary and reproductive functions Neuromusculoskeletal and movement-related functions Functions of the skin and related structures
Activity is the execution of a task or action by an individual. **Activity limitations** are difficulties an individual may have in executing activities.	Learning and applying knowledge General tasks and demands Communication Mobility Self-care Domestic life Interpersonal interactions and relationships Major life areas Community, social, and civic life
Participation is involvement in a life situation. **Participation restrictions** are problems an individual may experience in involvement in life situations.	
Environmental factors make up the physical, social, and attitudinal environment in which people live and conduct their lives.	Products and technology Natural environment and human-made changes to environment Support and relationships Attitudes Services, systems, and policies
Personal factors are the individual's internal factors.	Demographics (sex, age, social background, education, profession, etc) Coping style Past and current experience Overall behavior pattern, character, and other factors that influence how disability is experienced by the individual

Adapted from International Classification of Functioning, Disability and Health (ICF). World Health Organization. http://www.who.int/classifications/icf/en/. Accessed December 4, 2012.

TABLE 2-2. BEHAVIORAL RISK FACTOR SURVEILLANCE RESULTS					
QUESTION: HOW IS YOUR GENERAL HEALTH?	EXCELLENT	VERY GOOD	GOOD	FAIR	POOR
Nationwide (states and DC)	18.8	33.4	30.9	12.5	4.4
Source: Prevalence and Trends Data: Health Status–2012. Centers for Disease Control and Prevention. http://apps.nccd.cdc.gov/brfss/list.asp?cat=HS&yr=2012&qkey=8001&state=All. Accessed December 4, 2012.					

TABLE 2-3. MENTAL ILLNESS SURVEILLANCE AMONG ADULTS IN THE UNITED STATES		
CHARACTERISTIC	NO. OF RESPONDENTS	MEAN NO. OF MENTALLY UNHEALTHY DAYS IN THE PAST 30 DAYS
Total	424,218	3.5
Male	161,046	2.9
Female	263,172	4.0
18 to 24 y	13,032	3.9
25 to 34 y	36,755	3.8
35 to 44 y	59,253	3.7
45 to 54 y	85,446	3.9
≥55 y	226,168	2.8
Source: Mental illness surveillance among adults in the United States. Centers for Disease Control and Prevention. http://www.cdc.gov/mmwr/preview/mmwrhtml/su6003a1.htm?s_%20cid=su6003a1_w#Tab10. Accessed May 20, 2014.		

will give birth to one or more children, and will determine the health of the next generation.[6] Maternal issues include tobacco use before and during pregnancy, prenatal care, pregnancy complications, and postpartum depression. Infant issues include preterm birth, sudden infant death syndrome (SIDS), and risks for infant mortality, such as birth defects, infections, prematurity, and maternal complications during the birth process.[6]

- *Mental health.* According to the Centers for Disease Control and Prevention,[7] "the burden of mental illness in the United States is among the highest of all diseases, and mental disorders are among the most common causes of disability. Recent figures suggest that approximately 1 in 4 adults in the United States have had a mental health disorder in the past year—most commonly anxiety or depression—and 1 in 17 had a serious mental illness."

Table 2-2 lists the data from the most recent Behavioral Risk Factor Surveillance System describing responses to the question: "How is your general health?" More than 15% of the respondents reported that they have poor health.[8]

Table 2-3 lists the mean number of mentally unhealthy days during the past 30 days among adults aged 18 years and older in response to the question: "Now thinking about your mental health, which includes stress, depression, and problems with emotions, for how many days during the past 30 days was your mental health not good?" The responses indicate that up to 4 days per month account for missed days of work.[8] The prevalence of mental health issues compounds the effect of physical impairments seen in both acute and chronic care settings. Certain mental illnesses tend to exacerbate morbidity from certain chronic diseases. Family members also carry the burden of mental health issues affecting their daily lives and the lives of those they love.

- *Nutrition, physical activity, and obesity.* A healthy diet and physical activity are essential for maintaining a healthy weight. Individuals who are overweight and obese experience a wide range of obesity-related medical conditions, including coronary artery disease, stroke, type 2 diabetes, and osteoarthritis. Indirectly, obesity significantly increases health care costs. According to the Food Research and Action Center, 68.8% of American adults are overweight or obese and 35.7% are obese.[9] According to research, "if obesity trends continue unchecked, obesity-related medical costs alone could rise by $48 to $66 billion a year in the United States by 2030."[10]
- *Oral health.* Oral health is essential for speaking, smiling, smelling, tasting, touching, chewing, swallowing, and expressing emotions.[10] Poor dental and oral hygiene can lead to oral diseases, including periodontal (gum) disease, which has been associated with several chronic diseases in adulthood as well as premature births and low birth weight.[11]
- *Reproductive and sexual health.* Reproductive and sexual health encompasses sexually transmitted diseases (STDs), reproductive health problems and infertility, fetal and perinatal health problems, and cancer. "An estimated 1.2 million Americans are living with the human immunodeficiency virus (HIV), and 1 out of 5 people with HIV do not know they have it."[12]
- *Social determinants.* According to the Healthy People 2020 website, social determinants are "personal, social, economic, and environmental factors" that contribute to individual and population health. These factors align with the Environmental Factors and Personal Factors listed in the ICF model, including education, employment, homes and neighborhood environments, and access to preventive services.
- *Substance abuse.* Substance abuse refers to the use of mind- and behavior-altering substances. Substance abuse contributes to cardiovascular conditions, pregnancy complications, teenage pregnancy, STDs, domestic violence, child abuse, motor vehicle crashes, homicide, and suicide.[13] Tragically, the overall cost of substance abuse in the United States, including lost productivity and health- and crime-related costs, is estimated at $600 billion annually.[14]
- *Tobacco.* Tobacco use is the single most preventable cause of disease, disability, and death in the United States, yet more deaths are caused each year by tobacco use than from HIV, illegal drug use, alcohol abuse, motor vehicle injuries, suicides, and murders combined.[15,16]

Addressing Health Care Risk Factors

Every health care provider should be aware of common health risks for any given population. For example, significant health disparities exist between different ethnic groups. Current national research has focused on health disparities between Whites, African Americans, Hispanics, American Indians, Alaska Natives, Asians, Native Hawaiians, and Pacific Islanders.[1] Although biological and sociological factors contribute to these disparities, most disparities are caused by multifactorial interactions involving genetic variation, sociocultural influences, environmental factors (including availability of healthy and nutritious food), and lifestyle behaviors. Table 2-4 illustrates the percentage of adults who are obese based on their racial status, as measured by the Racial and Ethnic Approaches to Community Health across the US (REACH U.S.) task force.

According to national statistics collected as part of Healthy People 2020, "heart disease death rates are more than 40 percent higher for African Americans than for Whites.[1] The death rate for all cancers is 30 percent higher for African Americans than for Whites; and for prostate cancer, the death rate is more than double that for Whites.[1] African American women have a higher death rate from breast cancer despite having a mammography screening rate that is nearly the same as

TABLE 2-4. MEDIAN PREVALENCE OF ADULT OBESITY BY RACIAL GROUP		
RACIAL GROUP	MEN	WOMEN
Black	28.50%	31.60%
Hispanic	26.60%	30.90%
Asian/Pacific Islander	23.60%	25.60%
American Indian	27.70%	26.30%
Source: Minority health surveillance–REACH US 2009. Centers for Disease Control and Prevention. http://www.cdc.gov/Features/dsREACHUS/. Accessed May 20, 2014.		

the rate for White women. The death rate from HIV/AIDS for African Americans is more than 7 times that for Whites, and the rate of homicide is 6 times that for Whites.[1] Although the nation's infant mortality rate is down, the infant death rate among African Americans is still more than double that of Whites."[1]

One study points out specific factors believed to contribute to the health disparities of African Americans as compared with other Americans.[17] These contributing factors include the following:

- Excessive cardiovascular risk factors, such as high blood pressure, diabetes, obesity, physical inactivity, and psychosocial stress
- Unfamiliarity with information linking personal risk factors to atherosclerosis and heart disease
- Cultural factors affecting an individual's desire to seek health care
- Economic factors limiting health care access
- Psychosocial stress, racism, and frustration dealing with health care providers
- Genetic predisposition to these pathologies[17]

The population of Hispanics is increasing in the United States, and this group is also suffering from health disparities. According to national health statistics, Hispanics are at an increased risk of dying from diabetes, developing high blood pressure, and becoming obese.[1] Incidences of diabetes in American Indians and Alaska Natives are twice that of Whites.[18] The Pima of Arizona have one of the highest rates of diabetes in the world. American Indians and Alaska Natives also have disproportionately high death rates from unintentional injuries and suicide, with factors contributing to this disparity including cultural barriers, geographic isolation, inadequate sewage disposal, and low income.[18] Although Asians and Pacific Islanders generally have good health, Vietnamese women have a five-fold increase in cervical cancer compared with White women. Also, Asians and Pacific Islanders living in the United States are at an increased risk of developing hepatitis and tuberculosis.[1]

Strategies to address health disparities for minorities include health promotion education, risk factor modification, culturally competent health care delivery, and continued research on factors contributing to racial and ethnic variances in disease and injury.[1] Income and education often go hand in hand as they relate to access to health care information, activities, and programming. Those with the greatest health disparities, regardless of sex or ethnicity, have the highest poverty rates and the least education. Individuals with low incomes and low levels of education are at increased risk for heart disease, diabetes, obesity, elevated blood lead level, and low birth weight. While wealthier populations make gains in their health, groups with lower socioeconomic status have increasing disparities in their health.[1] A recent study examining factors linked to men's mortality found that childhood conditions, including lower socioeconomic status, family living arrangements, mother's work status, rural residence, and parents' nativity, played key roles in causing earlier mortality.[19] These findings suggest that economic and educational policies that are targeted at children's well-being are implicitly health policies with effects that reach far into the adult life course. Health care professionals must acknowledge their role in promoting health education, particularly to disadvantaged children.

The importance of a national health promotion initiative such as Healthy People 2020 cannot be overstated. Although individual lifestyle behaviors contribute significantly to overall health, various settings, including the home setting, the work environment, and community settings (eg, leisure, commerce, religious, government) can play a key role in health. Each setting poses various risks and opportunities for health promotion. For example, it is well known that secondhand smoke is associated with significant morbidity and mortality; many communities have enacted laws to restrict exposure to secondhand smoke in public places to limit exposure to smoke toxins and to prevent illness.[20]

Although both environmental and socioeconomic factors affect an individual's health, so do collective attitudes, beliefs, and perceptions related to health, fitness, and wellness. In one study examining factors influencing health behaviors in a rural community, researchers found that low reimbursement, poor community attitudes, inpatient priorities, personnel shortages, low educational levels, weak local economies, and large older populations were often barriers to health promotion and disease prevention services.[21] Researchers determined that the implementation of an effective health initiative requires a collaborative effort beyond the local community and health care providers. Organizations within and beyond communities trying to develop health initiatives are essential for expanding and leveraging facilities, acquiring needed equipment, establishing legitimacy, securing adequate funding, developing interpersonal connections, and expanding resources. Health care providers must partner with philanthropists and grant writers to secure funding for health promotion activities.

Political advocacy is also essential for establishing adequate national funding to support the Healthy People 2020 initiative. Implementing the needed programs for a healthy nation requires effective leadership, communication, interpersonal relations, and trust building. A collective effort to promote national health should provide a positive effect on all Americans seeking a healthier lifestyle.

Ideally, preventive screenings and health education can contribute to national efforts to address leading health indicators. Once individual needs are assessed, treatments can be developed that maximize the individual's function. Health care providers working together in the same community can identify facility and community resources to meet common health care needs and plan preventive strategies for that community. The ICF model can be applied to comprehensive services that involve the individual and the context in which the person functions. Applications of the ICF model are listed in Table 2-5.

The Community Health Assessment aNd Group Evaluation (CHANGE): Building a Foundation of Knowledge to Prioritize Community Health Needs—An Action[22] is a community-oriented planning guide based on Healthy People 2020 with the purpose of encouraging individuals to participate in achieving the overarching goals of the national initiative. "This action guide provides step-by-step instructions for successfully completing the CHANGE tool. CHANGE can be used to gain a picture of the policy, systems, and environmental change strategies currently in place throughout the community; develop a community action plan for improving policies, systems, and the environment to support healthy lifestyles; and assist with prioritizing community needs and allocating available resources. The action steps for the CHANGE plan include the following[22]:

- *Action Step 1*: Identify and assemble a diverse team of 10 to 12 individuals
- *Action Step 2*: Develop team strategy to complete CHANGE as a whole team or divide into subgroups
- *Action Step 3*: Review all CHANGE sectors
- *Action Step 4*: Gather data from individual sites or locations within each sector

TABLE 2-5. INTERNATIONAL CLASSIFICATION OF FUNCTIONING, DISABILITY AND HEALTH APPLICATIONS

LEVEL	APPLICATION
Individual	1. For the assessment of individuals: What is the person's level of functioning? 2. For individual treatment planning: What treatments or interventions can maximize functioning? 3. For the evaluation of treatment and other interventions: What are the outcomes of the treatment? How useful were the interventions? 4. For communication among physicians, nurses, physical therapists, occupational therapists and other health works, social service works, and community agencies 5. For self-evaluation by consumers: How would I rate my capacity in mobility or communication?
Institutional	1. For educational and training purposes 2. For resource planning and development: What health care and other services will be needed? 3. For quality improvement: How well do we serve our clients? What basic indicators for quality assurance are valid and reliable? 4. For management and outcome evaluation: How useful are the services we are providing? 5. For managed care models of health care delivery: How cost-effective are the services we provide? How can the service be improved for better outcomes at a lower cost?
Society	1. For eligibility criteria for state entitlements such as social security benefits, disability pensions, workers' compensation, and insurance: Are the criteria for eligibility for disability benefits evidence based, appropriate to social goals, and justifiable? 2. For social policy development, including legislative reviews, model legislation, regulations and guidelines, and definitions for anti-discrimination legislation: Will guaranteeing rights improve functioning at the societal level? Can we measure this improvement and adjust our policy and law accordingly? 3. For needs assessments: What are the needs of persons with various levels of disability—impairments, activity limitations, and participation restrictions? 4. For environmental assessment for universal design, implementation of mandated accessibility, identification of environmental facilitators and barriers, and changes to social policy: How can we make the social and built environment more accessible for all people, those with and those without disabilities? Can we assess and measure improvement?

Adapted from Towards a Common Language for Functioning, Disability and Health–ICF. World Health Organization. http://www.who.int/classifications/icf/training/icfbeginnersguide.pdf?ua=1. Accessed May 20, 2014.

- *Action Step 5*: Review data gathered with the community team
- *Action Step 6*: Enter data
- *Action Step 7*: Review consolidated data to determine areas of improvement
- *Action Step 8*: Build the Community Action Plan by developing and organizing annual objectives that reflect the collected data"

Whereas some individuals may be more capable of affecting health care policy for communities, others may implement health care screening programs or provide health promotion activities for a specific at-risk population. As health care professionals, it is important to work in concert with others in achieving Healthy People 2020 goals. Helpful resources, such as those offered by Healthy People 2020, the Center for Disease Control and Prevention, and US Preventive Services Task Force, can guide both individual and community efforts to improve national health.

Educators of health care professionals have unique opportunities for offering health education in their local community. One example of how college students can affect community health is through service learning, such as promoting healthy lifestyle behaviors and providing educational materials about healthy choices. According to one researcher, "the values, methods, and intended results of service learning are closely related to effective health promotion and disease prevention. Service learning focuses on personal and civic responsibility, thus providing students with opportunities for enhancing individual and community health. Service learning also espouses social justice and provides a vehicle for students to learn about, reflect on, and address health disparities."[23]

Healthy People 2020 provides a useful framework for improving the health of individuals, the health of communities, and the health of the nation. This health initiative, in conjunction with Healthy People in Healthy Communities, focuses on the overriding goals of increasing the quality and years of healthy life and eliminating health disparities between various populations. These comprehensive resources can guide the development of needed health and wellness programs for underserved populations and populations at risk for injury and illness.

Education is a key factor in health care. According to data collected for Healthy People 2020, the overall death rate for those with less than 12 years of education is more than twice that for people with 13 or more years of education.[24] The infant mortality rate is almost double for infants of mothers with less than 12 years of education compared with those with 13 or more years of education.[24] These statistics suggest that health promotion and usable health education must be provided early and targeted to those with limited education to substantially affect lifestyle behaviors.[1]

People with disabilities have health disparities related to their levels of physical activity. In addition, individuals with chronic illness or injury generally have higher levels of obesity, possibly due to their having activity limitations or their needing assistance to access health care services and facilities.[25] Research has shown that people with disabilities generally report more anxiety, pain, sleeplessness, and days of depression, leading to diminished quality of life.[23] Our role as health care providers includes advocating for access and facilities that will enable those with disabilities to engage in meaningful physical activity and to maintain a physically and mentally healthy lifestyle.

Unfortunately, individuals living in rural areas have even greater risks for injuries, heart disease, cancer, and diabetes.[25] To further complicate this problem, fewer preventive care services and emergency care facilities are available to those living in isolated rural areas. New technology that can reach out to rural communities needs to be used to improve access to services and to enhance education for preventive care.

Homosexual and bisexual individuals also experience disparate health problems.[26] Gay men have an increased incidence of STDs, substance abuse, depression, and suicide, particularly male adolescents.[27] Lesbians reportedly have higher rates of smoking, obesity, alcohol abuse, and stress than heterosexual women. Furthermore, lesbians and bisexual women evidenced higher behavioral risks and lower rates of preventive care than heterosexual women.[27] Family and social acceptance of sexual orientation affect an individual's mental health and could help reduce this health disparity.

The role of health care providers encompasses the provision of preventive practices to ensure optimal health for all populations. The Healthy People 2020 initiative provides a framework for addressing these issues by identifying populations at risk for poor health and health disparities. These challenges must be addressed in each community to improve the health of our nation. A multidisciplinary approach that incorporates strategies to address barriers to each population at risk is needed to achieve health equity. Not only must health care providers deliver education, resources, and access to health care, but we must also empower individuals to make their own informed decisions for embracing a healthy lifestyle.

Objectives to Improve Health

Healthy People 2020 contains a wide range of specific objectives to improve health, organized into focus areas related to the leading health indicators.[1] These focus areas include, but are not limited to, the following:

- Access to quality health services
- Arthritis
- Osteoporosis
- Chronic back conditions
- Cancer
- Chronic kidney disease
- Diabetes
- Disability and secondary conditions
- Educational and community-based programs
- Environmental health
- Family planning
- Food safety
- Health communication
- Heart disease and stroke
- HIV
- Immunization and infectious diseases
- Injury and violence prevention
- Maternal, infant, and child health
- Medical product safety
- Mental health and mental disorders
- Nutrition and overweight
- Occupational safety and health
- Oral health
- Physical activity and fitness
- Public health infrastructure
- Respiratory diseases
- STDs

- Substance abuse
- Tobacco use
- Vision and hearing

Health care professionals are uniquely qualified to address specific foci outlined by Healthy People 2020, particularly those related to healthy lifestyles incorporating healthy nutrition, physical activity, and fitness.

With the opportunities to directly provide therapy services through direct access, physical therapists provide a new avenue for accessibility to health care, especially for younger populations engaging in physical activity.[28] During initial screening of patients or health screenings for populations at risk, physical therapists, along with physicians and physician assistants, are capable of screening multiple body systems for potential disease and risks for injury. Familiarity with pathologies and risks for disease enable all trained health care professionals to screen for risk factors associated with pathology, as well as signs and symptoms of arthritis, osteoporosis, chronic back conditions, cancer, chronic kidney disease, diabetes, heart disease, stroke, respiratory diseases, obesity, signs and symptoms of HIV, mental health problems, and sensory losses, including hearing and visual impairments. The prevalence of these pathologies could be reduced with appropriate health and wellness screenings, referrals, and health education to reduce risk factors contributing to illness.

The role of health care focuses on enhancing health, fitness, and wellness to reduce disability and secondary conditions associated with common pathologies. This role is broadened through providing health screenings for health risks; encouraging individuals to maintain updated immunizations; informing clients of potential work-related injuries and risks of physical inactivity; educating clients about healthy lifestyle behaviors exclusive of tobacco use and abuse of drugs and alcohol; promoting good nutrition; and discussing other potential health hazards.

The national goals for Healthy People 2020 provide guidelines for affecting the leading health indicators and promoting a healthier nation.[1] Although the overarching goals are to increase the quality and years of healthy life and to eliminate health disparities between various populations, more measurable outcomes have been developed to focus on national health concerns and means to address these 2 primary goals. The national goals for Healthy People 2020 directly related to health care professional practice include the following[1]:

- Increase the quality and years of healthy life
- Increase incidence of people reporting healthy days
- Increase incidence of people reporting active days
- Reduce activity limitations, especially for older adults
- Reduce days of pain for those with arthritis, osteoporosis, and chronic back pain
- Increase the adoption and maintenance of daily physical activity
- Increase leisure time physical activity
- Increase proportion of people who regularly perform exercises for flexibility and muscle fitness
- Reduce the incidence of and deaths from cancer
- Increase the diagnosis of and reduce the incidence of type 2 diabetes
- Decrease the incidence of depression
- Decrease the incidence of heart diseases, including stroke and high blood pressure
- Decrease the incidence of high cholesterol levels among adults
- Eliminate health disparities
- Decrease personal stress levels and mental health problems

- Reduce steroid use, especially among youth
- Reduce accidents, destructive habits, and environmental pollution.
- Increase access of health information and services for all people
- Increase the proportion of all people who eat well (meet dietary guidelines, eat no more than 30% fat calories, eat no more than 10% saturated fat, eat 5 servings of vegetables and fruits daily, eat 6 portions of grain, consume needed calcium and iron, and avoid excess sodium)
- Increase the prevalence of healthy weight and reduce the prevalence of overweight

Health care providers need to be aware of all the goals contributing to national health because working in collaboration with others ensures a more comprehensive and collaborative approach to good health. The ultimate outcome of these collaborative efforts is tracked by the Centers for Disease Control and Prevention and those involved with Healthy People 2020. The efficacy of health promotion and injury prevention activities is monitored by federal agencies involved in tracking health-related statistics, such as disparities in access to health care and individual differences that influence health, fitness, and wellness. Certain factors are identified as key variables for monitoring health and serve as leading health indicators of the nation's health status. For example, physical activity is the health indicator that is most appropriately addressed by physical therapists. With backgrounds in anatomy, physiology, pathophysiology, exercise physiology, kinesiology, biomechanics, and related sciences, health care professionals can design optimal exercise programs for both healthy and ill clients. A recent Surgeon General's report on physical activity and health concluded that moderate physical activity can reduce substantially the risk of developing or dying from heart disease, diabetes, colon cancer, and high blood pressure.[10]

According to Healthy People 2020, *physical activity* is "bodily movement that is produced by the contraction of skeletal muscle and that substantially increases energy expenditure."[1] *Moderate physical activity* includes "activities that use large muscle groups," such as walking, swimming, housework, bicycling, and occupational activities.[1] *Vigorous physical activity* refers to "rhythmic, repetitive physical activities that use large muscle groups at 70% or more of maximum heart rate for age."[1] An exercise heart rate of 70% of maximum heart rate for age is approximately 60% of maximal cardiorespiratory capacity and is sufficient for cardiorespiratory conditioning.[1] Maximum heart rate equals approximately 220 beats per minute minus age. Examples of vigorous physical activities include jogging/running, lap swimming, cycling, aerobic dancing, skating, rowing, jumping rope, cross-country skiing, hiking/backpacking, racquet sports, and competitive group sports (eg, soccer and basketball).

Physical activity plays an important role in primary and secondary prevention of conditions such as coronary heart disease (CHD), a leading cause of death and disability in the United States.[1] Risks posed by physical inactivity are almost as high as several well-known CHD risk factors, such as cigarette smoking, high blood pressure, and high blood cholesterol. According to measures by Healthy People 2020, physical inactivity is more prevalent than any one of these other risk factors.[1,29] The prevalence of overweight people and those with type 2 diabetes has increased over the past few decades.[1] Additionally, physical activity levels generally decline during adolescence. Recent research has shown that physical fitness and physical activity during adolescence can serve as predictors of cardiovascular disease risk in young adulthood. One study concluded that changes in the levels of physical activity and physical fitness between adolescence and young adulthood, especially in aerobic fitness, seemed to be the best predictor of cardiovascular risk factor levels in young adulthood.[28] These findings suggest that both health care professionals and physical educators can play an important role in the identification of inactive youth and the development of appropriate aerobic exercises to reduce cardiovascular risks.

People with musculoskeletal problems affecting bones and joints also benefit from physical activity. Individuals with arthritis and osteoporosis significantly benefit from weight-bearing activities that increase bone mineral density, improve aerobic fitness, and increase muscle strength.[30] Bone health benefits from sustained exercise that is properly prescribed to minimize risks of side effects.

The majority of adults in the United States are not involved in vigorous physical activity. According to Healthy People 2020, "only about 28.4 percent of adults in the United States report regular, vigorous physical activity that involves large muscle groups in dynamic movement for 20 minutes or longer 3 or more days per week. Only 15 percent of adults report physical activity for 5 or more days per week for 30 minutes or longer, and another 40 percent do not participate in any regular physical activity."[1] Health care professionals must address the issues confronting those who remain inactive. Some barriers to activity include limited access to facilities for exercising or safe environments. For example, older adults may have concerns about safety when walking in their neighborhoods, wearing proper attire, and tolerating conditions warranting special attention, such as hot weather and icy conditions. The goal to increase physical activity and fitness is a cooperative effort between public efforts and professional organizations devoted to improving national health. Physical activity programs in recreation centers, worksites, health care settings, and schools can be developed and monitored by health care professionals who are best equipped to customize programs for the needs of special populations.

Disparities in Levels of Physical Activity

Various cultural and ethnic groups experience disparities in their leisure time physical activity. According to the Surgeon General,[13] "the proportion of the population reporting no leisure-time physical activity is higher among women than men, higher among African-Americans and Hispanics than Whites, higher among older adults than younger adults, and higher among the less affluent than the more affluent. Participation in all types of physical activity declines, strikingly, as age or grade in school increases. In general, persons with lower levels of education and income are least active in their leisure time. Adults in North Central and Western States tend to be more active than those in the Northeastern and Southern States. People with disabilities and certain health conditions are less likely to engage in moderate or vigorous physical activity than are people without disabilities. Health promotion efforts need to identify barriers to physical activity faced by particular population groups and provide interventions that address these barriers."[31]

In a study examining the levels of physical activity and obesity in low-income populations, especially women of African American and Hispanic heritage, a low-fat diet and moderate/vigorous physical activity program were found to be beneficial. Interestingly, interventions were delivered through Internet and video, encouraging those most at risk to consume 30% or less calories from fat and to engage in moderate and vigorous physical activity.[31]

Health Education Resources

Health care providers must provide education that identifies risk factors for poor health in target populations and discuss effective strategies that can positively affect the well-being of both that individual and the community at large. Although it is important to emphasize the importance of self-responsibility in managing lifestyle behaviors and optimizing wellness through healthy habits, using a team approach to health education and social support can expand access to needed resources for populations at the greatest risk for health disparities. The following topics target common health concerns for at-risk populations:

- Parents of young children
  - Good nutrition
  - Fitness activities

  - Protection from preventable injuries
  - Effective discipline
  - Protection against childhood illness
  - Protection in childhood sports activities
  - Proper nutrition for physical activity
  - Reducing childhood obesity
  - Safety when swimming (including protection against skin cancer)
- Children aged 8 to 12 years
  - Good nutrition
  - Fitness activities
  - Safety issues
  - Playing it safe (protection in sports activities)
  - Proper nutrition for physical activity
  - Getting in shape (managing childhood obesity)
  - Safety when swimming/protection against skin cancer
  - Ergonomics (including wearing backpacks and sitting at the computer)
- Adolescents
  - Good nutrition
  - Fitness activities
  - Principles of fitness training
  - Safety issues for athletes
  - Protection against infections
  - Proper nutrition for physical activity
  - Screening for fitness
  - Red flags for depression
  - Prevention and management of obesity
  - Pregnancy (healthy behaviors for a healthy baby)
  - Pregnancy (ways to reduce back pain)
  - Child development for teenage mothers/pregnant teenagers
  - Screening for poor posture (including scoliosis)
  - Changes leading to healthy lifestyle habits (starting exercise programs and/or quitting smoking or other risky behaviors)
  - Screening for stress
  - Stress management
  - Ergonomics for the workplace (computer users)
  - Ergonomics for the workplace (manual labor)
- Young and middle-aged adults
  - Good nutrition
  - Fitness activities

  - Principles of fitness training
  - Choosing the right shoes for fitness training
  - Proper nutrition for physical activity
  - Screening for fitness
  - Ergonomics for the workplace (computer users)
  - Ergonomics for the workplace (manual labor)
  - Red flags for depression
  - Prevention and management of obesity
  - Pregnancy (ways to reduce back pain)
  - Child development for new mothers
  - Screening for poor posture
  - Healthy lifestyle habits (quitting smoking or other risky behaviors)
  - Screening for diabetes
  - Screening for heart disease
  - Screening for stress
  - Stress management
  - Prevention of low back pain
  - Medications (benefits and risks of commonly used over-the-counter drugs)
  - Prevention of skin cancer
  - Prevention of osteoporosis
- Older adults
  - Reducing the risks of falls
  - Good nutrition
  - Physical activities for health and wellness
  - Principles of fitness training for older adults
  - Choosing the right shoes for fitness training
  - Proper nutrition for physical activity
  - Red flags for depression
  - How to maintain healthy bones
  - Ergonomics for computer users
  - Ergonomics for the home
  - Screening for stress
  - Stress management
  - Medications (the more you take, the more you need to know)

As advocates for good health and improved quality of life, health care professionals must carefully screen for potential health risks, clearly explain these risks in an understandable manner, and help individuals develop strategies to maintain healthy lifestyle behaviors that reduce the risk of disease and injuries. This book provides resources for identifying health risks, locating reliable health education resources, and developing strategies to promote general health and well-being.

In addition, the role of advocacy for prevention practice and the management of health promotion businesses are discussed.

Summary

Health care professionals can play a key role in meeting the national health goals of Healthy People 2020. In particular, health care professionals are well prepared to identify risk factors for pathology and develop appropriate and evidence-based strategies to promote a healthy society. While recognizing the importance of self-responsibility in lifestyle behaviors, health care professionals can work collaboratively with others interested in health, fitness, and wellness to encourage universal access to health care, engagement in physical activity, and reduction in unhealthy habits.

References

1. Healthy People 2020. US Department of Health and Human Services. http://www.healthypeople.gov. Accessed December 4, 2012.
2. International Classification of Functioning, Disability and Health (ICF). World Health Organization. http://www.who.int/classifications/icf/en/. Accessed December 4, 2012.
3. Clinical preventive services. Centers for Disease Control and Prevention. http://www.cdc.gov/aging/services/index.htm. Accessed December 4, 2012.
4. Towards a Common Language for Functioning, Disability and Health. World Health Organization. http://www.who.int/classifications/icf/training/icfbeginnersguide.pdf. Accessed December 4, 2012.
5. Injury and violence. Healthy People 2020. http://www.healthypeople.gov/2020/LHI/injuryViolence.aspx. Accessed December 4, 2012.
6. Recommendations to improve preconception health and health care—United States. Centers for Disease Control and Prevention. http://www.cdc.gov/mmwr/preview/mmwrhtml/rr5506a1.htm. Accessed December 13, 2013.
7. Preterm birth. Centers for Disease Control and Prevention. http://www.cdc.gov/reproductivehealth/MaternalInfantHealth/PretermBirth.htm. Accessed December 13, 2013.
8. Reeves WC, Strine TW, Pratt LA, et al. Mental illness surveillance among adults in the United States. *MMWR*. 2011;60(3):1-32.
9. Overweight and obesity in the US. Food Research and Action Center. http://frac.org/initiatives/hunger-and-obesity/obesity-in-the-us/. Accessed December 4, 2013.
10. Wang CY, McPherson K, Marsh T, Gortmaker S, Brown M. Health and economic burden of the projected obesity trends in the USA and the UK. *Lancet*. 2011;378:815-825.
11. Oral health in America: a report of the Surgeon General. National Institute of Dental and Craniofacial Research. National Institutes of Health. http://www2.nidcr.nih.gov/sgr/sgrohweb/home.htm. Accessed December 13, 2013.
12. HIV/AIDS policy #3029-12. The Henry J. Kaiser Family Foundation. www.kff.org. Accessed December 4, 2012.
13. Substance abuse. Healthy People 2020. http://www.healthypeople.gov/2020/LHI/substanceAbuse.aspx. Accessed December 4, 2012.
14. DrugFacts: Understanding drug abuse and addiction. National Institute on Drug Abuse. National Institute of Health. http://www.drugabuse.gov/publications/drugfacts/understanding-drug-abuse-addiction. Accessed December 4, 2012.
15. Centers for Disease Control and Prevention. Annual smoking—attributable mortality, years of potential life lost, and productivity losses—United States, 2000-2004. *MMWR*. 2008;57(45):1226-1228.
16. Mokdad AH, Marks JS, Stroup DF, et al. Actual causes of death in the United States. *JAMA*. 2004;291(10):1238-1245.
17. Borrell LN, Diez Roux AV, Rose K, Catellier D, Clark BL. Neighborhood characteristics and mortality in the Atherosclerosis Risk in Communities Study. *Int J Epidemiol*. 2004;33(2):398-407.
18. American Indian/Alaska Native profile. US Department of Health and Human Services Office of Minority Health. http://minorityhealth.hhs.gov/templates/browse.aspx?lvl=2&lvlID=52. Accessed December 4, 2012.
19. Hayward MD, Gorman BK. The long arm of childhood: the influence of early-life social conditions on men's mortality. *Demography*. 2004;41(1):87-107.
20. Chan S, Lam TH. Preventing exposure to secondhand smoke. *Semin Oncol Nurs*. 2003;19(4):284-290.
21. Carter D. Healthy People 2010: a blueprint for the decade ahead. *Body Positive*. December 2010. http://www.thebody.com/content/art31138.html. Accessed May 20, 2014.

22. Community Health Assessment and Group Evaluation (CHANGE): building a foundation of knowledge to prioritize community health needs—an action. Centers for Disease Control and Prevention. http://www.cdc.gov/healthycommunitiesprogram/tools/change/pdf/changeactionguide.pdf. Accessed December 4, 2012.
23. Ottenritter NW. Service learning, social justice, and campus health. *J Am Coll Health.* 2004;52(4):189-191.
24. Life expectancy. Centers for Disease Control and Prevention. http://www.cdc.gov/nchs/fastats/lifexpec.htm. Accessed October 15, 2005.
25. Moriarty D, Zack M, Kobau R. The Centers for Disease Control and Prevention's Healthy Days Measures: population tracking of perceived physical and mental health over time. *Health Qual Life Outcomes.* 2003;1:37.
26. Mays VM, Yancey AK, Cochran SD, Weber M, Fielding JE. Heterogeneity of health disparities among African American, Hispanic, and Asian American women: unrecognized influences of sexual orientation. *Am J Public Health.* 2002;92(4):632-639.
27. Klose M, Jacobi F. Can gender differences in the prevalence of mental disorders be explained by sociodemographic factors? *Arch Women's Ment Health.* 2004;7(2):133-148.
28. Hasselstrom H, Hansen SE, Froberg K, Andersen LB. Physical fitness and physical activity during adolescence as predictors of cardiovascular disease risk in young adulthood. Danish Youth and Sports Study. An eight-year follow-up study. *Int J Sports Med.* 2002;23 Suppl 1:S27-S31.
29. Physical activity and health: a report of the Surgeon General. US Department of Health and Human Services. http://www.cdc.gov/nccdphp/sgr/pdf/execsumm.pdf. Accessed October 15, 2013.
30. Singh MA. Physical activity and bone health. *Aust Fam Physician.* 2004;33(3):125.
31. Ofili E. Ethnic disparities in cardiovascular health. *Ethnic Disparities.* 2001;11(4):838-840.

3

Key Components of Fitness

Catherine Rush Thompson, PT, PhD, MS

"True enjoyment comes from activity of the mind and exercise of the body; the two are united."
—Alexander Von Humboldt, as quoted in Tryon Edwards' *A Dictionary of Thoughts*, 1908

Fitness, or the state of being fit, is essential to mental and physical health. Whereas *mental fitness* includes self-acceptance, open-mindedness, self-direction, and calculated risk-taking, *physical fitness* is reflected in an individual's *metabolic fitness* (physiological measures at rest) and *performance-based fitness* (measures of movement and physical skill). Overall, fitness involves commitment, motivation, and responsibility for one's physical and mental well-being. Both mental fitness and physical fitness are integral to maintaining a healthy mind and body.

Mental Health, Fitness, and Wellness

Mental health is far more than the absence of mental illness; it involves an individual's self-perception, a realistic perception of others, and the ability to meet the demands of daily living. Mental health infers a mental condition characterized by good judgment. According to the *International Index and Dictionary of Rehabilitation and Social Integration*,[1] mental fitness involves habits related to the maintenance, improvement, and recovery of mental health. These habits include mental relaxation, reflection, meditation, intellectual stimulation, and creativity.

Mental fitness is a state of mind involving enjoyment of one's social and physical environment, belief in one's creativity and imagination, and using one's mental abilities to the fullest extent by taking risks, asking questions, accepting alternative points of view, and having an openness to continual growth and change.[1] Mental fitness combined with an optimistic life perspective offers the hope for achieving happiness and sustained health.

Maintaining mental fitness requires paying attention to one's lifestyle by balancing work and leisure, maintaining social contact with those who provide enjoyment, reviewing one's aims and goals in life, and planning to meet those goals. In addition, it is essential to be aware of the mind-body interaction and the need to get adequate diet, sleep, and exercise. Other key factors for maintaining

Thompson CR.
Prevention Practice and Health Promotion: A Health Care Professional's Guide to Health, Fitness, and Wellness, Second Edition (pp 37-50).

mental fitness include relationships with trusted friends and family members for advice and support when problems arise, as well as having an awareness of potential problems that arise from poor health and other risk factors in one's life. Finally, mental fitness relies on problem-solving abilities that incorporate the identification of problems, using personal and other resources judiciously, and taking the needed steps to resolve those problems. When serious problems arise and are handled ineffectively, an individual's mental health is jeopardized by the chronic stress these problems may cause.

Mental fitness allows a person to develop self-appreciation or the ability to assess both personal strengths and weaknesses. At the same time, mental fitness allows the individual to appreciate one's own and other people's unique and individual contributions. This appreciation helps to build strong affiliations with others that provide mutually supportive social networks.

Mental wellness, the more holistic concept of well-being, includes mental fitness and physical fitness as well as *resilience*, which is the ability to "bounce forward" from hardship. Some experts suggest that resilience is the overriding characteristic that predicts how well individuals handle both physical and mental challenges.[2] Mentally aware individuals accept that all the answers to life's challenges are not self-evident and often require assistance from others and reflection on personal experiences. Mental wellness involves handling stressors through appropriate stress management techniques, such as relaxation and exercise. According to *Mental Health: A Report of the Surgeon General*,[3] protective factors for mental health include interpersonal forgiveness.

Although tools are being developed to assess mental fitness and wellness, no standardized tool is currently available. A simple visual analog scale for each of the characteristics of mental fitness (including self-acceptance, open-mindedness, self-direction, and calculated risk taking) may provide some indication of an individual's personal perspective of mental fitness. The health professional's observations or inquiries of key traits (commitment, motivation, and responsibility for one's physical and mental well-being) could also be included in a subjective evaluation of an individual.

Stress assessments, such as the Holmes and Rahe Social Readjustment Rating Scale,[4] provide valuable information about an individual's life changes and potential stressors that could affect mental fitness. Often, patients who are injured or ill, particularly those in a hospital setting, are under significant stress related to their illness, their social isolation, the financial burden of hospitalization, and other significant life changes. Appropriate referrals to resources for social, financial, or psychological support in times of need are important for managing stressors that affect mental fitness.

Health care professionals can play an important role in promoting mental health through exercise and physical activity. Numerous studies support the benefits of exercise and physical activity, including improving mood state and self-esteem.[5-7] Acute aerobic exercise for 20 to 40 minutes can elevate mood and anxiety for several hours subsequent to activity. For healthy individuals, exercise is preventive, but for those with mild-to-moderate illness, well-controlled exercise can serve to promote both physical and mental health. The only cases where exercise has proven detrimental involve individuals who exercise excessively, as often observed in females with anorexia[8]; therefore, the guidance of a health care professional can help prevent any problems arising from inappropriate levels of exercise. Later chapters discuss exercise prescription based on individualized needs.

Physical Fitness

Whereas mental fitness reflects an individual's ability to handle mental stress, physical fitness enables an individual to withstand physiological stressors and extreme demands on the body. Individuals with preexisting levels of physical fitness are less vulnerable to illness and recover from injury and disease more readily than individuals who are *hypokinetic* (physically inactive or sedentary).

Physical fitness is evident with the body at rest and in action. Physical fitness at rest is defined as *metabolic fitness* (involving bodily functions at rest, including vital signs and blood tests).

TABLE 3-1. TARGET TOTAL CHOLESTEROL AND LOW-DENSITY LIPOPROTEIN CHOLESTEROL LEVELS	
TOTAL CHOLESTEROL LEVEL	**TOTAL CHOLESTEROL CATEGORY**
< 200 mg/dL	424,218
200 to 239 mg/dL	161,046
≥ 240 mg/dL	263,172
LDL CHOLESTEROL LEVEL	**LDL CHOLESTEROL CATEGORY**
< 100 mg/dL	36,755
100 to 129 mg/dL	59,253
130 to 159 mg/dL	85,446
160 to 189 mg/dL	226,168
≥ 190 mg/dL	Very high

Note: Cholesterol levels are measured in milligrams (mg) of cholesterol per deciliter (dL) of blood.

Source: High blood cholesterol: what you need to know. NIH Publication No. 05-3290. US Department of Health and Human Services. http://www.nhlbi.nih.gov/health/public/heart/chol/wyntk.pdf. Accessed May 20, 2014.

Performance-based or *motor fitness* relates to the body in action. Motor fitness can be divided into the following 2 categories:

1. *Health-related fitness* (cardiorespiratory fitness, muscle strength, muscle endurance, flexibility, posture and body composition), and
2. *Motor skill* (balance, coordination, reaction time, power, speed, and agility).

The remainder of this chapter provides an overview of these physical fitness concepts and how they relate to health, wellness, and preventive care.

Metabolic Fitness

Metabolic fitness reflects the health status of physiological systems at rest. Measures of metabolic fitness include standard blood and urine tests, such as blood lipid profiles, blood sugar, resting blood pressure, and insulin levels. Metabolic fitness shows positive responses to mild to moderate physical activity related to maintaining and building muscle tissue for glucose and fat metabolism, increasing maximum oxygen uptake, and reducing the risk of diabetes and heart disease.[9,10]

Lipid Profile

A *lipid profile* involves a series of blood tests including total cholesterol, *high-density lipoprotein* (HDL) cholesterol (good cholesterol that can increase with exercise), *low-density lipoprotein* (LDL) cholesterol (damaging cholesterol), and *triglycerides* (another type of fatty material found in the blood). Sometimes the laboratory report will provide ratio or risk scores based on lipid profile results and other risk factors, such as smoking, high blood pressure, low HDL cholesterol, diabetes, personal or family history of heart disease or vascular disease, older age, male sex, and other blood lipids. These laboratory values are often used to determine the risk for coronary heart disease or stroke. Treatment is based on overall risk of coronary heart disease. Target LDL cholesterol levels are listed in Table 3-1.

Although their role in heart disease is not entirely clear, it appears that as triglyceride levels rise, levels of HDL cholesterol fall. It is the complex interaction of these 3 types of lipids that is altered when a person has *hypercholesterolemia* (high blood cholesterol). Certain genetic causes of abnormal cholesterol and triglycerides, known as *hereditary hyperlipidemias*, are often difficult to treat. High cholesterol or triglycerides can also be associated with other diseases a person may have, such as diabetes. In most cases, however, elevated cholesterol levels are associated with an overly fatty diet coupled with an inactive lifestyle. It is also more common in those who are obese. Although individual lipid values are important to note, the 2 most important values are HDL cholesterol and total cholesterol.[11,12] According to the American Heart Association, the goal is to have a total cholesterol-to-HDL cholesterol ratio of 5-to-1 or better; an optimum ratio is 3.5-to-1.[13] Individuals with abnormal lipid levels need a referral to their physician for appropriate medical management.

Glucose Tests

The *oral glucose tolerance test* (OGTT or GTT) is a test sampling venous blood and is used to measure glucose use over time. It helps to identify individuals with diabetes or those at risk for diabetes. Another glucose test is the fasting plasma glucose test (FPG), which requires fasting prior to the blood sampling. The American Diabetes Association (ADA) recommends FPG as the screening test of choice "because FPG is easier and faster to perform, more convenient and acceptable to patients, and less expensive."[14] In healthy individuals, glucose levels rarely rise above 140 mg/dL (7.8 mmol/L) following meals. However, in individuals with increasing impairment of glucose tolerance, glucose levels rise following meals. According to the American Diabetes Association's Diagnosis and Classification of Diabetes Mellitus, fasting glucose levels in individuals with impairments in glucose tolerance often fall below 126 mg/dL.[15] The health care provider should be aware of test differences and their implications for diabetes risk screening.

Blood Insulin

The *blood insulin test*, or *insulin test*, measures blood samples for the amount of circulating insulin, a hormone released from the beta cells of the pancreas and responsible for regulating blood glucose usage by surrounding tissue. This blood test provides information about how effectively the body can use glucose and synthesize and store triglycerides and proteins. High blood glucose following a meal stimulates the release of insulin, whereas low blood glucose inhibits insulin release. Normal values are 5 to 20 μm/mL while fasting. Lower-than-normal values suggest type 1 or 2 diabetes, and above-normal levels suggest possible type 2 diabetes, obesity (secondary to the insulin resistance syndrome), or other insulin-related disease processes.[14] Obesity decreases the sensitivity of various tissues to insulin, which normally results in the pancreas overcompensating and making excess insulin. A person with potential diabetes or other insulin-related pathologies requires an appropriate medical referral.

Pulse Rate

The *pulse rate* is the number of throbbing sensations felt over a peripheral artery when the heart beats. This rate normally ranges from 60 to 100 pulses per minute and indirectly assesses the heart's activity, as well as the status of blood flow through peripheral arteries. Assessment includes counting the number of pulsations, noting the quality of pulsations, and determining the rhythm of heartbeats. When counting the pulse rate, the examiner places a fingertip over an artery and senses the pulse through gentle pressure over the artery. Regular rhythms or pulse sensations may be counted for 30 seconds and multiplied by 2 for a 1-minute pulse rate. The quality of the pulse is reflected in pulse strength. Numerous factors influence pulse rate, including age, activity preceding measurements, increased temperature, medications, sex, stress, pain, emotions, blood volume, and body build. Although age, sex, and body build tend to remain constant for an individual, other factors should be controlled as much as possible to improve reliability of the test. It is important that the tested individual be in a resting position, supine or sitting, for at least 5 minutes for resting pulse rates. Pulse examinations may have interobserver variation. Individuals who lack both *pedal pulses* (pulses measured at the top of the foot above the ankle) have a high risk of peripheral artery disease and should be referred for a thorough cardiovascular examination. Also, a *bruit* (high-pitched sound during auscultation of vessels) suggests possible vascular problems, such as an aneurysm, arteriovenous fistula, or stenosis, and also indicates the need for referral.

Blood Pressure

Blood pressure involves indirectly measuring the effectiveness of the heartbeat, the adequacy of blood volume, and the presence of any obstruction to vascular flow through the use of a sphygmomanometer and a stethoscope. Pressure measurements include systolic, diastolic, and pulse pressure. Sites for placement of the stethoscope include the brachial artery, the popliteal artery, and the radial artery. Normal blood pressure is 120/80, with the top number representing the systolic pressure and the lower number representing the diastolic pressure. Systolic blood pressure is the rhythmic contraction of the heart, especially of the ventricles, driving blood through the aorta and pulmonary artery after each dilation (relaxation) or diastole. Blood pressure varies with age, sex, and body size. It is important to listen for Korotkoff sounds. The 5 Korotkoff sounds are noted as the pressure in the syphgmomanometer cuff is released during the measurement of arterial pressure. They are described as follows: Korotkoff I is a sharp thud, Korotkoff II is a loud blowing sound, Korotkoff III is a soft thud, Korotkoff IV is a soft blowing sound, and Korotkoff V is silence or the diastole.[16] These sounds help the clinician identify systolic blood pressure, diastolic pressure, and possible abnormalities in blood flow.

Blood pressure can also be obtained by palpation or by Doppler (an ultrasound method of examining blood vessels). Abnormal blood pressure readings include hypertension (high blood pressure) and hypotension (low blood pressure). Orthostatic hypotension is commonly seen in patients with low blood pressure. *Orthostasis* means upright posture, and *hypotension* means low blood pressure.[16] Thus, orthostatic hypotension consists of symptoms of dizziness, faintness, or lightheadedness that appear only on standing and are caused by low blood pressure. Orthostatic hypotension may be caused by anemia, hypovolemia (low blood volume), medications, dialysis, neurological problems, or cardiac problems.[16]

The American Heart Association categorized blood pressure as follows:

- Normal: less than 120/less than 80
- Prehypertension: 120 to 139/80 to 89
- High blood pressure–stage 1: 140 to 159/90 to 99
- High blood pressure–stage 2: 160 or higher/100 to 110
- Hypertensive crisis: higher than 180/higher than 110

Altered blood pressure may require a referral for further examination, and a hypertensive crisis requires immediate medical care.

Health-Related Fitness

Health-related fitness, also known as *physiological fitness*, is generally associated with a reduced risk of disease. Components of physiological or health-related fitness include cardiorespiratory fitness, muscular strength, muscular endurance, flexibility, and posture. Although many view body composition as a component of physical fitness, it may also be considered a component of metabolic fitness as a nonperformance measure of fitness.

Cardiorespiratory Fitness

Cardiorespiratory fitness is the individual's aerobic capacity to perform large-muscle, *whole-body* (gross motor) physical activity of moderate to high intensity over extended periods of time. This type of physical fitness is particularly important for the prevention of heart disease and metabolic syndrome, which is a condition that predisposes individuals to heart disease, stroke, and diabetes.

Cardiorespiratory fitness is assessed by a variety of measures that examine oxygen use and endurance while the individual performs functional movement, such as walking and running. The best measure of cardiorespiratory fitness is *VO_2 max*, representing the volume (V) of oxygen used when a person reaches his or her maximum (max) ability to supply oxygen (O_2) to muscle tissue during exercise. This value may be compared with a resting value of oxygen usage, known as VO_2 resting. One *MET* (metabolic equivalent) is another unit of measure representing resting oxygen uptake. One MET equals approximately 3.5 mg of oxygen consumed per minute per kg of body weight. Because MET levels may vary between males and females, it is important to find current MET tables for reference. A helpful table for MET values can be found at http://www.instituteoflifestylemedicine.org/file/doc/tools_resources/METValues.pdf.

Another indicator of cardiorespiratory fitness is *respiratory reserve* (VO_2R), or the difference between the maximum oxygen uptake and resting oxygen uptake (VO_2 max − VO_2 resting). A percentage of this value is often used to determine appropriate intensities for physical activity. When testing an individual during exercise, the examiner can gauge the individual's perception of the physical effort needed to perform the activity by using *ratings of perceived exertion* (RPE). This subjective assessment of exercise intensity is based on how the individual feels during various levels of physical exertion over time. Although RPE is considered a reliable tool, clinicians need to consider that clients, particularly those with brain injury, may interpret the words on the scale differently and should be cautious of other observations when evaluating exercise tolerance.[17]

The Rockport 1-mile walk test, the YMCA 3-minute step test, and distance walks/runs can be used to determine functional cardiovascular fitness or endurance. Other measures of cardiovascular endurance include maximal exercise performance (on a treadmill or cycle ergometer) while mechanically measuring the individual's oxygen consumption at moderate to high intensities of exercise.

Another factor used to assess cardiovascular fitness is the speed at which the heart rate returns to pre-exercise levels after performing extended exercise. In determining cardiovascular fitness, it is important to measure an individual's resting and maximum heart rate to know safe ranges of exercise. Various formulas are used to calculate an individual's maximum heart rate. Evidence-based calculations for determining maximum heart rate include the following 2 formulas:

- $HR_{max} = 206.9 - (0.67 \times \text{age})$ for men
- $HR_{max} = 206 - (0.88 \times \text{age})$ for women[18]

Resting heart rate is the individual's lowest heart rate, measured at rest. The heart rate recovery is measured immediately after performing strenuous exercise, then remeasured after a period of rest. A quick heart rate recovery indicates good cardiovascular fitness.

Muscular Strength

Muscular strength is the ability of muscles to produce force at high intensities over short periods of time. Muscle strength is essential for the performance of daily activities of living and key to preventive care. *Sarcopenia*, or age-related loss of muscle mass, can be prevented with regular exercise. According to the Centers for Disease Control and Prevention, sarcopenia resulting from decreased physical activity is one of the top 5 health risks for older adults.[19] Sarcopenia is likely a multifactorial condition that impairs physical function and predisposes an individual to disability.[19] This disabling condition may be reduced with lifestyle interventions that include increased muscle strengthening. The following chapter discusses the principles of fitness training designed to increase muscular strength.

Muscular Endurance

Muscular endurance is the ability to perform gross motor activity of moderate to high intensity over a long period of time. Quality of life is affected by reduced strength and endurance that limit a person's ability to remain physically active. When combined together vs alone, muscle endurance training and strength training have a greater effect on walking distance, endurance exercise time, and the quality of life of patients with chronic obstructive pulmonary disease (COPD). It is estimated that 16 million people in the United States have COPD, including emphysema, chronic bronchitis, and chronic asthma.[19] These individuals could benefit from exercise that improves both their strength and muscular endurance for activities of daily living.

Computer-controlled equipment can measure the muscular force used in generating an *isometric contraction* (involving no movement of body parts) *and isokinetic contractions* (involving controlled movement). These types of equipment are costly, may require specialized expertise, and are not always available in community or clinical settings. Although these highly reliable types of quantitative assessments of muscle strength are desirable, there are a number of other options available to the clinician:

- *Manual muscle testing* (MMT) is used to evaluate the strength of individual muscles and muscle groups based on palpating muscle contractions or having the individual perform specific movements (either gravity eliminated or with resistance provided by either gravity or manual resistance).
- *Handheld dynamometry* can be a reliable assessment technique when used by an experienced clinician. The handheld dynamometer consists of a simple, adjustable gripping device capable of measuring muscular force and sensitive to detection of neuromuscular weakness. The grip strength is a useful measure for overall arm strength and can be a helpful screening tool for fitness.
- *The one-repetition maximum strength test (1-RM)* is a popular method of measuring muscle strength. This test provides a measure of the maximal force (generally using free weights) an individual can lift with one repetition.
- *The YMCA bench press test* is used to evaluate strength and muscular endurance using a relatively light load. This test has separate loads for males and females (males are required to lift an 80-lb barbell and females are required to lift a 35-lb barbell).
- *The push-up test* involves performing standard push-ups while positioned with hands and feet touching the floor, the body and legs well-aligned, and the arms extended and at right angles to the body. This test is primarily used for assessing upper body strength.

Muscular endurance may be tested by examining the ability of muscles to repeatedly contract over time. All of the muscle strength assessments with repeated muscular contractions include a muscle endurance component and can be used to determine muscular endurance.

Flexibility

Flexibility is the ability to move muscles and joints (including soft tissue) through their full range of motion (ROM). Without flexibility, joints cannot move to their fullest extent, despite having full muscle strength to complete the movement. Limited spinal flexibility can lead to functional limitations that impair independent living, such as functional reaching and maintaining balance. Spinal flexibility is a contributor to *functional reach*, a measure of functional limitation and an established measure of balance control. Because older adults are at an increased risk for losing balance and falling, maintaining joint flexibility across the lifespan is important for maintaining functional independence and one's quality of life. The *sit and reach test* is commonly used to measure the overall flexibility of the body but primarily tests the flexibility of the posterior legs, back, shoulders, arms, head, and neck.[20] ROM measurements also provide information about the individual's ability to either actively or passively move specific joints in all planes of motion. It is essential that the clinician be familiar with anatomy and well trained in the use of a goniometer, patient positioning, and the "end-feels" of the joint to assess ROM accurately. Many factors influence joint ROM, including disease processes or injuries affecting joint tissue, bone or surrounding tissues, inactivity or immobility, age (older adults tend to be less flexible), hormonal status (pregnant women tend to be more lax), and sex (men tend to be less flexible). *Joint play* is the normal looseness within a joint that allows movement to occur. The joint play movements are very small but precise in range. Movements of joint play are independent of the action of voluntary muscles, yet the summation of normal joint play movements allow pain-free and fluid motion. If muscles are imbalanced, impaired, or inactive, they may cause limitations in joint play movements, unless the joint is passively moved to maintain joint motion.

Posture

Posture is the maintenance of correct alignment of body parts. Although many think of posture as maintaining static or unmoving positions, postural adjustments responsible for maintenance of good posture during rest and during activity involve continuous muscle adjustments and awareness of where the body is in space. Poor postural habits commonly lead to body malalignment and chronic musculoskeletal problems, such as low back pain. According to the Centers for Disease Control and Prevention, 15% of adult physician visits are related to back pain. Interestingly, the incidence of low back pain is highest in 2 groups: (1) sedentary individuals with poor sitting posture and weakened muscles, and (2) individuals who injure their backs doing manual labor.[21] In both instances, proper posture while sitting or lifting large objects plays a key role in reducing the risk of low back pain and disability. Photographs are particularly useful for documenting postural problems or asymmetries. The forward bending test is a classic screening for spinal malalignment. Lordosis, commonly referred to as sway back, or an increased curve in the lower spine, is commonly detected and often leads to low back pain later in life. Proper exercise and postural alignment can alleviate some of the contributors to chronic back pain.

Body Composition

Body composition is the final aspect of health-related fitness. Body composition is often represented as 2 components: lean body weight and fat weight. The National Institutes of Health (NIH) uses body mass index (BMI) to define normal weight, overweight, and obesity because it correlates strongly (in adults) with the total body fat content. According to the NIH, overweight is defined as a BMI of 25 to 29.9 kg/m^2, depending on sex, whereas obesity is generally defined as a BMI of 30 kg/m^2 and above.[22] It is important to note that muscular people may have a high BMI without undue health risks. Body composition often focuses on body fat because a high percentage of Americans are obese and at risk for significant health problems.

Assessing body fat and monitoring changes in body fat with exercise can be helpful in identifying changes in body composition over time. Health and fitness professionals use a wide range of tests to determine body composition, depending on their clinical setting and available equipment. Some measures are sophisticated and costly, whereas others involve low-cost equipment and precise measurement techniques for increased reliability:

- *Skinfold thickness* measurements involve measuring skin and subcutaneous adipose tissues at several different standard anatomical sites around the body and converting these measures to percentage body fat. One calculation for the percent body fat is % body fat = (fat weight/total body weight) × 100.
- BMI is the key index for relating a person's body weight to height. The BMI equation is as follows: BMI = M/(H × H), where M = body mass in kilograms and H = height in meters. A higher BMI score usually indicates higher levels of body fat. This calculation is accurate for normal populations but is not valid for elderly populations, pregnant women, or muscular athletes. A helpful site for locating BMI calculators for both children and adults can be found at http://www.cdc.gov/healthyweight/assessing/bmi/index.html.
- *Waist-to-hip ratio* is measured using a tape measure around the waist and the largest hip circumference. The ratio is a simple calculation of the waist girth divided by the hip girth. Table 3-2 gives general guidelines for acceptable levels for waist-to-hip ratio.

When combining BMI with waist measurements, the health professional can determine an individual's risk for disease, particularly cardiac pathology. Table 3-3 lists BMI scores with hip-to-waist ratios and associated risks for disease.

Table 3-2. Hip-to-Waist Ratios					
	ACCEPTABLE		**UNACCEPTABLE**		
	Excellent	*Good*	*Average*	*High*	*Extreme*
Male	< 0.85	0.85 to 0.90	0.90 to 0.95	0.95 to 1.00	> 1.00
Female	< 0.75	0.75 to 0.80	0.80 to 0.85	0.85 to 0.90	> 0.90

Adapted from Waist circumference and waist-hip ratio: report of a WHO expert consultation. World Health Organization. http://whqlibdoc.who.int/publications/2011/9789241501491_eng.pdf. Accessed May 20, 2014.

Table 3-3. Body Mass Index and Risk of Associated Disease				
			DISEASE RISK* RELATIVE TO NORMAL WEIGHT AND WAIST CIRCUMFERENCE	
	BMI, kg/m²	*Obesity Class*	*Men ≤ 102 cm (40 in); Women ≤ 88 cm (35 in)*	*Men > 102 cm (40 in); Women > 88 cm (35 in)*
Underweight	< 18.5			
Normal	18.5 to 24.9			
Overweight	25.0 to 29.9		Increased	High
Obesity	30.0 to 34.9	I	High	Very high
	35.0 to 39.9	II	Very high	Very high
Extreme obesity	40.0+	III	Extremely high	Extremely high

*Disease risk for type 2 diabetes, hypertension, and cardiovascular disease.

+Increased waist circumference also can be a marker for increased risk, even in persons of normal weight.

Source: Classification of overweight and obesity by BMI, waist circumference, and associated disease risks. National Heart, Lung, and Blood Institute. National Institutes of Health. http://www.nhlbi.nih.gov/health/public/heart/obesity/lose_wt/bmi_dis.htm. Accessed May 20, 2014.

- *Girth measurements and body breadth measurements* are additional measures of the body's size and shape. Girth measurements, or circumferential measures of various body parts, indicate growth, nutritional status, and fat patterning. Body breadth measurements (used to determine body type and frame size) are taken at the hips, shoulders, extremities, and other areas of concern. The clinician can use these measurements over time to monitor changes in the body proportion and size.
- *Hydrostatic weighing* has been called the gold standard for measuring body composition. For this assessment, the individual, dressed in minimal clothing, is weighed for the dry weight; the fully submerged underwater weight is then determined. Body density is then calculated, taking into account the body weight, the density of water, the residual lung volume, and corrections for air trapped in the gastrointestinal tract.
- *Bioelectric impedance* involves measurement of the conduction of electrical currents through the body. It is important to consider that body hydration, body temperature, and other variables affect the body's conductivity and should be held constant for all measurements for improved reliability. The device measures the amount of fat-free mass that allows current flow. Bioelectric impedance analysis is based on the principle that the resistance to an applied electric current is inversely related to the amount of fat-free mass within the body.[23]

- *Dual-energy x-ray absorptiometry (DEXA)* uses radiographs to differentiate the components of soft tissue (fat and lean) and bone. DEXA also has the ability to determine body composition in defined regions (ie, in the arms, legs, and trunk). DEXA measurements are based in part on the assumption that the hydration of fat-free mass remains constant at 73%. Hydration, however, can vary from 67% to 85% and can be variable in certain disease states.[24] This assessment tool is highly expensive, but offers accurate body composition analysis that can screen for additional problems, such as osteoporosis. Individuals may have total body scans for total body composition or regional body scans of areas at risk for osteoporosis. Total body scans may be helpful in diagnosing and monitoring the following conditions: obesity, growth hormone abnormalities and treatment effects, primary hyperparathyroidism, secondary hyperparathyroidism, anabolic steroids therapy, anorexia nervosa, Cushing's syndrome, muscular dystrophy, cachexic or wasting disorders (AIDS, cancer), chronic kidney disease, and malabsorptive syndromes.[25]
- *Near infrared interactance (NIR)* is based on light penetration using a fiber optic probe into various tissues with reflection off the bone. The NIR contains a digital analyzer that indirectly measures the tissue composition (fat and water) at various sites on the body. The NIR data are entered into a prediction equation with the person's height, weight, frame size, and level of activity to estimate the percent body fat. This assessment of body fat, although simple, fast, and noninvasive, is costly and not reliable for very lean or very obese individuals.
- *Magnetic resonance imaging (MRI)* is a diagnostic imaging tool that uses contrast materials to help provide a clear picture of body structure. It uses magnets and computers to create images of certain areas inside the body. Unlike radiographs, MRI does not involve ionizing radiation. The person lies within the magnet as a computer scans the body. High-quality images show the amount of fat and where it is distributed. MRI takes approximately 30 minutes, but its use is limited due to the high cost of equipment and analysis.
- *Computed tomography (CT)* scans the body, providing cross-sectional images of each scan. A radiograph tube sends a beam of photons toward a detector. As the beam rotates around a person, data are collected, stored, and applied to calculations that determine body composition. CT is particularly useful in giving a ratio of intra-abdominal fat to extra-abdominal fat. Although CT scans are noninvasive, they subject individuals to radiation and are extremely costly.
- The *BOD POD* (COSMED, Rome, Italy), instead of using water to measure body volume, uses air displacement. The BOD POD uses computerized sensors to measure how much air is displaced while a person sits within the capsule, then calculates the body density and estimated body fat.[25] This new equipment is expensive and limited in availability but provides values highly correlated ($r = .93$) with hydrostatic weighing.[25]

Although these measures provide a variety of indices for physical fitness, it is important to consider that physical fitness is influenced by genetics, environmental influences, and the individual's activity levels. Many factors offer insight regarding the individual's disease risk and health habits, including patterns of growth and development, a history of exercise and good nutrition, a medical and psychosocial history, and a history of significant others in that individual's environment. For example, genetic information can be used to trace potential health problems or to predict family characteristics, such as typical growth and developmental patterns.

Motor fitness provides another array of tests offering insight regarding an individual's physical capabilities for performing complex motor tasks.

Skill-Related or Motor Fitness

Motor fitness is often associated with athletic competition but should be considered in the overall fitness of all individuals. Motor fitness is essential for effectively, efficiently, and safely performing activities of daily living and participating in the community. Components of motor fitness include postural balance, coordination, reaction time, power, speed, and agility.

Postural Balance

Postural balance, or equilibrium, can be described as the body's ability to maintain an intended position (*static balance*) or progress through various movements without losing postural control (*dynamic balance*). Although equilibrium normally develops in the first 2 years of life, various factors may affect an individual's ability to maintain balance. These factors include visual input, normal functioning of the vestibular system (responsible for sensing movement and head position in space), adequate muscle strength and joint ROM to assume and maintain postures, and normal somatosensory or sensations regarding the body's position in space. This information is integrated in the central nervous system to coordinate all the inputs responsible for the maintenance of equilibrium at rest and while moving.

Some assessments of balance involve sophisticated equipment that can isolate the various factors contributing to balance problems, whereas other measures focus on functional skills for independent living. Athletes performing in high-level competition require tests designed to meet specific criteria that exceed normative values of the general population. Tests for highly skilled athletes are not included in this listing of postural balance tests. Various tests for postural balance include the following:

- *Dynamic posturography*: This measure of balance requires equipment that can isolate the various factors contributing to standing balance. The individual stands on a platform in an enclosed space that obscures vision. For safety purposes, the person wears a harness to prevent falls. During the test, the platform is moved to elicit equilibrium reactions or the visual field is altered to isolate possible deficits in balance. By isolating the various factors that contribute to the maintenance of standing balance, this test assesses movement coordination and the organization of visual, somatosensory, and vestibular information relevant to postural control.
- *One-legged stance test*: The individual is asked to stand on 1 leg while the examiner times the duration of stance on each leg (with eyes opened or closed).
- *Sharpened Romberg's test*: The individual stands with both feet in tandem (feet touching heel-to-toe), while both arms are crossed at chest level as the examiner stands nearby for safety. This test is performed with eyes open and eyes closed to isolate visual input that can mask problems with balance.

The following are standardized tests that have a wide range of functional tasks and balance criteria used to determine the balance capabilities of populations at risk, including older adults and individuals with motor problems.

- *Berg Balance Scale*: This standardized scale is a 14-item test that focuses on reaching, bending, transferring, standing, rising, and other functional tasks for a total of 56 points.
- *Clinical Test of Sensory Interaction and Balance*: This standardized assessment measures static balance under 3 visual and 2 supported conditions.
- *Functional reach test*: This test measures the difference in inches between a person's arm position at rest (with the shoulder flexed to 90 degrees) and the distance reached forward, while maintaining a fixed base of support while standing.
- *Tinetti Balance Test of the Performance-Oriented Assessment of Mobility Problems*: This test consists of 28 items related to balance while standing and moving.
- *Timed Up and Go Test*: This balance test measures the time needed to rise to standing from a chair, walk 3 meters, turn, walk back to the chair, and sit down.
- *Physical performance test*: This test measures standing and moving balance, feeding, and writing; the majority of these items are timed.

Coordination

Coordination is harmonious movement reflecting the coordination of muscle contractions and their timing for desired movement. Coordinated movement includes the smooth and controlled lay-up for a basketball goal performed by a skilled athlete and the graceful movement of a figure skater performing on ice. Likewise, coordinated movement can include placing blocks into a tower without error, as well as performing jumping jacks with ease. Tests for coordination include the following:

- *Finger-to-nose test*: This test is designed to observe the smoothness and timing of arm movement. The individual is asked to repetitively touch the nose using the index finger and then to touch the clinician's outstretched finger.
- *Dysdiadokinesis or rapidly alternating movements*: For this test, the individual alternately taps the palm then the back of one hand on the thigh. The examiner observes this movement for smoothness and speed.
- *Lower extremity coordination*: For coordination in the lower extremities or legs, the individual is tested for smoothness and speed of movement while trying to make precise movements with each leg, such as sliding the heel down the shin of the opposite leg.

Individuals with poor coordination may need a more thorough examination to determine if fatigue, neurological insult, or other factors may contribute to poorly coordinated movement.

Reaction Time

Reaction time is the amount of time needed to produce movement in response to a stimulus. Reaction time is especially important for completing movements within a safe time frame for effective function. For example, reaction time is critical when driving a car, such as quickly pressing on the brakes at a red light. Computers, the more expensive option, can test reaction times to various visual stimuli with specialized programs and equipment providing the appropriate stimuli for the desired motor response. *The ruler test*, a quick and readily available test for reaction time, measures the response when a ruler is dropped over the individual's head. The aim is to catch the ruler before it drops onto the floor.

Power

Power is the ability to generate force (measured in force units/time units [ie, watts]) or the ability to exert maximum muscular contraction instantly in an explosive burst of movements. Power is important for lifting objects and pushing objects, as observed in competitive football and weightlifting. The *PWC-170 test* is used to predict the power output (watts) at a projected heart rate of 170 beats per minute (bpm). The individual is asked to perform 2 consecutive 6-minute bicycle ergometer rides with workloads selected to produce a heart rate between 120 and 140 bpm on the first session and 150 and 170 bpm on the second session. For each session, the average heart rate (bpm) and power output (watts) are recorded.[26]

Speed

Speed is the rate of movement and is essential for performing daily activities in a timely manner. Speed is often a convenient measure used to determine the amount of time a person needs to ambulate from one point to another or to perform work-related tasks, such as typing. Timed tests for skilled motor performance determine an individual's speed. Examples of timed tests include the *60-meter speed test*,[27,28] which assesses gross motor speed for normal or athletic populations; and the *Jebsen hand function test*,[29] which is a standardized assessment used to measure dexterity or the speed of fine motor movements. With 7 subtests, this tool evaluates a broad range of hand functions used in daily activities, using common items such as paper clips, cans, pencils, and other functional objects.

Agility

Agility is the ability to move in a quick and easy fashion or the ability to perform a series of explosive power movements in rapid succession in opposing directions. Agility is often demonstrated by maneuvering around other objects, such as going through an obstacle course as quickly as possible without falling or losing control of movement. Agility may be measured by observing how an individual navigates an environment or may include a battery of standardized tests that assess movement in multiple directions. Tests of agility generally involve the ability to rapidly and easily change directions. Tests of agility include the *hexagonal obstacle agility test*, the *Illinois agility run test*, and the *lateral changing of direction test*.[30]

The *Bruninks-Oseretsky Test of Motor Proficiency*[31] is a useful test that can be used to screen for multiple areas of motor fitness for pediatric populations. This measure is a norm-referenced, standardized test composed of 8 subtests designed to evaluate the following skills: gross motor development, running speed and agility, balance, bilateral coordination, strength (arm, shoulder, abdominal, and leg), upper-limb coordination, fine motor development, response speed, visual-motor control, upper-limb speed, and dexterity. The examiner can select measures that best match the functional skills associated with the individual's occupation or leisure function for a customized screening test for any of these areas of motor fitness.

Summary

The aim of Healthy People 2020 is to build a society in which all people live long, healthy lives. Both mental health and physical fitness are foundational to optimizing each individual's participation in all that life offers. Whereas mental fitness includes self-acceptance, open-mindedness, self-direction, and calculated risk-taking, physical fitness is reflected in an individual's metabolic fitness (physiological measures at rest) and performance-based fitness (measures of movement and physical skill). Overall, fitness involves commitment, motivation, and responsibility for one's physical and mental well-being.

Health care professionals should enhance all types of fitness when working with populations ranging in age from young infants to older adults. How can the health care professional enhance mental and physical fitness? Chapter 4 provides information about physical activity and fitness training designed for various populations. Chapter 5 outlines the screening process for identifying health, fitness, and wellness concerns. Chapter 6 focuses on issues in childhood and adolescence and how they can be addressed, and Chapters 7 through 9 discuss common issues in adulthood affecting adults and older adults and appropriate management. As additional resources for healthy lifestyle habits affecting mental and physical fitness, Chapter 10 provides suggestions for stress management and Chapter 11 offers basic nutritional guidelines and suggestions for healthy diets. Finally, Chapter 12 discusses health protection screening that enables health care experts to determine whether individuals are both physically and mentally able to meet the challenges of everyday life or whether a referral to an expert is needed. Additional chapters consider health conditions affecting various body systems and offer suggestions for preventing problems as well as addressing chronic illness. Using the World Health Organization model of disability, the health care professional can identify impairments affecting body systems and body functions, consider how activities are limited by these impairments, and explore resources to enable those in their care to have both mental and physical fitness and improved quality of life.

References

1. "mental fitness." International Index and Dictionary of Rehabilitation and Social Integration. http://www.med.univ-rennes1.fr/iidris/index.php?action=contexte&num=1487&mode=mu&lg=an. Accessed May 20, 2014.
2. Doll B, Lyon M. Risk and resilience: implications for the delivery of educational and mental health services in schools. *School Psychology Review.* 1998;27:3.
3. Mental health: a report of the Surgeon General. US Department of Health and Human Services. http://www.surgeongeneral.gov/library/mentalhealth/home.html#forward. Accessed October 15, 2005.
4. Holmes TH, Rahe RH. The social readjustment rating scale. *J Psychosom Res.* 1967;11:213-218.

5. Vance DE, Wadley VG, Ball KK, Roenker DL, Rizzo M. The effects of physical activity and sedentary behavior on cognitive health in older adults. *J Aging Phys Act.* 2005;13(3):294-313.
6. Elavsky S, McAuley E, Motl RW, et al. Physical activity enhances long-term quality of life in older adults: efficacy, esteem, and affective influences. *Ann Behav Med.* 2005;30(2):138-145.
7. Sacker A, Cable N. Do adolescent leisure-time physical activities foster health and well-being in adulthood? Evidence from two British birth cohorts. *Eur J Public Health.* 2006;16(3):332-336.
8. Hughes CS, Hughes S. The female athlete syndrome. Anorexia nervosa: reflections on a personal journey. *Orthop Nurs.* 2004;23(4):252-260.
9. Saltin B, Pilgaard H. Metabolic fitness: physical activity and health [in Danish]. *Ugeskr Laeger.* 2002;164(16):2156-2162.
10. Horvath P, Eagen C, Nadine M, et al. The effects of varying dietary fat on performance and metabolism in trained male and female runners. *J Am Coll Nutr.* 2000;19(1):52-60.
11. Behrenbeck T. How important is cholesterol ratio? Mayo Clinic. http://www.mayoclinic.com/health/cholesterol-ratio/AN01761. Accessed May 25, 2003.
12. McLaughlin T, Abbasi F, Cheal K, Chu J, Lamendola C, Reaven G. Use of metabolic markers to identify overweight individuals who are insulin resistant. *Ann Intern Med.* 2003;139:802-809.
13. Page IH, Berrettoni JN, Butkus A, Sones FM Jr. Prediction of coronary artery disease based on clinical suspicion, age, total cholesterol, and triglyceride. *Circulation.* 1970;42(4):625-645.
14. Report of the Expert Committee on the Diagnosis and Classification of Diabetes Mellitus. *Diabetes Care.* 1997;20(7):1183-1197.
15. Diagnosis and classification of diabetes mellitus. American Diabetes Association. http://care.diabetesjournals.org/content/31/Supplement_1/S55.short. Accessed May 20, 2014.
16. Pickering TG, Hall JE, Appel LJ, et al. Recommendations for blood pressure measurement in humans and experimental animals: part 1: blood pressure measurement in humans: a statement for professionals from the subcommittee of professional and public education of the American Heart Association council on high blood pressure research. *Circulation.* 2005;111(5):697-716.
17. Dawes HN, Barker KL, Cockburn J, Roach N, Scott O, Wade D. Borg's rating of perceived exertion scales: Do the verbal anchors mean the same for different clinical groups? *Arch Phys Med Rehab.* 2005;86(5):912-916.
18. Gulati M, Shaw L, Thisted R, et al. Heart rate response to exercise stress testing in asymptomatic women. *Circulation.* 2010;122:130-137.
19. Newman AB, Lee JS, Visser M, et al. Weight change and the conservation of lean mass in old age: the Health, Aging and Body Composition Study. *Am J Clin Nutr.* 2005;82(4):872-878.
20. Wells KF, Dillon EK. The sit and reach—a test of back and leg flexibility. *Research Quarterly.* American Association for Health, Physical Education and Recreation. http://www.tandfonline.com/doi/abs/10.1080/10671188.1952.10761965?journalCode=urqe17#.U3twfygngTI. Accessed May 20, 2014.
21. Healthy People 2020. US Department of Health and Human Services. http://www.healthypeople.gov/. Accessed April 20, 2013.
22. Calculate your body mass index. National Institutes of Health. http://www.nhlbi.nih.gov/guidelines/obesity/BMI/bmicalc.htm. Accessed December 29, 2013.
23. Williamson DF. Descriptive epidemiology of body weight and weight change in US adults. *Ann Intern Med.* 1993;119(7 Pt 2):646-649.
24. Whole body dual x-ray absorptiometry (DEXA) to determine body composition. Blue Cross Blue Shield of Mississippi. http://www.bcbsms.com/index.php/index.php?q=provider-medical-policy-search.html&action=viewPolicy&path=%2Fpolicy%2Femed%2FWhole+Body+DEXA.html. Accessed May 20, 2014.
25. Buchholz A, Bartok C, Schoeller D. The validity of bioelectrical impedance models in clinical populations. *Nutr Clin Pract.* 2004;19(5):433-446.
26. McCrory MA, Gomez TD, Bernauer EM, Mole PA. Evaluation of a new air displacement plethysmograph for measuring human body composition. *Med Sci Sports Exerc.* 1995;27(12):1686-1691.
27. Gore C, Booth M, Bauman A, Neville O. Utility of pwc75% as an estimate of aerobic power in epidemiological and population-based studies. *Med Sc Sports Exerc.* 1999;31(2):348-351.
28. Mackenzie B. 60 metre speed test. http://www.brianmac.co.uk/speed60.htm. Accessed April 4, 2013.
29. Davis Sears E, Chung KC. Validity and responsiveness of the Jebsen-Taylor Hand Function Test. *J Hand Surg Am.* 2010;35(1):30-37.
30. Fitness testing: agility. Fitnessforworld. http://www.fitnessforworld.com/fitness_testing/agility.htm. Accessed September 30, 2012.
31. Wilson BN, Polatajko HJ, Kaplan BJ, Faris P. Use of the Bruininks-Oseretsky test of motor proficiency in occupational therapy. *Am J Occup Ther.* 1995;49(1):8-17.

4

Fitness Training

Catherine Rush Thompson, PT, PhD, MS

"Physical fitness is not only one of the most important keys to a healthy body, it is the basis of dynamic and creative intellectual activity."—John F. Kennedy, *Sports Illustrated*, December 26, 1960

Improving Fitness

A healthy lifestyle involving physical activity positively affects fitness and well-being. Physical fitness can involve any physical exertion that improves mental and physical health, including the prevention or correction of impairments. Physical activity must be performed to a certain extent (number of repetitions or minutes) to reap any benefits. According to the Surgeon General's report, "significant health benefits can be obtained by including a moderate amount of physical activity (eg, 30 minutes of brisk walking or raking leaves, 15 minutes of running, or 45 minutes of playing volleyball) on most, if not all, days of the week. Through a modest increase in daily activity, most Americans can improve their health and quality of life...Additional benefits can be gained through greater amounts of physical activity. Regular physical activity is one of the most potent and least expensive preventive measures for mental health, physical health and well-being...People who maintain a regular regimen of physical activity [that is, of longer duration or of more vigorous intensity] are likely to derive greater benefit."[1] Table 4-1 lists both the physical and mental benefits of physical activity.

Considerations for Exercise and Physical Activity

Numerous factors need to be taken into consideration when engaging in exercise or physical activity. These factors relate to the individual, the environment, and the type of exercise or physical activity selected.

Thompson CR.
Prevention Practice and Health Promotion: A Health Care Professional's Guide to Health, Fitness, and Wellness, Second Edition (pp 51-70).

Table 4-1. Benefits of Physical Activity
• Lower overall mortality. Benefits are greatest among the most active persons but are also evident for individuals who reported only moderate activity.
• Lower risk of coronary heart disease. The cardiac risk of being inactive is comparable to the risk from smoking cigarettes.
• Lower risk of cancers, including colon cancer and breast cancer
• Lower risk of diabetes
• Lower risk of developing high blood pressure. Exercise also lowers blood pressure in individuals who have hypertension.
• Lower risk of obesity
• Lower risk of developing depression
• Improved mood and relief of symptoms of depression
• Improved quality of life and improved functioning
• Improved function in persons with arthritis
• Lower risk of falls and injury
• Prevention of bone loss and fracture after the menopause
• Improved quality of sleep
• Improved sleep
• Improved memory
• Increased endurance
• Increased strength
• Reduced stress and tension
• Increased energy
• Slowed aging process
• Boosted confidence

The Individual

For the individual, general health is the key consideration. Anyone initiating a new exercise program should be screened for potential health problems. Screening should include past and current medical information, medications (over the counter and prescription), family history of medical conditions, and lifestyle considerations: nutritional habits, exercise habits, stress, smoking, and alcohol consumption. Any contraindications to exercise indicate the need for a referral to the appropriate health professional. A helpful fitness screening test is the *Physical Activity Readiness Questionnaire (PAR-Q)*, which can be used to identify existing cardiovascular problems, orthopedic problems, and neurological problems.[2] Questions from the PAR-Q are listed in Table 4-2.

If the individual answers "yes" to one or more questions, he or she should be seen by a physician before initiating a standard exercise program. If there are no positive responses, then this person is more likely to be safe starting an appropriate exercise program under supervision. If the individual has a cold and no other medical conditions, low-intensity exercise is generally safe, unless symptoms include fever, sore muscles or joints, vomiting or diarrhea, or a productive cough. These symptoms should resolve before resuming physical exercise.

Table 4-2. PAR-Q Questions
1. Has your doctor ever said you have heart trouble?
2. Do you frequently have pains in your heart and chest?
3. Do you often feel faint or have spells of severe dizziness?
4. Has a doctor ever said your blood pressure was too high?
5. Has your doctor ever told you that you have a bone or joint problem such as arthritis that has been aggravated by exercise or might be made worse with exercise?
6. Is there a good physical reason not mentioned here why you should not follow an activity program even if you wanted to?
7. Are you over age 65 and not accustomed to vigorous exercise?
Adapted from Thomas S, Reading J, Shephard RJ. Revision of the Physical Activity Readiness Questionnaire (PAR-Q). *Can J Spt Sci.* 1992;17(4):338-345.

Healthy individuals of all ages may engage in physical activity with little, if any, risk. Individuals with chronic illness or diseases need therapeutic exercise programs specifically designed to meet their needs. Any questions about an individual's health should be discussed with the patient's physician, then proper precautions should be addressed in a customized exercise program. Chapters 13 through 16 address health issues and special considerations affecting exercise prescription for individuals with pathology or special needs.

Eating a balanced diet improves general health and reduces the risk of many diseases. The food pyramid illustrated at the website for the United States Department of Agriculture (www.MyPyramid.gov) provides general guidelines for proper nutrition to maintain good health. This website offers specific nutritional guidelines based on an individual's age, sex, and level of physical activity.

Hydration is a key factor to address during exercise because body sweat can dehydrate the body, regardless of weather conditions. Individuals should drink approximately 400 to 600 mL of water 2 to 3 hours before exercise, 150 to 350 mL during exercise (approximately every 15 to 20 minutes), and 450 to 675 mL after exercise for every 0.5 kg of weight lost during exercise, according to the American Dietetics Association.[3]

Small meals should be consumed approximately 4 hours prior to exercise to allow time for digestion. Examples of healthy meals prior to exercise include (1) cereal, fruit, milk, and toast; (2) yogurt, muffin, and fruit; (3) pasta with tomato sauce; or (4) soup, a sandwich with lean meat, and milk. In general, individuals who are engaged in endurance activities need increased complex carbohydrates (whole grains, fruits, and vegetables) to maintain adequate energy sources for muscle contraction.[3]

Athletes in particular demand a ready source of carbohydrates and fats for sustaining muscle contractions. Glycogen, available in the liver and skeletal muscles, also contributes energy sources for physical activity. During exercise, however, muscle glycogen reserves can be used up when activities last more than 90 minutes. Gradually decreasing the amount of training during the last 6 to 7 days before an important game and simultaneously increasing the amount of dietary carbohydrates results in higher physical performance.[3] Also, a combination of carbohydrates and proteins is effective for accelerating recovery after exhausting exercise.

Older adults should monitor nutrient intakes to insure adequacy, especially carbohydrates and proteins. Carbohydrates promote glucose storage and provide an energy source during exercise. Protein promotes strength training–induced muscle hypertrophy or muscle building. Supplementation of certain vitamins and minerals (including the vitamins B_2, B_6, B_{12}, D, E, and folate, as well as calcium and iron) is recommended. Nutrition is an essential tool that older adults should use to enhance exercise performance and health.[3] Additional information about healthy nutrition is provided in Chapter 11.

Pregnancy

Many pregnant women benefit when performing regular, moderate physical activity when compared with those who remain sedentary over the course of their pregnancies. Chapter 8 provides an overview of women's health, with a focus on pregnancy. This chapter provides updated information from the American College of Obstetricians and Gynecologists outlining guidelines and precautions for exercise during pregnancy.

Aging

Aging is a universal experience and is often accompanied by loss of strength, endurance, and flexibility. Chapter 9 is dedicated to prevention practice for older adults, including assessment of physical fitness and appropriate exercises for the unique needs of aging populations.

Medications

Individuals taking medications should consult with the appropriate health care professional before engaging in exercise. Exercise increases heart rate, so stimulants (such as caffeine, cold medications, diet pills, allergy remedies and herbal teas) may contain compounds that can further elevate heart rate. Any ingested medication, food, or beverage with significant stimulating effects should be carefully monitored before engaging in exercise.

Some medications have side effects that result in impaired coordination, poor judgment, drowsiness, and dehydration. Antihistamines can cause an individual to feel drowsy, resulting in increased reaction time (slower response), poor balance, and incoordination, and should be avoided during certain exercises. These side effects pose a significant risk for individuals on treadmills, bicycles, or other similar sports equipment.

Certain types of medications may enhance performance, although often at some risk. The International Olympic Committee has banned the use of certain stimulants, pain relievers, steroids, diuretics and hormones, over-the-counter preparations (such as Actifed, Sudafed, Dexatrim, Metabolife, Midol, Alka-Seltzer Plus, Vicks Inhaler) and herbal teas with ephedrine.[4] Most of these drugs have acceptable alternatives. One class of drugs called fluoroquinolones has been linked to serious tendon injuries, often in the ankle, shoulder joint, or hand. When used in high doses, Cipro (a fluoroquinolone prescribed for infections) may have severe effects, including tendon rupture.[5]

Anti-inflammatory drugs (available by prescription and over the counter) are commonly used to treat musculoskeletal pain and inflammation. These drugs are effective for relieving pain and inflammation but can cause stomach bleeding and ulcers, as well as permanent tissue damage with chronic use.[5] Antianginal medications used to control cardiovascular problems may also affect exercise tolerance. Beta blockers, commonly used for high blood pressure and certain heart conditions, effectively lower the heart rate both at rest and during exercise.[5] Some eye drops used to treat glaucoma contain beta blockers. Beta blockers tend to keep the heart rate slower, so pulse rates do not reflect the level of exertion the body is experiencing. Measures other than pulse rate should be used to gauge exercise tolerance when working with individuals taking beta blockers.

Exercise and Alcohol

Alcohol should be avoided when an individual is engaged in aerobic exercise because of potential fluid loss and dehydration. Alcohol consumed during exercise decreases coordination and masks the warning signs of fatigue, resulting in subsequent injury.

The Environment

Environmental factors can include both physical and psychosocial factors. Wearing the proper attire for a given activity; considering the surface used for exercise; using well-maintained, safe equipment; tending to the temperature; and monitoring physical activity are all physical factors that can contribute to a positive experience. In many cases, engaging in activity with others can offer needed support for maintaining a regular routine of physical activity.

Poor weather or temperature control can pose a significant health hazard to those seeking physical activity. Unless the body is conditioned to exercise in hot weather, it is not advisable to perform vigorous exercise when it is over 98°F, especially if the humidity is high.[6] In hot environments, water loss can cause dehydration, so plenty of water is needed for exercise. Electrolyte replacements, such as Gatorade or diluted fruit juice, can limit dehydration, but caffeinated beverages (such as coffee and cola drinks) are diuretics and will cause the body to lose more fluid. Age-associated changes in thermoregulation and an increased susceptibility to dehydration underscore the critical importance of adequate fluid intake by older adults.

Proper clothing allows the body to breathe yet protects the body from excessive sunlight. Wearing light-colored clothing reflects sunlight; however, exercising early in the morning or late in the afternoon avoids exposure to harmful midday sun rays. Likewise, exercise should be limited when the temperature is below freezing accompanied by wind speed, contributing to the wind chill factor. During cold weather, individuals should wear layered clothing. Ideally, clothing should be made of fabrics that fit close to the skin and pull moisture away from the body. A porous windbreaker keeps the body warm while blocking wind, and a hat prevents significant heat loss.[7] Hands can be protected by mittens. Petroleum jelly can also be used to insulate the skin, keeping the exposed hands, nose, and ears warm.[7] To avoid unnecessary chill, individuals should avoid getting wet.

For outdoor exercise, it is advisable to avoid times of peak sunlight to prevent increased risk for skin cancer (unless a suitable sunscreen is used). The individual should wait at least 2 to 3 hours after a meal before exercising to avoid cramps, nausea, or vomiting.[7] To fully recover from physical activity, a 30-minute break postexercise is suggested.

Several studies tout the benefits of using music during exercise. Music can serve as a distraction to physical exertion and discomfort, increase physical effort, improve motivation and physical performance, stimulate the brain to match movements to its rhythm, and elevate mood.[8] Other environmental factors, such as the use of a mirror, can provide visual feedback, allowing exercisers to self-correct movements for improve performance. Finally, group activities offer social support that can encourage participation, socialization, and exercise adherence.

Types of Exercise

Various types of physical activity strengthen muscles, increase cardiorespiratory endurance, increase bone strength, and improve flexibility. The following are common types of exercise and physical activity use to improve fitness:

- *Aerobic exercise* requires the continual use of oxygen, uses large muscle groups, can be maintained continuously, and is rhythmic in nature. Types of aerobic exercise include bicycling, cross-country skiing, inline skating, fitness walking, jumping rope, running, stair climbing, and swimming. Low-intensity aerobic exercise generally demands a small, yet continual, level of oxygen, so the body can sustain exercise for a longer period of time. Individuals should be able to carry on a conversation while performing aerobic exercise. Aerobic fitness levels can improve with as little as 10 minutes of aerobic exercise, as long as exercise is performed often (2 to 3 times a day, 5 days a week).[1] To balance general fitness, health, body composition, and scheduling concerns, 30 minutes is optimal for many people. Benefits of aerobic exercise include improved cardiovascular fitness, muscular strength, endurance, body composition, and mental fitness. With sustained aerobic exercise, the cardiac muscle becomes more efficient at pumping blood, the skeletal muscles build endurance and become more toned, the body increases lean body mass and reduces fatty tissue, and the individual can experience better sleep, less depression, and improved mood.

- *Anaerobic exercise* is performed in the absence of a continual oxygen source. Anaerobic activities are short in duration and high in intensity, involving short bursts of exertion followed by periods of rest. Examples of anaerobic exercise include activities with variable—yet demanding—physical activity, such as racquetball, downhill skiing, weight lifting, sprinting, softball, soccer, and football. The benefits of anaerobic exercise include increased calorie consumption, increased metabolism, shorter workouts, improved brain function, and increased lean muscle tissue.[9]
- *Isometric exercise* is active exercise performed against stable resistance without change in the muscle length. Strength can be increased if the isometric contraction is sustained for 6 to 8 seconds; however, any one isometric exercise will only increase muscle strength at one joint angle. Strengthening the other joint positions requires repetition of alternative exercises involving those joints. If an individual has cardiac disease or high blood pressure, isometric exercises can pose problems. Muscle contractions involving the upper body can increase intrathoracic pressure or pressure in the chest. Taking a deep breath and performing a contraction against a closed glottis causes a problematic effect on the body called the Valsalva effect. This increase in intrathoracic pressure is combined with the intrathoracic pressure caused by the weight of the specific lift. During the muscular contractions in this form of exercise, blood pressure can rise quite dramatically. Arterial hypertension produced during heavy weight lifting with the Valsalva effect is extreme. The resultant elevated blood pressure may be dramatically reduced when the exercise is performed with an open glottis, facilitated by proper breathing during heavy resistance isometric exercises.
- *Isotonic exercise* involves muscle shortening to generate force. As each muscle moves through its range of motion (ROM), isotonic contractions tone muscles. Isotonic training provides a broad variety of movements, allowing the individual to exercise all major muscle groups. The disadvantages include uneven forces throughout the range of movement and unequal muscle tension for muscle groups.
- *Isokinetic exercise* involves constant-velocity muscle actions that may be either *concentric* (muscle tension is generated as the muscle length decreases or shortens) or *eccentric* (muscle tension is generated as the muscle length increases or lengthens). Unlike isotonic exercise, isokinetic exercise provides muscular overload at a constant speed while the muscle mobilizes its force through the full ROM. Cybex (Medway, Massachusetts) and Biodex (Shirley, New York) manufacture a variety of isokinetic exercise machines designed to vary the resistance to muscle contraction throughout the ROM. Table 4-3 compares isometric, isotonic, and isokinetic exercises, outlining the advantages and disadvantages of each type of exercise.
- *Sports exercise* is any type of exercise involving physical games and competition. Extensive scientific research shows that regular physical activity and playing sports are among the best forms of preventive medicine.[10] Participation in sports and fitness activities offers potential health benefits for individuals of all ages, such as combating obesity and osteoporosis and enhancing cardiovascular fitness. Psychological benefits of sports include the development of a positive self-image and increased support for exercise adherence.[9] However, negative consequences of musculoskeletal injuries sustained during sports participation pose long-term health problems. Sports with the highest risks of injury per 1000 hours of activity include skating, basketball, running or jogging, racquetball, and any competitive sport involving athletes who are nonprofessional.[11,12] Proper exercise equipment and prevention of injury through proper training can reduce injuries from high-risk sports.

Table 4-3. Comparison of Isometric, Isotonic, and Isokinetic Exercises

	ADVANTAGES	DISADVANTAGES
Isometric	Does not aggravate sensitive joint surfaces Easy to perform and remember Reproducible Easy to measure Convenient Cost effective	Not functional Any improvements are speed and angle specific Many contraindications Not efficient in terms of strength No endurance enhancements
Isotonic	Functional Easy to monitor Minimal equipment needed Convenient Best strength and endurance enhancements	Maximal loading only at specific angles Momentum key factor Synergists either limit progress or are undertrained Unsafe for joints Highest likelihood of injuries Gives delayed-onset muscle soreness Many contraindications Difficult to monitor accurately
Isokinetic	Maximal loading throughout whole range of motion Objective, reproducible, and easily quantifiable Muscles easily isolated Safest form of exercise Few contraindications	Time consuming Requires a lot of training and skill to use Costly Not functional

Adapted from Carter G. Muscle training. PopularFitness.com. http://www.popularfitness.com/articles/muscle-training.html. Accessed May 20, 2014.

- *Therapeutic exercise,* sometimes referred to as *corrective exercise,* is designed to use bodily movements to restore normal function in diseased or injured tissues and to maintain well-being. The goals of therapeutic exercise include enabling or improving ambulation; releasing contracted muscles, tendons, and fasciae; mobilizing joints; improving circulation; enhancing respiratory capacity; improving coordination; reducing rigidity; increasing balance; promoting relaxation; increasing muscle strength; and improving exercise performance and functional capacity. Therapeutic exercise is prescribed to address individualized needs based on health status and fitness goals. Clinicians educate their clients regarding key concerns and goals for health and wellness, then subsequently design an exercise program, prevention strategies, and/or physical activities that meet the specific needs and personal goals of that individual.
- *Active exercise* is exercise performed independently. When an individual is unable to perform active exercise, assistance is provided. This assistance is referred to as *active-assisted exercise*

(when the patient assists in the movement) or *passive exercise* (when the patient does not provide any assistance in the movement). Generally, active-assisted range of motion (AAROM) or passive range of motion (PROM) exercises are provided to those who are debilitated by injury or illness. These types of exercises are not recommended for individuals who have unstable tissue (such as a broken bone or dislocation) requiring stabilization.

- *Physical activity* generally refers to all forms of large muscle movements, including sports, dance, games, work, and lifestyle activities. Physical activity is often measured by examining activities of daily living necessary for independent functioning. Popular physical activities among adults in the United States are walking, gardening (yard work), stretching exercise, resistance exercise, and jogging or running.
- *Aquatic therapy*, or *aquatherapy*, refers to therapeutic intervention using the water as an environment for performing aerobic exercise or relaxation activities. Aquatic immersion provides various types of stimulation, including hydrostatic pressure, buoyancy, resistance, and heat (if the pool is properly thermoregulated for the individual's medical condition). These various simultaneous inputs affect the cardiopulmonary, neurological, and musculoskeletal systems in individuals with and without impairments. According to the Halliwick Concept,[13] as learners adjust to the water environment, they develop control in rotation, improve balance, and execute movements more smoothly. Aquatic therapy with its buoyant effect is also used to support individuals with conditions impairing upright posture and/or weight bearing (eg, muscular dystrophy, spinal cord injuries, and rheumatoid arthritis).
- *Hippotherapy* (from the Greek word *hippos* meaning *horse*), according to the American Hippotherapy Association, refers to activities performed on a horse designed to improve sensorimotor processing. Neurological processing and movement of the client is stimulated by the variable, rhythmic, and repetitive movement of the horse's gait, facilitated through input similar to human pelvic patterns while walking.[14] Specific riding skills are not taught (as in therapeutic riding); however, hippotherapy can positively improve the balance, posture, mobility, and function of the client. Individuals who engage in hippotherapy include those with cerebral palsy, developmental delay, learning disabilities, multiple sclerosis, traumatic brain injury, and stroke. "A general psychotherapeutic and psychohygienic effect is created by joy, change and a new impetus in rehabilitation and by the emotional contact with the 'comrade animal.'"[14]
- *T'ai chi* is an ancient Chinese practice designed to exercise body, mind, and spirit. Over 100 exercises include t'ai chi postures that gently work muscles, requiring the motor control to maintain balance while transitioning into a new posture. The slow, controlled movements are gentle, continuous, and circular. One study of middle-aged women found that a form of this exercise effectively induced improved physical fitness, psychological relaxation, and mental concentration, as measured by subjective reports and physiological measures of respiratory rate, heart rate, electroencephalography, surface electromyography, and exercise tolerance.[15] T'ai chi exercise is particularly effective in balance training and fall prevention for older adults.[16-18]
- *Yoga* has many connotations but is used in this text to describe a type of exercise involved in attaining bodily or mental control through a variety of postures. *Yog*, the root of yoga, means to bind or to connect, referring to the spiritual aspect of these exercises, suggesting a connection with the soul of God. Yoga exercises have been practiced for more than 5000 years and are designed to incorporate breathing and meditation to calm the mind. Hatha yoga is the physical path of yoga and uses physical poses and breathing techniques designed to develop a strong, healthy, and flexible body.[19] Recent studies have shown that yoga training optimizes the sympathetic response to stressful stimuli and restores the autonomic regulatory reflex mechanisms in hypertensive patients.[20] Furthermore, yoga-based intervention may benefit individuals with chronic low back pain, reducing levels of depression and disability, as sug-

gested by a pilot study[21] featuring participants (between the ages of 30 and 65) with chronic low back pain.[21] Finally, a study examining the use of yoga for adult patients with asthma demonstrated that those practicing yoga techniques reported a significant degree of relaxation, positive attitude, and better yoga exercise tolerance. There was also a tendency toward lesser usage of beta-adrenergic inhalers, although pulmonary function tests did not vary significantly between yoga and control groups.[22] Overall, practicing the breathing and postures of Hatha yoga offer beneficial effects for both healthy and chronically ill populations.

- *Weight Training*: Discretion should be used in selecting equipment used in weight training. There are advantages and disadvantages to various types of equipment selected for muscle strengthening and endurance. Free weights and resistance machines vary in the requirements of the individual using the equipment, the benefits, the risks, and the costs. Free weights require adequate strength, balance, and coordination to handle and stabilize the weights without loss of postural control or dropping the weight. A spotter is indicated for safety purposes when using heavier weights. Free weights are more adaptive than resistance machines in terms of allowing free movement patterns and more activities closely resembling daily activities. As a low-cost alternative to weight machines, free weights tend to be durable but also take more time for a complete workout than many weight machines. They can also create clutter if not stored properly. Resistance machines, the more costly alternative to free weights, can isolate muscle activity and provide a safe environment for weight training. No spotter is needed, and changing weights on the machine is generally simple. However, movement is generally restricted to certain ROMs and angles of movement. The equipment is often too expensive for an individual to own, so membership to a fitness club is an additional cost.

There is a wide range of exercises and physical activities that can be adapted to each individual's health needs and preferred environment.

Preparation for Physical Activity

Warming up muscles prior to exercise can prevent delayed-onset muscle soreness (DOMS), the pain and discomfort felt in muscles following exercise.[23] Methods to decrease DOMS include (1) beginning exercise gradually, (2) performing concentric (shortening) contractions before building in eccentric (lengthening) contractions, (3) performing a regular warm-up, and (4) performing moderate exercise whenever soreness is experienced.[23]

Stretching warm-up exercises have the most benefit for activities involving bouncing and jumping activities with a high intensity of stretch-shortening cycles (SSCs).[24] These types of activities, such as soccer and football, require a muscle-tendon unit that is compliant enough to store and release high amounts of elastic energy needed for powerful movements. With insufficient compliance, the muscle-tendon unit is easily injured. In activities with low intensity or limited SSCs, such as jogging, cycling, or swimming, there is less need for a compliant muscle-tendon unit. Stretching has little, if any, benefit as part of a warm-up exercise prior to participating in low-intensity aerobic exercise.[24]

Various types of muscle stretching can be used to prepare for exercise. *Static stretch* involves placing the muscle at the end of its range and holding it for 15 to 30 seconds.[24] When performed correctly, static stretch effectively lengthens a tight muscle without injury. It can also be used to relieve muscle soreness and muscle spasms. *Proprioceptive neuromuscular facilitation* (PNF) is a technique that can optimize flexibility. With PNF, there is little danger of overstretching a muscle, and strength can be developed. Like static stretch, PNF may be used to relieve muscle soreness and cramps, but it uses a reflex rather than pressure to relax the muscle prior to elongating it. PNF uses a contract-relax technique that helps to relax the opposing muscle before contracting the desired muscle. With continuous repetitions, this technique is the most effective for lengthening muscle.[25] *Ballistic stretch* involves a rapid movement to quickly stretch a muscle to its full range. This technique prepares the muscle for sports involving vigorous movement, power, and speed. Once the ballistic stretch lengthens the muscle maximally, the individual holds the position for 15 to 30 seconds for optimal lengthening of the muscle.[25]

Balance of Activity

The *physical activity pyramid*[26,27] provides useful guidelines for balancing physical activity. The pyramid has 4 levels based on the frequency of desired physical activity. The bottom, widest tier is described as *daily physical activity or incidental activity.* It is recommended that each individual perform 30 to 60 minutes of daily exercise, including stretching, walking, stair climbing, shopping, dancing, housework, gardening, and other light work. According to the pyramid, this is how most people should spend the majority of their time. The second tier, *aerobic activity,* should be performed 3 to 5 days per week at moderate-to-high intensities for an average of 30 minutes each day. Activity categories in this tier include brisk walking, running, jumping rope, swimming, bicycling, step aerobics, and other exercises of similar intensity. The third tier includes *sports and active leisure activities*, such as tennis, touch football, swimming, weight training, and gardening. This level of exercise should be performed 2 to 3 nonconsecutive days per week. For weight training, an individual should perform 1 to 3 sets of 8 to 12 repetitions of resistance exercise, using body weight, free weights, tubing, bands, or weight machines. The top tier of the physical activity pyramid lists watching television, working at the computer, and playing board games, all sedentary activities that contribute little to physical fitness but can contribute to mental fitness. In terms of physical activity, sedentary activities should be limited to allow time for more demanding types of exercise and activity (Figure 4-1).

Exercise Prescription: The FITTE Formula

Exercises should be developed using the FITTE formula, designed to progress an exercise program from appropriate levels of intensity and duration to more demanding exercises for improved fitness. The letters in the FITTE formula represent the following:

F = frequency of exercise (how often)
I = intensity of exercise (how hard)
T = time or duration of exercise (how long)
T = type of training (specificity of activity)
E = level of enjoyment

Ideally, the individual selects a favorite or highly enjoyable type of activity or sport (T = type, E = enjoyment) that can be performed at regular intervals (F = frequency), at a comfortable level of intensity (I = intensity based on heart rate or 1 RM), for a desired duration (T = time). Using the FITTE formula in conjunction with the physical activity pyramid allows the clinician to design well-balanced and easy-to-follow exercise programs. The metabolic demands of each type of physical activity should also be taken into consideration when developing an exercise program. The *Compendium of Physical Activities Tracking Guide* lists metabolic equivalent values for over 600 different activities.[28]

Level of Activity	Frequency	Type of Exercise	Examples
I	Occasional	Sedentary activity	Watching television Playing computer games
II	2-3 times per week	Sports activities Leisure activities	Playing tennis Playing football Playing soccer Swimming Gardening Weight-lifting
III	5-6 days per week	Planned aerobic activities	30 minutes total per day Walking 3-4 km Biking 12-16 km Stair Climbing Skiing Cross-Country Running
IV	Increased incidental activity	Continual movement throughout the day	Walking the dog Using the stairs rather than the elevator Getting up regularly from seated work or leisure activities

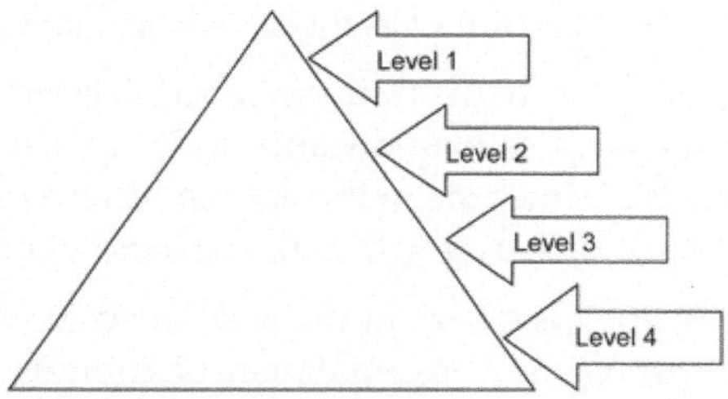

Figure 4-1. Levels of physical activity pyramid. (Adapted from Physical activity. The Exercise and Physical Fitness Page. Georgia State University. http://www2.gsu.edu/~wwwfit/physicalactivity.html. Accessed May 20, 2014; and There are a lot of ways to get the physical activity you need! Centers for Disease Control and Prevention. http://www.cdc.gov/physicalactivity/downloads/pa_examples.pdf. Accessed May 20, 2014.)

General Exercise Principles

When prescribing an exercise program, lower levels of exertion are used to determine the body's tolerance to physical stress. Exercise tolerance must develop over time as the body builds the stamina and strength to perform regular exercise with sufficient intensity and duration to increase cardiovascular endurance and strength. Baseline levels of exercise may be 3 times per week at 5% to 60% intensity (maximum heart rate) for 30 minutes' duration. At this level, the individual should become familiar with the desired level of activity and determine the types of exercise that best suit his or her personal needs and interests. Although it is not advisable to begin an exercise program with vigorous exercise, the ultimate outcome should be moderate to vigorous activity most days of the week, according to the Surgeon General. There are key principles to consider when setting up an exercise program, including the following[29]:

- The *principle of individuality* requires that exercise prescription be designed to meet the individual's needs, taking into account mental status, physiological status, unique environmental considerations, and other personal factors. This principle is key for individuals who are interested in athletic training or who have risk factors that could be exacerbated by exercise. The program that will be the most successful is one that takes individuality into account from the beginning.

- The *principle of overload* refers to the progressive increase in the amount of exercise needed to improve fitness levels. To experience overload, the individual must increase the frequency, intensity, or duration of exercise or modify the type of exercise to increase physiological demand (ie, to progress the exercise from lower frequencies, intensities, and durations to progressively higher demands in all 3 areas). Exercise prescription must be designed to optimally challenge the individual with sufficient frequency, intensity, and duration to promote improvement in muscular strength and endurance along with cardiovascular fitness. When determining a safe range of exercise, it is recommended that the health care provider use the *threshold of training heart rate*. The threshold of training heart rate may vary between individuals and sports but can generally be calculated using the following formula: threshold of training heart rate = $HR_{max} \times 55\%$). For the intermediate athlete, exercise would be increased to 3 to 5 times per week at 60% to 75% maximum heart rate for 40 to 60 minutes. Higher levels of athletic performance require increased training, such as increasing exercise to 5 to 6 times per week at 65% to 90% maximum heart rate for 60 to 120 minutes. Higher levels of performance would develop over time because the overload on muscles and the cardiovascular system would result in changes in both aerobic and anaerobic capacity, depending on the type of exercise performed. The level of exercise an individual can tolerate can be judged using the Borg Scale of Perceived Exertion,[30] as discussed in Chapter 3 and illustrated in Table 4-4.
- The *principle of specificity* refers to the training effects derived from different types of exercise. Low-resistance activities, such as long-distance walking, performed with increasing repetitions or for longer periods of time tend to increase endurance; on the other hand, progressively higher resistance activities, such as weight training, tend to build muscle strength.
- The *principle of periodization* is based on the need to avoid overtraining yet enhance performance accomplished through the manipulation of training frequency, intensity, duration, type of exercise, and enjoyment. Generally reserved for elite athletes, periodization involves alternating training loads to produce peak performance for a specific activity, or training that involves progressive cycling of various aspects of a training program during a specific period of time. For example, periodization may be used in a resistance program to alternate high-resistance training with low-resistance training to improve different components of muscular fitness (eg, strength with higher resistance versus endurance with lower resistance). This system of training is typically divided up into cycles that may last as little as 7 days to as long as months, according to the need to prepare for immediate competition vs the need to maintain fitness for subsequent seasons of competition. One benefit of periodization is reducing the boredom and monotony of performing the same exercise routine on a regular basis. The various types of health-related fitness (ie, cardiovascular endurance, muscle strength, muscular endurance, musculoskeletal flexibility, and body composition) and skill-related fitness (ie, agility, speed, power, balance, and coordination) can be addressed using the principles of overload, specificity, and periodization.
- The *principle of reversibility* refers to the tendency of the body to lose strength, endurance, flexibility, and power when exercise is not maintained. The body adapts to increasing levels of physical activity and "detrains" when exercise is not maintained over time. Just as the body upregulates to manage the overload of strenuous exercise, it downregulates when the body demands less energy. For this reason, among others, regular exercise is recommended to keep the body healthy.
- The *principle of progression* refers to the need to build muscular strength and endurance over time rather than try to reach an exercise on the initial attempt. Exercise progression follows a slow and steady incremental change in exercise routine that gives the body time to adapt to the increased demands of physical activity.
- The *principle of adaptation* is the counterpart to progression. As the body gains strength and endurance and becomes more fit, it also becomes more efficient, relying on less effort and

Table 4-4. Borg Scale of Perceived Exertion

Instructions for Borg Scale of Perceived Exertion: The following scale is used to rate perception of physical exertion during physical activity. The perceived exertion should incorporate all feelings during exercise, including physical effort, fatigue, muscle pain, shortness of breath, and stress. Choose the number from the chart below that best reflects your level of physical exertion. Performing activities at level 13 helps to build endurance, and working up to levels 15 to 17 result in greater muscle strength.

6	No exertion at all
7	Extremely light (7.5)
8	Very light
9	Very light exercise, like walking at a comfortable pace
10	Light
11	
12	
13	Somewhat hard
14	Somewhat hard to exercise, but it still feels okay
15	Hard (heavy)
16	
17	Very hard
18	Very strenuous, really pushing hard, feeling very heavy and very tired
19	Extremely hard
20	Maximal exertion, the most strenuous exercise they have ever experienced.

9 corresponds to "very light" exercise. For a healthy person, it is like walking slowly at his or her own pace for some minutes.

13 on the scale is "somewhat hard" exercise, but it still feels okay to continue.

17 "very hard" is very strenuous. A healthy person can still go on, but he or she really has to push him- or herself. It feels very heavy, and the person is very tired.

19 on the scale is an extremely strenuous exercise level. For most people, this is the most strenuous exercise they have ever experienced.

Adapted from Perceived exertion (Borg Rating of Perceived Exertion Scale). Centers for Disease Control and Prevention. http://www.cdc.gov/physicalactivity/everyone/measuring/exertion.html. Accessed May 20, 2014.

energy to perform the same physical activity. With time, as the body adapts to increasing demands, the individual needs to increase the parameters of physical activity (duration, frequency, and/or intensity) to gain fitness, as described in the principle of overload.

- The *principle of recovery* describes the need to give the body time to repair from any increased demands from strenuous physical activity. For a marathon runner, it may require a day of rest between training sessions. For highly motivated athletes, it is difficult to take a break from activity, but it is essential for restoration of healthy muscle tissue. A debilitated individual may require minutes to hours of rest between shorter bouts of physical activity. It may be as simple as catching one's breath when initially performing a new task.

Exercises That Can Cause Injury

Certain exercises can predispose people to injury, including the following:

- Hyperextending or overextending any joint
- Placing excessive stress on joints, such as performing double leg lifts
- Performing ballistic movements with the spine—either the low back or cervical spine
- Performing excessive hyperflexion of joints, which potentially damages ligaments, bursae, cartilage, and other joint structures
- Moving into positions that can pinch the nerves in the head, neck, trunk, and extremities

Before suggesting any specific exercises, all involved movements should be analyzed for stresses imposed on joints and soft tissue.

Hyperkinetic Conditions

Certain individuals are at risk of too much exercise. These individuals have a condition called *activity nervosa*, characterized by too much activity and too little rest; this condition is often seen in conjunction with *anorexia nervosa* and *bulimia nervosa* (pathological eating disorders characterized by too little or too much eating, respectively).[31] Too much activity can result in joint injuries of the foot, ankle, or knee; stress fractures of the extremities; and muscle or connective tissue injuries, such as shin splints, strained hamstring muscles, and calf pain. Individuals with psychological disorders, such as anorexia nervosa and body neurosis, also have an obsessive concern for an attractive body, often leading to excessive exercise accompanied by poor eating habits.

Special Considerations Before Prescribing an Exercise Program

Given the risks associated with exercise, it is advisable to get an informed consent from individuals who are receiving exercise advice or counseling. An informed consent provides sufficient information to enable individuals to make a well-informed decision about fitness testing and training. The informed consent form should provide clear explanations of the purpose, procedures, and risks associated with testing and exercise prescription, as well as inclusion and exclusion criteria. Certain individuals may be precluded from exercise based on their medical history, whereas other individuals may be at risk because of their age. Each individual should be screened for his or her risk of harm from fitness training. The American College of Sports Medicine offers helpful information for screening and prescribing specific exercise programs for patients with chronic or debilitating disease in its book, *Exercise Management of Persons With Chronic Diseases and Disabilities*.[32]

Individuals with high risk factors, as described by the American College of Sports Medicine, are those with unstable medical conditions that should result in exclusion from regular exercise, including cardiopulmonary disease and metabolic disease.[32] Other individuals who are excluded from exercise are those for whom the risk of exercise outweighs benefits of exercise or those with pathologies exacerbated or worsened by exercise. Men who are 45 years and older and women who are 55 years or older are at moderate risk for exercise complications.[32] Also, younger individuals with 2 or more risk factors for coronary artery disease are at moderate risk for complications from exercise.[32] Physical therapists can modify exercise regimens to meet the needs of individuals at moderate risk for complications from exercise. Men younger than 45 years and women younger than 55 years, provided they have no more than one cardiovascular risk factor, are at little risk of cardiac problems associated with regular exercise, provided it is properly prescribed for that individual.[32] Risks associated with exercise testing include the risk of death (less than 0.01%), myocardial infarction (0.04% or less), and complications requiring hospitalization (0.02% or less).[32]

If fitness testing and training are conducted in a clinic or recreation center, emergency information should be clearly written in posted emergency plans. In addition, the room layout should be designed for a safe exit, limiting the risk of accidents. Personnel should be certified in cardiopulmonary resuscitation in case of a medical emergency. If equipment is in use, it should be maintained, positioned for maximal visual supervision, and kept clean between uses.

Once the examiner has attained the desired performance on a fitness test, it is appropriate to discontinue testing, allowing the individual time to recover. Also, testing or exercise should be discontinued if the individual shows signs of distress, such as angina or chest pain; an excessive rise in blood pressure (systolic blood pressure higher than 260 mm Hg and diastolic blood pressure higher than 115 mm Hg); dizziness; lightheadedness; nausea; confusion; poor coordination; a pale complexion; cold, clammy hands; bluish skin tone; severe fatigue; or changes in heart rhythm.[32] If there is a life-threatening situation, the emergency plan should be put into action. If the situation is non–life threatening, the individual should be given time to cool down from the activity by slow, steady movement, such as walking.

The range of mental and physical tests needed to assess an individual's fitness depends on the goals and types of fitness the person chooses to pursue. A health care professional has the knowledge and skills to provide appropriate assessments and resources for both the mental and physical fitness of the people seeking their services. Referrals may be made to physicians or other health care providers, when appropriate. Fitness involves an individual's commitment, motivation, and responsibility for his or her own well-being. One key fitness goal is to ensure that all individuals have the needed resources for maintaining fit minds and bodies.

Factors Influencing Maintenance of Physical Activity

Despite the proven benefits of physical activity, more than 50% of American adults do not get enough physical activity to provide health benefits; 26% are not active at all in their leisure time.[1] Activity decreases with age, and sufficient activity is less common among women than men, and among those with lower incomes and less education. Insufficient physical activity is not limited to adults. More than one-third of young people in grades 9 through 12 do not regularly engage in vigorous physical activity.[1] Initiating an exercise program at any age requires significant contemplation and decision making, while maintaining a program of physical activity requires some level of motivation.

The health belief model developed in 1952 by Hochbaum, Kegels, and Rosenstock was designed to test the hypothesis that health-related behaviors could be predicted based on an individual's beliefs about risks to his or her health and wellness.[33] This model has been used extensively in research exploring preventive health behavior. This theory has implications for providing health education about the benefits of exercise, the risks of not exercising, and the appropriate actions to take for age-appropriate exercise; however, little evidence supports this theory in terms of exercise adherence.

The theory of reasoned action was developed by Ajzen[34] as an explanation of how attitudes or intentions are reflected in behavior. According to this theory, the most important determinant of a person's behavior is behavior intent. The individual's intention to perform a behavior, such as exercise, is a combination of attitude toward performing the behavior (ie, beliefs about the outcomes of the behavior and the value of these outcomes) and the subjective norm (ie, beliefs about what other people think the person should do, as well as the person's motivation to comply with the opinions of others). Two assumptions of this theory are (1) human beings are rational and make systematic use of information available to them, and (2) people consider the implications of their actions before they decide to engage or not engage in certain behaviors. Given these 2 assumptions, the theory does not hold true for exercise behavior because the knowledge about the benefits of exercise is pervasive, yet not everyone engages in regular physical activity, as evidenced by the growing population of sedentary children and adults.

Social learning theory,[35] also known as social cognitive theory, suggests that behavior change, such as exercising, is affected by environmental influences, personal factors, and attributes of the behavior itself. A person must believe in his or her capability to perform the behavior (ie, the person must possess self-efficacy) and must perceive an incentive to do so (ie, the person's positive expectations from performing the behavior must outweigh the negative expectations). Additionally, a person must value the outcomes or consequences that he or she believes will occur as a result of performing a specific behavior or action. Several studies point to self-efficacy as the single most important characteristic that determines a person's behavior change, including exercise program participation. An individual's self-efficacy can be increased by providing clear instructions; providing adequate opportunities for skill development, training, and practice; and modeling the desired (and achievable) behavior in such a way that it evokes trust and respect from the individual.[35,36]

Factors that contribute to relapse include negative emotional or physiologic states, limited coping skills, social pressure, interpersonal conflict, limited social support, low motivation, high-risk situations, and stress. Principles of relapse prevention include identifying high-risk situations for relapse (eg, change in season, program location, instructor) and developing appropriate solutions (eg, finding a place to walk inside during bad weather, finding a stable location, or maintaining the same instructor).[35,36] Helping people distinguish between a *lapse* (eg, a few days of not participating in exercise) and a *relapse* (eg, an extended period of not exercising) is thought to improve adherence.

The transtheoretical model of change provides a continuum of change from precontemplation to contemplation, preparation, action, and maintenance.[37] According to this theory, tailoring interventions to match a person's readiness or stage of change is essential. For example, for people who are not yet contemplating becoming more active, encouraging a step-by-step movement along the continuum of change may be more effective than encouraging them to move directly into action. Relapses are not uncommon, and maintaining a new action over a prolonged time may require motivators that are meaningful to the individual. The following questions can be used to guide others through the process of healthy exercise habits:

- *Precontemplation stage—Goal: Individual will begin thinking about change.*

  "What would have to happen for you to begin exercising?"

  "What warning signs would let you know that you need to begin exercising?"

  "Have you tried to exercise in the past?"

- *Contemplation stage—Goal: Individual will examine benefits and barriers to change.*

  "Why do you want to exercise at this time?"

  "What were the reasons for not exercising?"

  "What would keep you from exercising at this time?"

  "What are the barriers today that keep you from exercising?"

  "What might help you with that aspect?"

  "What people, programs, and behaviors have helped you exercise in the past?"

- *Preparation stage—Goal: Individual will have needed resources to initiate exercise.*

  "Do you have the proper attire for your selected exercise?"

  "What resources or equipment do you think you need to safely exercise?"

  "What would help you begin exercising at this time?"

- *Action stage—Goal: Individual will develop self-efficacy in physical activity.*

  "What questions do you have about exercise?"

  "Do you understand my explanations about exercise?"

  "Does my showing you how to do this exercise help you understand how it is done?"

  "Do you understand that repeated performance of this activity will help you learn it more easily? Practice is essential."

  "Do you feel comfortable performing exercise without any assistance?"
- *Maintenance stage: Goal: Individual will integrate physical activity (exercise) into lifestyle.*

  "Are you familiar with how to modify your physical activity for variation?"

  "Are you progressing or varying your exercises for interest?"

  "Would you like to do this activity with your friends and family?"

  "Does your community offer programs to support this activity?"

  "What motivates you to maintain your physical activity?"

A criticism of most theories and models of behavior change is that they emphasize individual behavior change processes and disregard psychosocial, cultural, and physical environmental influences on behavior. A health-promoting environment is sensitive to cultural issues, offers psychosocial support as appropriate, and is conducive to a wide variety of activities, including outdoor recreational activities (bike paths, parks with walking paths) and indoor facilities for times of inclement weather. Social support for physical activity or participation in an exercise program includes having a friend or family member provide company while walking, offer a ride to the activity, or provide emotional support during participation in the program. Sources of social support for physical activity include family members, friends, neighbors, coworkers, and exercise program leaders and participants. When developing exercise programs for each population, ecological perspectives should be considered as they influence health behaviors.

What motivates individuals to exercise? Some suggest that those who exercise regularly have either *intrinsic motivation* (ie, engaging in an activity for pleasure with no expectation of material rewards or external constraints) or *extrinsic motivation* (ie, engaging in the behavior as a means to an end and not for the sake of the activity itself).[38] However, relying exclusively on external influences can undermine intrinsic motivation, making it more difficult to maintain physical activity once the external influences are removed.[38] According to Dishman,[39] who summarized the findings of numerous studies in his book, *Advances in Exercise Adherence*, there are a number of diverse nonhealth-related participation motives for exercise. Individuals are motivated to exercise by the desire to look good, lose weight, feel healthy, and improve fitness levels. Others have reported that individuals engage in regular exercise for fun because they enjoy the sensations that accompany the experience or the joy of being with other people. Motivators for exercise can be simply determined by asking the individual why he or she exercises. In addition to reinforcing motivators, as appropriate, the health care professional should try to reduce the number of perceived barriers for maintaining adherence.

Personal and environmental barriers that could interfere with exercise adherence are listed in Table 4-5.[40]

When prescribing exercises, health care providers should be aware of potential barriers to exercise adherence and consider addressing any barriers that might interfere with their client's success in both initiating and maintaining regular physical activity.

Community Support for Physical Activity

The most effective health behavior interventions occur on multiple levels: intrapersonal factors, interpersonal and group factors, institutional factors, community factors, and public policy.[40] Interventions that simultaneously influence these multiple levels and multiple settings may be

Table 4-5. Barriers to Exercise Adherence	
PERSONAL BARRIERS	**ENVIRONMENTAL BARRIERS**
• Lack of time • Lack of motivation • Injury • Rapid fatigability • Misconceptions about exercise: "Animals sweat, men perspire, women do neither." • Physical discomfort (physical ailments including low-back injuries, knee joint degeneration, or restrictive and obstructive lung or heart disease, obesity, diabetes, peripheral neuropathies, other chronic illnesses) • Emotional discomfort (fear of injury, especially fear of falling in older adults) • Control in life • Attitude toward exercise • Assessment of the benefits of exercise • Self-efficacy in performing exercises • Inertia: difficulty changing lifestyle behaviors • Isolation	• Access: Some individuals do not have access to facilities to exercise. • Cost: Health clubs are too expensive for many people. • Climate: In northern climates, inclement weather and unsafe outdoor conditions due to ice and snow may cause many individuals, especially the elderly, to go without regular physical activity for 6 months. For those living in warmer regions, extremes of heat and humidity are obstacles to activity.

expected to lead to greater and longer-lasting changes and maintenance of existing health-promoting habits. Examples of how communities can meet the growing need for physical activity include the following:

- Provide safe, accessible, and attractive trails for walking and bicycling, and sidewalks with curb cuts. This will make getting physical activity more enjoyable for everyone, including people with disabilities.
- Involve the widest possible variety of people, including people with disabilities, at all stages of planning and implementing community physical activity programs.
- Provide community-based physical activity programs that include aerobics, strength building and flexibility. These programs should meet the needs of specific populations, including racial and ethnic minority groups, women, older adults, people with disabilities, and low-income groups.
- Open schools for community recreation, form neighborhood watch groups to enhance safety, and encourage malls and other indoor or protected locations to provide safe places for walking in any weather.
- Ensure that facilities accommodate and encourage participation by people of all racial, ethnic, and income groups as well as women, older adults, and people with disabilities.

- Allow health care providers to encourage people to add more physical activity into their lives.
- Encourage employers to provide supportive worksite environments and policies that allow employees to incorporate moderate physical activity into their lives.

This is a promising area for the design of future intervention research to promote physical activity.

Summary

Physical activity is essential to good health and maintenance of both mental and physical fitness. Key factors to consider when helping others engage in healthy lifestyle behaviors include the individual, the environment, and the physical activity or exercise best suited to meet the individual's needs. Along with healthy nutrition and proper precautions, physical activity can progressively improve the health of most individuals. While recognizing the basic principles of fitness training, health care professionals must be realistic about issues of exercise adherence and barriers to maintaining lifestyle habits that incorporate regular physical activity. Subsequent chapters provide information about exercise designed for specific populations, including children, adults, pregnant women, individuals performing manual labor, older adults, and individuals with impairments affecting their musculoskeletal, neuromuscular, and cardiopulmonary systems. Using key concepts of fitness training with a holistic health care approach can optimize preventive care and improve the quality of life for those served.

References

1. US Department of Health and Human Services. Physical Activity and Health: A Report of the Surgeon General. Available at: http://www.cdc.gov/nccdphp/sgr/pdf/execsumm.pdf. Retrieved on March 18, 2014..
2. Thomas S, Reading J, Shephard RJ. Revision of the Physical Activity Readiness Questionnaire (PAR-Q). *J Canad Sci Sport*. 1992;17(4):338-345.
3. American Dietetic Association. Nutrition and athletic performance: position of the American Dietetic Association, Dietitians of Canada, and the American College of Sports Medicine. *J Am Diet Assoc*. 2002;100:1543-1556.
4. Silver M. Use of ergogenic aids by athletes. *Ergogenic Aids in Athletics*. 2001;9(1):61-70.
5. Khaliq Y, Zhanel GG. Musculoskeletal injury associated with fluoroquinolone antibiotics. *Clin Plast Surg*. 2005;32(4):495-502.
6. Tucker R, Rauch L, Harley YX, Noakes TD. Impaired exercise performance in the heat is associated with an anticipatory reduction in skeletal muscle recruitment. *Pflugers Arch*. 2004;448(4):422-430.
7. Gavhed D, Mäkinen T, Holmér I, Rintamäki H. Face cooling by cold wind in walking subjects. *Int J Biometeorol*. 2003;47(3):148-155.
8. Fritz T, Hardikar S, Demoucron M, et al. Musical agency reduces perceived exertion during strenuous physical performance. *Proc Natl Acad Sci U S A*. 2013;110(44):17784-17789.
9. Cotman C, Engesser-Cesar C. Exercise enhances and protects brain function. *Exerc Sport Sci Rev*. 2002;30(2):75-79.
10. Tofler IR, Butterbaugh GJ. Developmental overview of child and youth sports for the twenty-first century. *Clin Sports Med*. 2005;24(4):783-804.
11. Koh JO, Cassidy JD, Watkinson EJ. Incidence of concussion in contact sports: a systematic review of the evidence. *Brain Inj*. 2003;17(10):901-917.
12. Kraus JF, Conroy C. Mortality and morbidity from injuries in sports and recreation. *Annu Rev Public Health*. 1984;5:163-192.
13. The Ten Point Programme. Halliwick Association of Swimming Therapy in the UK. http://www.halliwick.org.uk/html/tenpoint.htm. Accessed May 20, 2014.
14. Barolin GS, Samborski R. The horse as an aid in therapy. *Wiener Medizinische Wochenschrift (1946)*. 1991;141(20):476-481.
15. Liu Y, Mimura K, Wang L, Ikuda K. Physiological benefits of 24-style Taijiquan exercise in middle-aged women. *J Physiol Anthropol Appl Human Sci*. 2003;22(5):219-225.

16. Fong SM, Ng GY. The effects on sensorimotor performance and balance with tai chi training. *Arch Phys Med Rehab.* 2006;87(1):82-87.
17. Zhang JG, Ishikawa-Takata K, Yamazaki H, Morita T, Ohta T. The effects of Tai Chi Chuan on physiological function and fear of falling in the less robust elderly: An intervention study for preventing falls. *Arch Gerontol Geriatr.* 2006;42(2):107-116.
18. Choi JH, Moon JS, Song R. Effects of Sun-style Tai Chi exercise on physical fitness and fall prevention in fall-prone older adults. *J Adv Nurs.* 2005;51(2):150-157.
19. Raub JA. Psychophysiologic effects of Hatha Yoga on musculoskeletal and cardiopulmonary function: a literature review. *J Altern Complement Med.* 2002;8(6):797-812.
20. Parshad O. Role of yoga in stress management. *West Indian Med J.* 2004;53(3):191-194.
21. Sherman KJ, Cherkin DC, Erro J, Miglioretti DL, Deyo RA. Comparing yoga, exercise, and a self-care book for chronic low back pain: a randomized, controlled trial. *Ann Intern Med.* 2005;143(12):849-856.
22. Vedanthan PK, Kesavalu LN, Murthy KC, et al. Clinical study of yoga techniques in university students with asthma: a controlled study. *Allergy Asthma Proc.* 1998;19(1):3-9.
23. Nie H, Kawczynski A, Madeleine P, Arendt-Nielsen L. Delayed onset muscle soreness in neck/shoulder muscles. *Eur J Pain.* 2005;9(6):653-660.
24. Witvrouw E, Mahieu N, Danneels L, McNair P. Stretching and injury prevention: an obscure relationship. *Sports Med.* 2004;34(7):443-449.
25. Etnyre BR, Abraham LD. Gains in range of ankle dorsiflexion using three popular stretching techniques. *Am J Phys Med.* 1996;65(4):189-196.
26. Physical activity pyramid. Division of Chronic Disease & Injury Prevention, Physical Activity & Cardiovascular Health Program. http://publichealth.lacounty.gov/physact/docs/Index%20Page/May2010/Newpyramid.pdf. Accessed May 25, 2013.
27. Physical activity guidelines for Americans. US Department of Health and Human Services. http://www.health.gov/paguidelines/guidelines/chapter1.aspx. Accessed May 25, 2013.
28. Ainsworth BE, Haskell WL, Herrmann SD, et al. 2011 Compendium of Physical Activities: a second update of codes and MET values. *Med Sci Sports Exerc.* 2011;43(8):1575-1581.
29. Gaal M. 7 principles of exercise and sports training. USA Triathlon. http://www.usatriathlon.org/about-multisport/multisport-zone/multisport-lab/articles/7-principles-of-training-082812.aspx. Accessed May 25, 2013.
30. Dawes HN, Barker KL, Cockburn J, Roach N, Scott O, Wade D. Borg's rating of perceived exertion scales: do the verbal anchors mean the same for different clinical groups? *Arch Phys Med Rehab.* 2005;86(5):912-916.
31. Solenberger SE. Exercise and eating disorders: a 3-year inpatient hospital record analysis. *Eat Behav.* 2001;2(2):151-168.
32. American College of Sports Medicine. *Exercise Management of Persons With Chronic Diseases and Disabilities.* Champaign, IL: Human Kinetics; 1997.
33. Rosenstock I. Historical origins of the health belief theory. Health Education Behavior. 1974;2(4):328-335.
34. Ajzen I. The theory of planned behaviour: reactions and reflections. *Psychol Health.* 2011;26(9):1113-1127.
35. Bandura A. Self-efficacy: toward a unifying theory of behavioral change. *Psychol Rev.* 1977;84(2):191-215.
36. Marcus BH, Selby VC, Niaura RS, Rossi JS. Self-efficacy and the stages of exercise behavior change. *Res Q Exerc Sport.* 1992;63(1):60-66.
37. Prochaska JO, Velicer WF. The transtheoretical model of health behavior change. *Am J Health Promot.* 1997;12(1):38-48.
38. King A, Friedman F, Marcus B, et al. Harnessing motivational forces in the promotion of physical activity: the Community Health Advice by Telephone (CHAT) project. *Health Educ Res.* 2002;17(5):627-636.
39. Dishman RK. *Advances in Exercise Adherence.* Champaign, IL: Human Kinetics; 1994.
40. Fletcher G, Trejo JF. Why and how to prescribe exercise: overcoming the barriers. *Cleve Clin J Med.* 2005;72(8):645-649, 653-654, 656.

5

Screening for Health, Fitness, and Wellness

Catherine Rush Thompson, PT, PhD, MS

"Healing is a matter of time, but it is sometimes also a matter of opportunity."—Hippocrates, *Precepts*

Health care professionals provide essential screening for the health, fitness, and wellness of the general public. Screening can lead to the early detection of illness and often more effective treatments for discovered maladies. With direct access, many health care professionals can play a key role in evaluating problems that would benefit from allied health care services versus those requiring the expertise of other professionals.

Screening vs Examination

Screening is essentially checking for pathology when there are no symptoms of disease. A screening often includes simple measures to identify risk factors for illness and is used to determine the need for further examination. Common screening activities include the following:

- Screening for lifestyle factors (eg, amount of exercise, stress, weight, and sports activities) leading to increased risk for serious health problems
- Screening posture for scoliosis
- Identifying high risk factors for slipping, tripping, or falling of older adults
- Performing prework screenings to identify risk factors in the workplace and the health status of potential workers

The initial examination of a client involves screening but also incorporates specific tests and measures that may lead to identification of a problem requiring further exploration and/or a referral to another practitioner. *Examination* includes taking the client's history, reviewing the body systems for potential pathology, and performing specific tests and measures guided by the initial screening, patient/client history, professional judgment, and relevant clinical findings. Thus, screening a patient is always the initial step in health care management to determine whether

Thompson CR.
Prevention Practice and Health Promotion: A Health Care Professional's Guide to Health, Fitness, and Wellness, Second Edition (pp 71-93).

further examination is needed or whether referral is more appropriate. Screening for health, fitness, and wellness provides health care professionals with opportunities to prevent illness and refer potential pathologies before they become complicated and difficult to manage. Primary prevention involves screening at-risk populations for conditions that are not evident and helping the client to develop and maintain healthy lifestyle habits to ward off disease. Once risks for physical or mental health problems are identified, qualified health care professionals can perform more extensive examinations to determine relevant needs and refer their clients for health issues outside their scopes of practice.

Interviewing the Client

Nonverbal Communication

Appropriate interpersonal skills are essential to developing rapport with an individual during the screening process. The interviewer must be a good listener and have the ability to focus energy, attention, and thoughts on what the individual is saying. Effective attending skills include displaying an appropriate level of energy, using nonverbal communication that invites an open conversation, using appropriate types of questions to initiate conversation, active listening, and projecting clinical competence. When interviewing a person, the health care professional needs to project a positive demeanor because first impressions are highly influential. The appropriate level of energy requires focusing both physical and mental energy on the individual speaking. Using a patient- or client-centered focus has been shown to be an effective interviewing skill.[1,2] Too much energy may be intimidating; too little energy may suggest disinterest. The interviewer must be able to read the patient's nonverbal communication to gauge what level of energy is optimal for interaction. Words have a 7% effect on interpersonal communication, the tone of voice used in asking questions has a 38% effect, and body language has a 55% effect.[3] The unconscious mind automatically understands the meaning of every gesture, posture, and voice inflection. The following 5 skills, if used effectively, can improve the enjoyment and outcome of interpersonal communication: (1) eye contact, (2) body position, (3) proper distance between the interviewer and interviewee, (4) gestures, and (5) facial expression.[4] There are some variations in communication across cultures, so the interviewer must develop some level of cultural competency to fully understand individuals with different ethnic backgrounds.

Eye Contact

Eye contact is the most common and powerful nonverbal behavior. Optimal eye contact involves looking directly at the interviewee when speaking or listening and conveying sincerity and respect for the other person. However, direct eye contact is not always culturally appropriate. People in other parts of the world, including Latin America, Africa, and Asia, may believe that direct eye contact is a sign of disrespect.[5] In Arab countries, prolonged direct eye contact is a gauge of trustworthiness.[6] Poor eye contact, excessive self-consciousness, negative self-evaluation, and self-preoccupation are common characteristics of shyness.[7] If the interviewer suspects that an individual is shy, sensitivity to shyness can be demonstrated by glancing briefly around the eyes instead of looking directly into the pupils. Because eye contact expresses intimacy, prolonged eye contact can provide the interviewee with a sense of safety when sharing private concerns.[8] However, uninterrupted eye contact may be too personal. It is important that the interviewer gauge the duration of eye contact based on other components of the interviewee's body language. Avoiding eye contact has negative implications, suggesting guilt, fear, or dishonesty. To make the interviewee more relaxed and comfortable, the interviewer must be careful to avoid staring, squinting, or excessively blinking during the interview.[8] Generally, more eye contact is experienced when topics are comfortable for both the interviewee and interviewer. Steady eye contact without staring indicates interest in the individual, and pupil dilation indicates keen interest. Eye shifts indicate that the individual may be processing or recalling information; however, darting eyes suggest that the individual is excited, worried, or wearing contact lenses. Furrowing of the brow implies that the individual is perplexed or trying to avoid a topic. Staring with the eyes fixed on an object or lowering the eyes down and away indicate preoccupation with another concern or discomfort discussing a topic. Finally, lack of eye contact projects many possible interpretations, including respect, avoidance of interaction, discomfort, embarrassment, or preoccupation with another concern.[8]

Body Position

Ideally, the interview should be conducted while both the interviewer and interviewee are comfortably seated, with the eyes at the same level and shoulders squarely facing each other. Certain body positions confer possible meanings that should be taken into account during the interview process. A more open body posture (arms relaxed at both sides) is more welcoming than a closed body posture (arms crossed over the chest).[9] Whereas a stiff posture indicates tension, anxiety, or concern, steady movement, such as rocking or squirming, suggests the person may be concerned, worried, or anxious. Leaning forward indicates eagerness, attentiveness, and openness to communication, but a person who is slouched, stooped, or turned away from the interviewer may be sad, ambivalent, or unreceptive to the interchange.[9] Good posture reflects confidence and assurance that the individual is paying attention to the information shared. Like eye contact, body posture can offer significant information regarding the interviewee's comfort level and general attitude during the screening process.

Distance

Physical distance between the physical therapist and interviewee is another key factor for interpersonal communication. Some individuals feel comfortable with physical proximity (an arm's length), whereas others may be offended. For example, southern Europeans (Italy and Greece) generally believe that touch is acceptable; however, individuals in northern Europe (England, France, and the Netherlands) expect little, if any, contact.[10]

Gestures

Gesturing is used instinctively to emphasize important points.[7,11,12] Although a lack of body gestures signals anger or lack of openness, gestures (such as playing with clothing, hair, or jewelry) are distracting. Again, cultural differences need to be considered. For example, Japanese men will tip the head backward and audibly suck air in through the teeth to signal "no" or that something is difficult. A Japanese gesture for "I do not know," "I don't understand," or "No, I am undeserving" is waving the hand back and forth in front of one's own face (palm outward).[7,11,12] The Taiwanese gesture to indicate "no" is to lift one's hand to face level, palm facing outward, and move it back and forth, sometimes with a smile.

Facial Expression

Incongruities between facial expression and verbal expression are not uncommon and often confound interpersonal communication. If facial expressions conflict with verbal messages, the listener will believe the nonverbal communication over what is said by the speaker. Certain facial expressions, such as wrinkling the forehead or speaking with a pursed or tight-lipped mouth, can indicate tension.[7,11,12] If someone says that she is fine but has a tense expression, more questions need to be asked to elicit additional information. Yawning is an obvious sign of boredom or tiredness. Rolling the eyes can be a dismissive expression that has a negative effect on communication. Any of these facial cues should be carefully noted. Again, cultural differences exist. Although many facial expressions tend to be universal, their interpretation may vary from one culture to the next. Generally, anxiety, fear, surprise, or joy can be easily observed in any individual, but this is not always the case.

Verbal Communication

Nonverbal communication plays a key role in the interview process, but verbal communication is critical for eliciting responses needed for a medical history and identification of health risks. It is helpful to initiate the interview using open, general questions, gently put, to elicit sincere behavior from interviewees, allowing them the freedom to respond with presupposed answers. Open-ended questions generally begin with words like "how" or "why" and cannot be answered by a simple "yes" or "no." For example, the interviewer might ask the individual, "How might your family health history affect your health status?" Responses to these broader questions provide an opportunity for the interviewee to express concerns and suggest safe issues to discuss. Closed-ended questions can be used to solicit simple "yes" or "no" responses related to specific screening questions. More direct questions are used to focus responses, such as identifying specific dates for previous health conditions. When the information is sensitive, the interviewer can provide an example that allows the respondent an opportunity to answer without embarrassment. For example, the therapist could state, "Women your age commonly have problems with controlling their bladder. Is this a problem that concerns you?"

Awareness of the individual's cultural background is critical to understanding his or her point of view and relevant issues. The LEARN model, which emphasizes listening and sharing similarities and differences, can be used to overcome cultural communication barriers.[13] The acronym LEARN represents the following key components of the model:

L = Listen with sympathy and understanding to the client's perception of the problem

E = Explain your perceptions of the problem

A = Acknowledge and discuss the differences and similarities

R = Recommend a course of action

N = Negotiate an agreement

Using the LEARN model enables the interviewer to systematically communicate in a culturally sensitive manner with a wide range of diverse individuals.

The purpose of active listening is to understand what the other person means. The meaning is conveyed in the content (who, what, when, where, how, and why), as well as the affect of the person (emotions and feelings accompanying the content). An effective listener can understand the meaning of what is said and communicate that the information is important. The listener must take into account the speaker's frame of reference, congruous or incongruous verbal and nonverbal communication, previous patterns or experiences with this individual, and key themes or patterns of what is said. For example, if the individual repeatedly complains of pain while forcibly smiling, this incongruity suggests further exploration of pain issues. If the meaning is understood, the listener should try to be empathetic to elicit additional information. Most people speak at the rate of 110 to 140 words a minute, yet they think at a significantly faster rate.[14] Full attention must be given to what is said. Throughout the interview, the interviewer may restate or summarize the interviewee's comments to confirm the meaning of what has been said. Both verbal and nonverbal agreement with these summary statements can give a clear indication of comprehension of what has been said by the interviewee. During the summation of discussion, the individual may be invited to elaborate on information shared to clarify any misunderstandings.

Projecting professionalism and clinical competence increases the sense of assurance during the interview process. Characteristics of professionalism include effective communication, professional appearance, timeliness, respect, tactful and courteous behavior, ethical and competent behavior, accountability, and good organizational skills.[15] Evidence of academic degrees, professional degrees, clinical specialist certifications, and professional memberships gives the individual more confidence of the interviewer's clinical competence and professionalism. A private area for the interview and a well-organized space for the screening process further provide the interviewee with a positive impression.

Screening for Mental Health

Mental health is directly or indirectly influenced by multiple factors, including memory, interpersonal relationships at work and at home, coping and stress management, social support, financial support, education, vocation, leisure activities, and personal values. Because genetics play a key role in mental health problems, family history of mental health dysfunction should be noted. Clues that suggest possible mental health problems include a negative affect, depression, anxiety, fear, aggression, or rage. Depressed patients tend to have reduced restlessness (leg and hand movements), reduced communication (less speech and gesturing), decreased active listening, and reduced eagerness (nodding and shaking the head).[16] In general, depressed individuals display slowness of thought and speech, impaired ability to concentrate, and decreased motor activity. According to the National Institutes of Mental Health,[17] an estimated 6.7% adults suffer from major depression disorders, with women 70% more likely to experience depression over their lifetimes. Depression is a significant psychosocial problem that affects an individual's health, fitness, and wellness and, ultimately, his or her quality of life. A 2-question initial screening test for depression has been developed and validated based on the *Diagnostic and Statistical Manual of Mental Disorders*[18,19] established criteria for the diagnosis of depression. The 2 questions are as follows:

1. During the past month, have you often been bothered by feeling down, depressed, or hopeless?
2. During the past month, have you often been bothered by little interest or pleasure in doing things?

A positive response to either of the questions is extremely sensitive and identifies more than 90% of patients with major depression. However, it is only approximately 60% specific and requires confirmation using a detailed clinical interview or more specific diagnostic tools.[18] If the screener suspects that the individual is experiencing mental health problems, it is appropriate to do a stress assessment and consider a referral for psychological or social services, as appropriate. Clear documentation of observations is useful for future reference.

Motor behaviors suggesting other types of mental health dysfunction include restlessness or performing unusual, purposeless movements. Those describing nonexistent sounds most likely have mental problems and need a referral for further examination. Additionally, those with memory problems or problems performing tasks that require concentration may need a more thorough psychological examination.[19,20] Normal individuals are motivated to survive, so those who suggest or exhibit self-harm may have mental illness. Signs of poor mental health include an obsession with negative thoughts and negative consequences, loss of creative and imaginative thoughts and ideas, unclear decision making, or a foggy mental state. Other characteristics of mental health disorders include unrealistic thoughts and perceptions, inappropriate emotions, and unpredictable behavior (as compared with the social norm).

Stress Assessment

During the interview, it is important to note stressors commonly affecting health status. Stressors include recent life changes or losses (eg, loss of family or friends, relocation of home and/or business), changes in marital status, or significant financial concerns. Responses to life changes vary because each individual's perception of a stressful situation differs. Some individuals may not show any symptoms of stress on the surface but may have emotional or physical changes that are not easily detectable. Other individuals may demonstrate more obvious problems, such as unusual behaviors or mannerisms, requiring further psychological examination. Convenient psychological measures of stress include the Holmes and Rahe Social Readjustment Rating Scale[21] (commonly used for adults) and Yeaworth's Adolescent Life Change Event Scale,[22] a questionnaire listing personal, social, and family changes believed to be stressful to adolescents. It is important to note that both positive and negative changes in a person's life may contribute to that individual's stress.

The perception of stress varies from person to person yet is ever-present in people's lives. All of these assessments provide the clinician with valuable information about the interviewee's recent stressors and the likelihood of illness.

Although minor psychological stress is ever-present, unrelenting stress can be extremely dangerous. Adrenaline, noradrenaline, and cortisol, released into the bloodstream, increase heart rate, increase respiration, dilate the pupils, and flush the skin. The body is aroused and rational thinking may be altered. This response is adaptive for primitive survival instincts but is not functional in inescapable stressful situations that can mount over time. Whereas acute stress responses may temporarily disable rational responses, chronic stress can impair both psychological and physiological functioning. Physiological stress measures for acute stress may be a part of a more extensive examination, including electrocardiography (ECG; measurement of heart electrical activity) and the galvanic skin response (GSR; measurement of the skin resistance to the passage of electric current).[23] Both of these measures can be useful in detecting the less dramatic physiological changes occurring with stress. Over time, increased blood pressure at rest may result from chronic stress. Individuals with hypertension need an immediate referral for appropriate intervention. Although stress measures are useful for identifying a variety of stress factors potentially contributing to illness, there are few comprehensive measures designed to identify how well individuals address the multiple dimensions of wellness.

Screening for a Balanced Lifestyle

Clinicians who anticipate a long-term relationship with clients may choose to conduct a wellness screening for a more holistic approach to health care and prevention practice. A wellness screening includes a broad range of questions reviewing social, physical, emotional, career/leisure, intellectual, environmental, and spiritual wellness. This type of screening tool could prove especially helpful in educating the client about balancing the multiple dimensions in life.

One general survey, entitled the 7 Dimensions of Wellness* (http://7dimensionsofwellness.com/quiz/) and developed at the University of Wisconsin-Seven Points, is brief, educational, and helpful in identifying potential risks or concerns affecting the individual's life. This survey may be administered as part of an interview or may be filled out by the individual independently, then discussed in the screening. This site also offers the option for professionals to create accounts to collect aggregate data. On this survey, overall wellness is accomplished when the individual's self-perception matches the criteria for each wellness dimension with an "always" response. If the individual is seeking ways to achieve a more balanced life for wellness, the site provides some ideas for reflection and guidance to promote well-being. The clinician may make referrals as needed to spiritual, social, psychological, or other professionals to ensure adequate resources for the individual to achieve wellness.

Screening for Physical Wellness

Health care professionals are experts in physical health and wellness and have a variety of tools to examine the musculoskeletal, neuromuscular, cardiopulmonary, and integumentary systems. It is helpful to have a comprehensive physical checklist to address possible risk factors for pathology affecting all body systems. After a quick review, the health care professional is alerted to potential risk factors and the need for a more complete examination to address areas of concern. Based on the client's history, age, and risk for pathology, the clinician can focus on the aspects most relevant to the client. For example, it is important to screen a young child for immunizations, a young adult for reproductive systems, and an older adult for factors that contribute to falls, such as poor vision and muscle weakness. The physical health screening checklist (Table 5-1) identifies risk factors

Table 5-1. Physical Health Screening	
• *Family history:*	Do you have a family history of: _____ Blood pressure _____ Stroke _____ Cancer _____ Diabetes _____ Allergies _____ Arthritis _____ Alcoholism _____ Mental illness _____ Seizure disorders _____ Kidney disease _____ Other
Physical Health	
• *General health:*	Weight: _____ (normal range _____ , overweight _____ underweight _____) _____ Fatigue _____ Weakness _____ Malaise _____ Fever _____ Illness
• *Immunizations:*	Are immunizations current? Yes _____ No _____ What is your travel history?
• *Birth history:*	Vaginal _________ C-section _________ Full-term? Yes _____ No _____ Any complications _______________
• *Medications:*	List prescription and over-the-counter drugs:
• *Medical history:*	Serious accidents (date, injury, length of care) Hospitalizations (date, injury, length of care) Surgeries (date, injury, length of care) _______________ Serious illness (date, injury, length of care) _______________
• *Skin:*	_____ Skin problems _____ Sun exposure _____ Any special needs for personal care for skin and hair
• *Vision:*	_____ Glasses _____ Any problems with vision
• *Ears:*	_____ Earaches _____ Infections _____ Discharge from ear _____ Ringing (tinnitis) _____ Dizziness (vertigo)
• *Nose and sinuses:*	_____ Discharge from the nose or sinuses _____ Sinus pain _____ Unusual and frequent colds _____ Change in sense of smell
• *Mouth and throat:*	_____ Pain _____ Toothache _____ Lesions or sores on the mouth or throat _____ Changes in the mouth or throat _____ Altered taste _____ Jaw pain
• *Neck:*	_____ Neck pain _____ Limitations in neck movement _____ Lumps, swelling, tenderness, or other discomfort

(continued)

Table 5-1 (continued). Physical Health Screening

• *Respiratory system:*	_____ History of asthma _____ Chest pain _____ Shortness of breath _____ Cough _____ Wheezing
• *Cardiovascular system:*	_____ Pain near heart with or without exertion _____ Dizziness when standing up _____ Personal history of any heart problems _____ Problems breathing when sleeping
• *Peripheral vascular system:*	_____ Coldness _____ Numbness _____ Tingling _____ Swelling of legs or hands _____ Pain in legs _____ Discolored hands or feet _____ Varicose veins _____ History of vascular problems
• *Gastrointestinal system:*	_____ Changes in appetite _____ Food intolerance _____ Heartburn _____ Abdominal pain _____ Nausea and vomiting _____ Flatulence (gas) Frequency of bowel movement _______________ _____ Recent changes in stool _____ Constipation or diarrhea _____ Rectal bleeding _____ Rectal conditions _____ Use of antacids or laxatives _____ High fiber in diet
• *Urinary system:*	_____ Frequency of urination _____ Problems with urgency _____ Pain with urination _____ Unusual color _____ Other problems _____ For women: Kegel exercises post-pregnancy
• *Male genital system:*	_____ Penis or testicular pain _____ Sores or lesions _____ Discharge _____ Lumps _____ Hernia
• *Female genital system:*	Menstrual history (last period, duration; cycle): _______________ Pregnancy history: _____ Vaginal itching _____ Discharge _____ Age of menopause _____ Menopausal signs or symptoms _____ Postmenopausal bleeding
• *Sexual history:*	_____ In relationship involving intercourse _____ Aspects of sex satisfactory _____ Contraception is satisfactory _____ Awareness of family planning _____ Awareness of sexually transmitted diseases (STDs) _____ Familiar with sex education _____ Presence of STDs

(continued)

Table 5-1 (continued). Physical Health Screening		
• *Musculoskeletal system:*	____ History of arthritis; gout; joint pain, swelling, or stiffness; deformity	
	____ Range of motion limitations	____ Muscular pain
	____ Muscle cramps	____ Muscle weakness
	____ Gait problems	____ Problems with coordination
	____ Back pain	____ Joint stiffness
	____ Limitations in movement	____ History of back/disk problems
• *Neurological system:*	____ History of seizures, blackouts, strokes, fainting; headaches	
	____ Motor problems: tics, tremors, paralysis, or coordination problems	
	____ Sensory: numbness, tingling	____ Memory: loss, disorientation
	____ Mood changes	____ Depression
	____ History of mental health dysfunction	
• *Hematologic system:*	____ Bleeding problems	____ Excessive bruising
	____ Lymph node swelling	____ Exposure to toxins and radiation
	____ Blood transfusions and reactions	
• *Endocrine system:*	____ History of diabetes	____ Thyroid disease
	____ Intolerance to heat and cold	____ Change in skin pigmentation and texture
	____ Excessive sweating	
	____ Abnormal relationship between appetite and weight (describe)	
	____ Abnormal hair distribution	____ Nervousness
	____ Tremors	____ Need for hormone therapy

for specific body systems, taking into consideration the individual's family history and personal health habits. The checklist may be done as part of an interview or completed by the individual before a physical screening. If a person completing the checklist does not understand the questions, this situation offers the clinician an opportunity to educate the client regarding those aspects that are not clearly understood.

The checklist notes the most common illnesses affecting Americans, including hypertension, stroke, metabolic syndrome, cancer, diabetes, allergies, arthritis, alcoholism, mental illness, seizure disorders, and kidney disease. Questions throughout the checklist provide additional opportunities to identify potential risk factors associated with specific body systems. This checklist can be used to survey an individual regarding potential health risks and current medical problems.

General Health

Observation of the individual's overall appearance provides various indicators of general health. If the person is obese, he or she is at risk for a variety of health conditions and needs a referral for a more extensive examination. The checklist offers common signs and symptoms indicating the need for a medical referral if they are chronic and unexplained. These clinical manifestations include fatigue, fever, weakness, and malaise and are commonly associated with a variety of systemic diseases.

Immunizations

Individuals who follow the prescribed schedule of immunizations are generally protected from a variety of common infectious illnesses. According to the Centers for Disease Control and Prevention,[24] the flu vaccine is now considered a standard vaccination for everyone 6 months and older. Those who travel, particularly outside of the country, may be unprotected from less common infective agents. For example, individuals who traveled to China during the severe acute respiratory syndrome (SARS) epidemic were at risk for developing this pathology even after leaving the country because of the incubation period of the virus. Individuals who have not been vaccinated should be advised of the risk of missing vaccinations.

Birth History

An individual's birth history is most relevant for those who are very young or who have developmental problems affecting their growth and development. The method of delivery (vaginal vs cesarean section), the length of gestation, and complications during the birth process can pose significant risks to normal development. The mother's health status throughout and following pregnancy is also important to note. Generally, a physician closely follows individuals with complications or problems during birth until health problems resolve.

Medications

People commonly take prescribed medications, vitamins, minerals, over-the-counter drugs, or diet supplements, or seek alternative therapies that could influence their health and wellness. Although physicians closely monitor prescribed medications, individuals may alter the effects of their medications by adding over-the-counter drugs, vitamins, minerals, herbs, or other extracts from natural sources. Pathology can develop when inappropriate dosages are used or incompatible drugs and agents are mixed. It is essential that the clinician request a comprehensive list of all agents the client is ingesting, applying to the skin, or administering via injection, whether or not they are prescribed. All ingested agents should be shared with the individual's primary physician. In addition, the clinician should ask the client if all medications are taken as prescribed to ensure that correct dosage is administered. Expiration dates of current drugs should be noted, if possible. If the individual is taking expired drugs or is not compliant with drug prescriptions, a referral should be made to the physician to ensure proper medical monitoring.

Medical History

A comprehensive medical history that includes serious accidents, hospitalizations, surgeries, and serious illnesses can identify individuals who are at risk for further pathology. Identifying the date and type of injury and the length of care for serious accidents allows the health care professional to appraise future risk. For example, individuals with a history of traumatic brain injury are at a higher risk for subsequent head injuries. A child with a history with frequent injuries may be either clumsy or a victim of abuse. Likewise, a history of hospitalizations, including the cause of hospitalization, the history of the disease or injury, surgeries performed, and the length of care, alerts the clinician to possible risk factors or medical conditions that require continual attention. A referral should be made as needed to monitor conditions that have worsened since the patient's discharge.

Skin

Skin problems can be identified through a visual screening process, noting the skin's color, texture (smooth or rough), thickness (visibility of vessels), and elasticity (presence of wrinkles), as well as the presence of birthmarks or evidence of bruising or scarring (suggestive of previous injury). Special products used for skin or hair care may be responsible for problems such as contact dermatitis. Individuals with chronic skin conditions, such as psoriasis and dermatitis, may need to be reminded to maintain their medical management if they are experiencing ongoing problems. If problems arise despite current medical management, a referral to the physician is needed.

The ABCDE rule of skin cancer helps to identify any abnormal skin lesions that are suspect and is outlined as follows[25]:

- "A" represents asymmetry in the lesion (ie, one half of the lesion is unlike the other half)
- "B" represents borders that are irregular or poorly circumscribed
- "C" represents color variation in the lesions (melanomas tend to have color variations that include tan, brown, black, white, red, and blue)
- "D" represents diameter greater than 6 mm (the size of a pencil eraser) because cancerous skin lesions tend to grow
- "E" represents elevation because normal skin lesions tend to be flat, so raised lesions may represent abnormal growth. (Some use "E" to represent evolving, or any change in the shape, size, color, height, or any other trait of a mole, or new symptoms, such as bleeding, crusting or itching).

The Center of Excellence for Medical Multimedia provides pictures illustrating suspect skin lesions at its website http://www.skincanceratoz.org/Resource-Center/ABCDE-Screening-Guidelines.aspx. Any suspected skin lesions should be reported to the physician immediately. Individuals at an increased risk for melanoma are those with fair complexions; excessive exposure to ultraviolet radiation from the sun or tanning booths; occupational exposure to coal tar, pitch, creosote, arsenic compounds, and radium; or HIV.

Vision

According to the American Medical Association,[26] "it is estimated that more than 14 million individuals in the United States aged 12 years and older are visually impaired (< 20/40). Of these cases, 11 million are attributable to refractive error. In the United States, the most common causes of nonrefractive visual impairment are age-related macular degeneration, cataract, diabetic retinopathy, glaucoma, and other retinal disorders." Obvious visual aids, such as glasses, are easy to identify; however, many individuals have had eye surgeries, such as LASIK, or wear contacts to improve their vision. The clinician should ask about any aids or surgeries to correct vision, as well as any problems with vision, including eye infections or soreness. Although an optometrist may examine visual acuity problems, infections or other visual impairments should be more thoroughly examined by a physician. During a screening, the interviewer should ask about visual problems and the need for visual aids to ensure adequate vision for daily functioning.

Ears

Ear problems are common across the lifespan. Young children are susceptible to ear infections, such as *otitis media*, because of the horizontal alignment of their eustachian tubes. Infants who drink from bottles while lying on their backs are at particular risk for ear infections. Other ear problems, such as earaches, discharges from the ear (thick drainage could indicate a ruptured eardrum or possible infection), *tinnitus* (ringing in the ear), *vertigo* (dizziness), or problems hearing may be reported and would warrant a medical referral.[25] Pain in the jaw just below the ear accompanied by an audible sound with opening and closing the mouth is commonly associated with *tempomandibular joint syndrome*. If the pain is severe, diagnostic imaging may be necessary to identify pathology.

Nose and Sinuses

A history of unusual or frequent colds, sinus pain, changes in smell, and any signs of discharge from the nose or sinuses suggests potential pathology. *Sinusitis* (inflammation of the sinus passages located behind the upper portion of the face) is one of the most common medical conditions affecting individuals. Up to 13% of the population experiences chronic sinusitis.[27] Morning headaches and pain or tenderness in the upper jaws, teeth, cheeks, ears, neck, eyes, and nose are common with sinusitis. In addition, the individual may have a stuffy nose, experience a loss of smell, and have swollen eyelids with pain between the eyes. Risks for sinusitis include nasal passage abnormalities, aspirin sensitivity, lung and immune disorders, allergies that affect sinuses, regular exposure to pollutants, using decongestant nasal sprays too often, and frequent swimming or diving, so it is helpful to ask follow-up questions about risk factors.[27]

Mouth and Throat

Risk factors for pathology of the mouth and throat include pain (such as a toothache, jaw pain, sore throat, or lesions in the mouth or throat), altered taste, or other changes in the mouth or throat region. All ages are susceptible to infections, such as strep throat, so complaints of a persistent sore throat need immediate medical attention. Other signs or symptoms that need attention include a painless lump on the inside of the lip (possible squamous cell skin cancer); a painless hard coating on the inside of the mouth or on the tongue (a precancerous condition common in smokers); small, open sores on the lips, tongue, sides or back of the mouth (cold sores or canker sores potentially caused by a virus); redness and swelling in gums or around a tooth (possible gingivitis or dental cavity); or sores around the mouth (possibly caused by a vitamin deficiency).[28]

Neck

Problems in the neck may present as neck pain or tenderness, limitations in movement, or swelling. Neck pain can indicate problems not only in neck tissue, but also in distant parts of the body. For example, neck pain may be referred pain from cardiac disease. The clinician can quickly determine if there are problems in blood flow, which are characterized by louder sounds on auscultation of the carotid arteries located on either side of the neck. Tenderness around the throat, especially accompanied by swelling, suggests inflammation of the lymph nodes along the jaw line. Although enlarged lymph nodes may simply indicate a normal body response to a cold, this condition may also be a sign of lymphoma or thyroid problems. If any of these problems exist, a physician referral should be made.

Respiratory and Cardiopulmonary Systems

The cardiopulmonary system may present with chest problems or other pain symptoms in the upper trunk, shortness of breath, coughing, or wheezing. Visual inspection may be used to note peripheral cyanosis (bluish coloring of the lips and extremities), use of the accessory muscles in lieu of abdominal muscles for breathing, atypical chest structure (eg, a barrel chest), abnormal breathing patterns, or atypical sounds. If these are new complaints, a physician referral is warranted.

Gastrointestinal System

Abdominal discomfort may be a sign of gastrointestinal problems, cardiovascular problems, or other possible pathologies. Generally, individuals with changes in appetite, food intolerance, possible heartburn (often confused with myocardial chest pain), nausea and vomiting, *flatulence* (gas), irregular bowel movements (constipation or diarrhea), or recent changes in stool are at risk for gastrointestinal pathology.[29] There is greater concern if there are complaints of rectal bleeding because this indicates likely pathology, possibly cancer. It is helpful to know about the individual's use of any antacids, laxatives, or fiber (dietary or herbal supplements) that may affect bowel function. One common condition, *gastroesophageal reflux disorder* (GERD), caused by excessive reverse flow of gastric acid, presents with persistent heartburn and acid regurgitation, as well as trouble swallowing, hoarseness in the morning, and chest pain.[30] There is an increased risk for GERD if individuals drink substances that weaken the sphincters controlling the flow of gastric juices, such as coffee and alcohol. Likewise, foods, such as spicy, fatty, and tomato-based foods, as well as chocolate, peppermint, garlic, onions, and citric fruit, have been associated with GERD. Additionally, conditions related to enlarged abdomens or being pregnant or overweight are contributors to GERD. This condition is chronic and can be controlled with lifestyle changes, as well as proper medical management under the supervision of a physician.

Urinary System

Screening the urinary system for pathology involves asking questions about the frequency of urination, problems with urgency, pain with urination, unusual color, or other problems. This topic is sensitive and may require open-ended questions that allow the individual to share any concerns. It is important to point out risk factors that warrant concern. A physician should address any problems with the urinary system that have not had prior medical attention to determine etiology and pathology.

Male Genital System

If talking to a man, it is best to follow up questions regarding continence with those related to the genital system. Prostate cancer, a silent but slow-growing disease, often develops with little early warning. Men with *benign prostate hyperplasia*, an enlarged yet noncancerous prostate, often have problems with increased frequency of urination, nighttime urination, pain with urination, inability to urinate, or trouble with ejaculation.[31] Although these signs and symptoms may be benign, they could also be related to prostate cancer, so a medical referral is needed. Other concerns related to the male reproductive system include penis or testicular pain, sores or lesions, any type of irregular discharge, lumps, or hernias. Because bladder cancer is the fifth leading cancer in the United States, any unusual signs or symptoms indicate a medical referral.

Female Genital System

When screening a woman, it is important to get a thorough menstrual history (last period, duration, and cycle), a pregnancy history, and information about vaginal itching or discharges. If a woman has already reached menopause, note the age of onset as well as menopausal signs and symptoms. Menopause manifestations include hot flashes (a hot sensation generally starting at the waistline and extending to the head), night sweats, irritability, insomnia, and vaginal dryness.[32] It is also important to check if women are engaged in regular exercise for their pelvic floor muscles. Kegel exercises, designed to tone pelvic floor muscles, are particularly important postpregnancy to restrengthen muscles stretched by a vaginal birth and to prevent incontinence. Although bleeding several years postmenopause is not unusual, this sign should be examined by a physician to ensure that any pathology is identified.[32] Additional issues related to women's health are described in Chapter 8.

Sexual History

History of a relationship involving intercourse may put an individual at risk for sexually transmitted diseases (STDs). Sexual history questions should delicately explore personal issues, including sexual satisfaction, contraception, and education about STDs, sex education, and family planning.[33] These concerns may be referred to professionals who commonly deal with sexual issues, including physicians, nurses, psychologists, and medical specialists in men's and women's health. The presence of STDs warrants an immediate medical referral.

Musculoskeletal System

Screening the musculoskeletal system can reveal conditions related to muscles, ligaments, tendons, and other joint structures, as well as other conditions that present with similar patterns of pain or dysfunction. An individual reporting a family history of musculoskeletal problems, such as arthritis or muscle pathology, is at an increased risk for developing similar problems. The classic signs of arthritis include joint pain, swelling, and stiffness. With pathological progression, the joints may have limited motion and, ultimately, deformity. Any of these clinical manifestations indicate a medical referral. The clinician should also inquire about complaints of muscle pain, muscle cramps, muscle or joint stiffness, or inflexibility to determine possible causes of these problems related to varying levels of physical activity. A more thorough musculoskeletal examination is in order if these signs and symptoms limit the individual's work, leisure, or other activities. Individuals should also be specifically asked about back pain or a history of back pain. If there are complaints of any pain, it is important to ask about current exercises or activities that tend to ameliorate or exacerbate (increase) the pain, noting the frequency, intensity, duration, and types of activities, as appropriate. On the other hand, bone pain is suggestive of something related to bone disease and should be examined carefully to eliminate the possibility of cancer. During the screening, the clinician may note problems with motor control, such as abnormalities in gait or incoordination. Movement should be observed with shoes removed to avoid the confounding possibility that footwear might contribute to any presenting problems. If motor control problems exist, a more extensive examination should be performed to determine possible causes of any problems.

Neurological System

Individuals with a history of seizures, blackouts, strokes, fainting, or headaches are at risk for possible neurological impairments that are transient or recurrent.[34] These problems, if persistent, need to be examined more thoroughly by a neurologist. Likewise, motor problems such as tics, tremors, paralysis, uncoordinated movement, or sensory changes (eg, numbness or tingling) may suggest more serious neurological pathology and should be referred for a more complete examination. Cognitive dysfunction, such as memory loss or disorientation, could be indicative of a progressive neurological problem or side effects of current medications. If the individual complains of these problems, medications and other agents taken by the individual may be suspect. Finally, emotional problems such as depression, mood changes, or mental health problems that interfere with function should be discussed with a psychologist or the primary physician to ensure that needs are met through appropriate exercise, proper counseling, and/or medication.

Hematologic and Lymphatic System

Individuals may have recent hematologic laboratory tests that prove valuable in determining possible pathology. If these values are available, they can guide the clinician in making appropriate recommendations for exercise and medical referrals. Of particular concern is excessive bruising, bleeding, vascular swelling, or lymph node swelling.[29] These problems suggest hematological or lymphatic pathology and should be medically managed. If an individual has received a blood transfusion, any adverse reactions to this transfusion should be noted. With the risk of HIV infections from transfusions, a screening test for this risk is also recommended. Chronic hematologic disorders may lead to observable changes to the skin (causing it to become more pale or yellow), may cause weakness (especially with physical exertion), and may contribute to *dyspnea* (shortness of breath). Individuals complaining of swelling, congestion, pain in their extremities unrelated to muscle or joint pain, or faintness may result from irregularities in the cardiovascular or lymphatic system.[29] All these conditions warrant a medical referral. Some individuals with lowered white blood cells are at risk for infection and may present with a sore throat, cough, or signs of infection (elevated temperature, chilling, sweating, or malaise). Additionally, these individuals may complain of painful urination.[35] These individuals need immediate medical attention if they present with these acute clinical manifestations.

Sickle cell anemia, a genetic (autosomal-dominant) disorder, is relatively common, particularly in Black individuals.[35] This pathology manifests in multiple body systems with sign and symptoms including joint pain, fatigue, breathlessness, rapid heart rate, delayed growth and puberty, ulcers on the lower legs (seen in adolescents and adults), jaundice or yellowing of the skin, attacks of abdominal pain, or fever.[36] Although sickle cell anemia is commonly diagnosed in childhood, complaints of *hematuria* (bloody urine), excessive urination, excessive thirst, chest pain, or poor eyesight/blindness suggest progression of the pathology.[36] A physician should more carefully examine any of these clinical manifestations.

Finally, individuals who have been exposed to toxins or radiation are at an increased risk for developing hematological pathology and should have laboratory tests to determine levels of toxicity.

Endocrine System

The endocrine system controls the pituitary, thyroid, parathyroids, adrenal gland, pancreas, and gonads. Dysfunction of these glands may be apparent in other portions of the screening but may also present with unique signs and symptoms. Growth and development of connective tissue is controlled by the endocrine system, so excessive or delayed growth is one indication of abnormalities. Also, signs associated with stress (increased respiration, increased perspiration, heart palpitations, changes in water retention or dehydration, increased blood pressure, increased pulse rate, or elevated body temperature) suggest potential problems with the endocrine glands. Signs and symptoms associated with musculoskeletal problems, including muscle weakness, fatigue, muscle pain, or muscle atrophy could be related to endocrine problems because these clinical manifestations are also associated with conditions such as Cushing's syndrome and thyroid disease.[29]

Clinicians should carefully screen for diabetes when screening the endocrine system. Diabetes insipidus is a pathology related to pituitary pathology, among other causes, and results from the kidney's inability to conserve water, leading to excessive urination and thirst.[37] Individuals with these symptoms or with a history of diabetes or thyroid disease need medical monitoring to ensure proper medical management. Diabetes mellitus type 1 classically presents with excessive urination, excessive thirst, weight loss, and blurred vision.[37] The risk of developing type 2 diabetes commonly increases with obesity, increased age, and lack of physical activity, presenting with similar signs and symptoms, but may also include foot pain, infections, and abnormal lipid profiles.[37] It is crucial to make an appropriate medical referral if any type of diabetes is suspected.

Other problems associated with endocrine pathology include intolerance to heat and cold, changes in skin pigmentation and texture, or abnormalities in appetite or weight. Neurological signs that are suspect for endocrine disease include nervousness and tremors.[29] Individuals with hyperthyroidism may also present with drowsiness, abnormal sensations or sensory loss, depression or personality changes, fatigue, or hyperactive reflexes. Likewise, hypothyroidism presents with personality changes and a risk for convulsions.[29] Individuals presenting with any clinical manifestations of possible endocrine pathology should be more thoroughly examined by a physician. In addition, women using hormone replacement therapy should be carefully monitored by a physician for effective and safe maintenance dosages.

Screening for Health Behaviors

Most pathological conditions are a combination of genetics and lifestyle behaviors. A thorough medical history provides some indication of genetic risk, but a comprehensive assessment of lifestyle behaviors offers equally important information. Areas to screen for lifestyle behaviors include activity and exercise (including activities of daily living and exercise behaviors), leisure activities, sleeping/resting behaviors, and nutrition. Nutrition screening includes both positive and negative health behaviors, such as healthy diet and smoking, caffeine, and alcohol use. The lifestyle behaviors screening tool (Table 5-2) is a quick and easy tool to determine general lifestyle behaviors. Additional age-related screening tools will be provided in subsequent chapters featuring specific populations with unique growth and development issues.

Screening for Alcohol Use Disorder

If alcohol use disorder is suspected, specific questions are recommended. Several screening tools are available, but the CAGE questionnaire is the most efficient and widely used.[38-40] CAGE is a mnemonic for a questionnaire that asks about attempts to *C*ut down on drinking, *A*nnoyance with criticisms about drinking, *G*uilt about drinking, and using alcohol as an *E*ye opener. The test takes approximately 1 minute to complete and, although it does not diagnose alcoholism or problem drinking, it should prompt further examination.

Another short screening test involves only 2 questions: "In the past year, have you ever drunk or used drugs more than you meant to?" and "Have you felt you wanted or needed to cut down on your drinking or drug use in the past year?" In one study, at least one positive response detected current substance-use disorders with nearly 80% sensitivity and specificity.[39] Additional screening tests include the Alcohol Use Disorders Identification Test (AUDIT) and the T-ACE, based on the CAGE test.[40] As with all screening tests, performance varies with the prevalence of substance abuse in the particular population screened.[40]

Assessment of Spiritual Beliefs

Current research supports the positive effects of spirituality for health and well-being. It is helpful to know whether an individual relies on a particular spiritual belief system for improved health, fitness, and wellness. Knowledge of this belief system can alert the clinician to values contributing to or contradicting traditional medical beliefs. Cultural sensitivity is particularly important whenever assessing a person's level of spirituality. A simple question might be, "How would you describe the role that spirituality plays in your health, fitness, and wellness?" It is inappropriate for

Table 5-2. Lifestyle Behaviors Screening Tool	
DESCRIBE EACH OF THE FOLLOWING:	
Activity and Exercise:	
Daily activities:	Do you have problems with your activities of daily living? Yes _____ No _____ If so, please describe: Dressing ____________________ Bathing ____________________ Hygiene ____________________ Self-care ____________________
Leisure activities: How would you describe the type, intensity, and duration of your physical activity (on a weekly basis). If you do a variety of activities, please note these activities separately.	
	Type ____________________ Duration ____________________ Frequency ____________________ Intensity ____________________
	Type ____________________ Duration ____________________ Frequency ____________________ Intensity ____________________
Sleep and Rest:	How would you describe your sleep behavior: Sleep patterns ____________________ Typical duration of sleep ____________________ Typical sleep posture ____________________ Does your partner interfere with your sleep? If so, how: Other comments:
Nutrition:	How would you describe your eating behavior? Overall diet ____________________ Alcohol intake ____________________ Caffeine (tea, coffee, cola drinks) intake ____________________ Smoking ____________________ Drugs (illicit) ____________________ Use of vitamins ____________________ Food allergies or intolerance ____________________ Mealtime habits ____________________

the interviewer to guide an individual into a personal religious belief system, but it is appropriate to suggest that the individual's personal belief system can contribute to wellness. Those with spiritual concerns or those seeking spiritual guidance should be referred to a hospital chaplain or advised to explore their spirituality through local centers of worship. People with strong beliefs should be encouraged to engage in meaningful spiritual activities. Additional information about spirituality is discussed in Chapter 10.

Screening for Intimate Partner Violence

Often, individuals come to a screening to get help but are embarrassed to admit that they are experiencing significant psychosocial problems. It is important to screen for possible violence because an individual may be experiencing significant stress in personal relationships. Because physical, sexual, and verbal abuse are prevalent in our society, a screening of intimate partner violence is essential.[41] Three questions that can open discussion about potentially life-threatening situations and address the issue of intimate partner violence are as follows[41]:

1. "Have you been hit, kicked, punched, or otherwise hurt by someone in the past year?"
2. "Do you feel safe in your current relationship?"
3. "Is there a partner from a previous relationship who is making you feel unsafe now?"

A positive screen is a "yes" answer to any of the 3 questions. This information should be shared with the individual's physician immediately.[41]

Screening for Holistic Health

A comprehensive screening for holistic health includes questions related to the mind, body, and spirit. The holistic health score sheet (Table 5-3) may be used to explore an individual's health more comprehensively, including the individual's physical and environmental health (body), mental and emotional health (mind), and social and spiritual health (spirit).[42] Scores on this survey categorize the individual as striving, nourishing, maintaining, sustaining, or surviving as indicators of the individual's overall health.

Regular Medical Screening Tests and Immunizations

During the screening, it is helpful to advise individuals to participate in other medical screenings for annual check-ups or as recommended by their physicians. Individuals should be reminded to follow the recommendations of the Centers for Disease Control and Prevention, including regular immunizations, laboratory tests, screening tests for cancer, and injury prevention. In addition, children and adults alike should be reminded to have regular dental examinations for preventive care.

Summary

Health care professionals play a key role in screening for primary, secondary, and tertiary prevention of pathology. Using simple screening tools in conjunction with effective communication skills can elicit key information leading to effective preventive care and management. Subsequent

TABLE 5-3. HOLISTIC HEALTH SCORE SHEET	
Each question requires a score, either 0 if the answer to the question is "never," 1 for "rarely," 2 for "sometimes," and 3 for "regularly." Questions in bold count double.	
BODY: PHYSICAL AND ENVIRONMENTAL HEALTH	
1. Do you maintain a healthy diet (high in fresh fruits, vegetables, grains, and fiber; low in fat and sugar)?	
2. Is your daily water intake adequate (at least 1/2 oz/lb of body weight: 160 lbs = 80 oz)?	
3. Do you live and work in a healthy environment with respect to clean air (both indoor and outdoor) and water?	
4. Do you make time to experience both sensual and sexual pleasure?	
5. Do you schedule regular massage to deep-tissue body work (at least once or twice/month)?	
6. **Do you engage in regular physical workouts (at least 3x/week for 30 minutes)?**	
7. Are you free of chronic aches and pains?	
8. Are you free of chronic ailments or diseases?	
9. Do you maintain physically challenging goals?	
10. Are you free of any drug or alcohol dependency?	
11. Are you within 20% of your ideal body weight?	
12. **Have you benefited in some way from understanding the causes of your chronic physical problems?**	
13. Are you physically strong?	
14. Is your body flexible?	
15. Do you have good endurance or aerobic capacity?	
16. Do you practice some form of body movement, such as yoga, t'ai chi, or a martial art?	
17. Do you have an awareness of life energy or chi?	
18. Do you feel physically attractive?	
19. Do you feel energized or empowered by nature?	
20. Are your 5 senses acute?	
21. Do you breathe abdominally?	
22. Do you sleep between 7 and 9 hours per day?	
23. Do you regularly awaken in the morning feeling well rested?	
24. Do you have daily, effortless bowel movements?	
25. Are you satisfied sexually, with regard to frequency and level of sexual energy?	
26. **Do you nurture and feel a strong sense of appreciation for your body?**	
Point Total = ________ BODY	

(continued)

Table 5-3 (continued). Holistic Health Score Sheet	
MIND: MENTAL AND EMOTIONAL HEALTH	
1. Do you have specific goals in your personal and professional life?	
2. Do you have the ability to concentrate for extended periods of time?	
3. Do you have a sense of humor?	
4. Is your outlook basically optimistic?	
5. Are you willing to take risks or make mistakes to succeed?	
6. **Does your job use all of your greatest talents?**	
7. Are you free from a strong need for control or the need to be right?	
8. Is your job enjoyable and fulfilling?	
9. Do you give yourself more supportive messages than critical messages in the course of a day?	
10. Is your sleep free from disturbing dreams?	
11. **Are you able to adjust beliefs and attitudes as a result of learning from painful experiences?**	
12. Are you able to fully experience your painful feelings such as fear, anger, sadness, and hopelessness?	
13. Are you aware of and able to express anger safely and nonviolently?	
14. Can you freely express sadness or cry?	
15. Do you use visualization or mental imagery to help you attain your goals or enhance your performance?	
16. Can you meet your financial needs and desires?	
17. Do you explore the symbolism and emotional content of your dreams?	
18. Do you believe it is possible to change?	
19. Do you have the ability to express fear?	
20. Do you enjoy high self-esteem?	
21. Do you maintain peace of mind and tranquility?	
22. Do you make time for spontaneous activities that constitute the abandon and absorption of play?	
23. Do you engage in meditation and contemplation to understand your feelings?	
24. Do you take time to "let down" and relax?	
25. Are you accepting of all your feelings?	
26. **Do you experience feelings of exhilaration?**	
Point Total=________ MIND	
SPIRIT: SOCIAL AND SPIRITUAL HEALTH	
1. **Do you actively commit time to your spiritual life?**	
2. **Do you listen to your intuition?**	
3. **Do you have an appreciation of nature?**	
4. **Do you have a regular place either in the house or in nature set aside for meditation, prayer, or reflection?**	

(continued)

Table 5-3 (continued). Holistic Health Score Sheet	
5. **Do you have a regular place either in the house or in nature set aside for meditation, prayer, or reflection?**	
6. **Do you make time to connect with young children, either your own or somebody else's?**	
7. **Are creative activities a regular part of your work or leisure?**	
8. **Have you demonstrated the willingness to commit to a marriage or comparable long-term relationship?**	
9. **Do you have one or more close friends to whom you talk openly?**	
10. **Are you free from anger toward God?**	
11. **Do you or did you feel close with your parents?**	
12. **Do you feel close with your children?**	
13. **If you have recently experienced the loss of a loved one, have you fully grieved that loss?**	
14. **Has your experience of pain enabled you to grow spiritually?**	
15. **Are you able to let go of your attachment to specific outcomes and embrace uncertainty?**	
16. **Do you act upon your intuition and take risks?**	
17. **Do you have faith in a God, spirit guides, or angels?**	
18. **Can you let go of self-interest in deciding the best course of action for a given situation?**	
19. **Are playfulness and humor important to you in your daily life?**	
20. **Do you have the ability to forgive yourself and others?**	
21. **Do you experience intimacy, besides sex, in your committed relationship?**	
22. **Do you routinely go out of your way or routinely give your time to help others?**	
23. **Do you feel a sense of belonging to a group or community?**	
24. **Are you grateful for the blessings in your life?**	
25. **Do you take walks or have daily contact with nature?**	
26. **Do you observe a day of rest completely away from work, dedicated to nurturing yourself and your family?**	
27. **Do you experience unconditional love?**	
Point Total=_______ SPIRIT **Holistic Health Total Score=_________________** **BODY, MIND, and SPIRIT OPTIMAL HEALTH SCALE:** 7=231 to 261 points=OPTIMAL 6=201 to 230 points=THRIVING 5=171 to 200 points=STRIVING 4=141 to 170 points=NOURISHING 3=111 to 140 points=MAINTAINING 2=81 to 110 points=SUSTAINING 1=80 or lower points=SURVIVING	
Adapted from Ivker RS, Zorensky EH. *Thriving: The Complete Mind/Body Guide for Optimal Health and Fitness for Men*. New York, NY: Crown; 1997.	

chapters will provide more details regarding age-appropriate screening tools and resources to help individuals manage their health and wellness needs.

REFERENCES

1. Heaven C, Maguire P, Green C. A patient-centred approach to defining and assessing interviewing competency. *Epidemiol Psyichiatr Soc.* 2003;12(2):86-91.
2. Thompson DW, Thompson NN. The art of interviewing your next CEO. *Trustee.* 2003;56(2):14-18.
3. O'Keefe M, Roberton D, Sawyer M, Baghurst P. Medical student interviewing: a randomized trial of patient-centredness and clinical competence. *Fam Pract.* 2003;20(2):213-219.
4. Meyerson H. Honing your nonverbal communication skills. *Vitality.* July 2001.
5. Stern MA. Communication tip: maintaining eye contact. Matthew Arnold Stern. http://www.matthewarnold-stern.com/tips/tipps16.html. Accessed August 6, 2004.
6. Carducci B. *Shyness: A Bold New Approach.* New York, NY: Harper Perennial; 2000.
7. Remland MS, Jones TS, Brinkman H. Interpersonal distance, body orientation, and touch: effects of culture, gender, and age. *J Soc Psychol.* 1995;135(3):281-297.
8. Goldin-Meadow S. The role of gesture in communication and thinking. *Trends Cogn Sci.* 1999;3(11):419-429.
9. Hale WW III, Jansen JH, Bouhuys AL, Jenner JA, van den Hoofdakker RH. Non-verbal behavioral interactions of depressed patients with partners and strangers: the role of behavioral social support and involvement in depression persistence. *J Affect Disord.* 1997;44(2-3):111-122.
10. Bouhuys AL, Jansen CJ, van den Hoofdakker RH. Analysis of observed behaviors displayed by depressed patients during a clinical interview: relationships between behavioral factors and clinical concepts of activation. *J Affect Disord.* 1991;21(2):79-88.
11. Goldin-Meadow S. The role of gesture in communication and thinking. *Trends Cogn Sci.* 1999;3(11):419-429.
12. LeBaron M. Cross-cultural communication. Beyond Intractability. http://www.beyondintractability.org/bi-essay/cross-cultural-communication. Accessed May 30, 2013.
13. Berlin E, Fowkes WA. A teaching framework for cross-cultural health care. *West J Med.* 1983;139:934-938.
14. Williams JR. Guidelines for the use of multimedia in instruction. Proceedings of the Human Factors and Ergonomics Society 42nd Annual Meeting; 1998; Chicago, IL.
15. Joseph C. 10 characteristics of professionalism. *Houston Chronicle.* http://smallbusiness.chron.com/10-characteristics-professionalism-708.html. Accessed May 30, 2013.
16. Clinical depression. University of Pittsburgh School of Medicine. http://www.medschool.pitt.edu/somsa/Depression.html. Accessed May 30, 2013.
17. Major depression disorder in adults. National Institutes of Health. http://www.nimh.nih.gov/statistics/1MDD_ADULT.shtml. Accessed May 30, 2013.
18. Arroll B, Khin K, Kerse K. Screening for depression in primary care with two verbally asked questions: cross sectional study. *BMJ.* 2003;327:1144.
19. Thibault JM, Steiner RW. Efficient identification of adults with depression and dementia. *Am Fam Physician.* 2004;70(6):1101-1110.
20. Hamilton M. Development of a rating scale for primary depressive illness. *Br J Soc Clin Psychol.* 1967;6:278-296.
21. Holmes T, Rahe R. The social readjustment rating scale. *J Psychosom Res.* 1967;11(2):213-218.
22. Yeaworth RC, York J, Hussey MA, Ingle ME, Goodwin T. The development of an adolescent life change event scale. *Adolescence.* 1980;15(57):91-97.
23. Sun F, Kuo C, Cheng H, Buthpitiya S, Collins P, Griss M. Activity-aware mental stress detection using physiological sensors. Carnegic Mellon University. http://repository.cmu.edu/cgi/viewcontent.cgi?article=1011&context=silicon_valley. Accessed May 30, 2013.
24. Flu vaccine effectiveness: questions and answers for health professionals. Centers for Disease Control and Prevention. http://www.cdc.gov/flu/professionals/vaccination/effectivenessqa.htm. Accessed May 30, 2013.
25. ABCDE screening guidelines. Center of Excellence for Medical Multimedia. http://www.skincanceratoz.org/Resource-Center/ABCDE-Screening-Guidelines.aspx. Accessed May 30, 2013.
26. Ko F, Vitale S, Chou CF, Cotch MF, Saaddine J, Friedman DS. Prevalence of non-refractive visual impairment in US adults and associated risk factors, 1999-2002 and 2005-2008. *JAMA.* 2012;308(22):2361.
27. Chronic sinusitis: mobility. Centers for Disease Control and Prevention. http://www.cdc.gov/nchs/fastats/sinuses.htm. Accessed May 30, 2013.
28. Swartz M. *Textbook of Physical Diagnosis.* 5th ed. New York, NY: Saunders-Elsevier; 2005.
29. Sinusitis: risk factors. Mayo Clinic. http://www.mayoclinic.com/health/chronic-sinusitis/DS00232/DSECTION=risk-factors. Accessed May 30, 2013.
30. GERD. Medline Plus. http://www.nlm.nih.gov/medlineplus/gerd.html. Accessed May 30, 2013.

31. Prostate enlargement: benign prostatic hyperplasia (NKUDIC). National Kidney and Urologic Diseases Information Clearinghouse. http://kidney.niddk.nih.gov/kudiseases/pubs/prostateenlargement/. Accessed May 30, 2013.
32. Menopause. National Institutes of Health. http://www.nlm.nih.gov/medlineplus/menopause.html. Accessed May 30, 2013.
33. Sexually transmitted diseases (STDs). Centers for Disease Control and Prevention. http://www.cdc.gov/std/. Accessed May 30, 2013.
34. Good DC. Episodic neurologic symptoms. In: Walker HK, Hall WD, Hurst JW, eds. *Clinical Methods: The History, Physical, and Laboratory Examinations*. 3rd ed. Boston, MA: Butterworths; 1990. http://www.ncbi.nlm.nih.gov/books/NBK374/. Accessed May 20, 2014.
35. Haiken M. Understanding white blood cell count. Caring.com. http://www.caring.com/articles/low-white-blood-cell-count. Accessed May 30, 2013.
36. What is sickle cell anemia? National Heart, Lung, and Blood Institute. http://www.nhlbi.nih.gov/health/health-topics/topics/sca/. Accessed May 30, 2013.
37. American Diabetes Association. Screening for diabetes. *Diabetes Care*. 2002;25(1): s21-s24.
38. Schulz JE, Parran T Jr. Principles of identification and intervention. In: Graham AW, Schultz TK, Wilford BB, eds. *Principles of Addiction Medicine*. 2nd ed. Chevy Chase, MD: American Society of Addiction Medicine; 1998:250-251.
39. Mayfield D, McLeod G, Hall P. The CAGE questionnaire: validation of a new alcoholism screening instrument. *Am J Psychiatry*. 1974;131(10):1121-1123.
40. Screening tests. National Institutes of Health, National Institute on Alcohol Abuse and Alcoholism. http://pubs.niaaa.nih.gov/publications/arh28-2/78-79.htm. Accessed May 30, 2013.
41. Feldhaus KM, Koziol-McLain J, Amsbury HL, et al. Accuracy of 3 brief screening questions for detecting partner violence in the emergency department. *JAMA*. 1977;277:1357-1361.
42. Ivker RS, Zorensky EH. *Thriving: The Complete Mind/Body Guide for Optimal Health and Fitness for Men*. New York, NY: Crown; 1997.

6

Health, Fitness, and Wellness Issues During Childhood and Adolescence

Catherine Rush Thompson, PT, PhD, MS

"It takes a village to raise a child."—African proverb

The Dynamic Process of Growth and Development

Neonates, infants, children, and adolescents face unique changes as they grow and develop into adults. Many people contribute to this dynamic process, including families, communities, educators, and health care professionals. Health care professionals should be aware of physical and psychosocial transformations taking place early in life. These changes play a key role in promoting health for infants, children, and adults in various practice settings, ranging from pediatric intensive care units to community fitness centers and sports fields. Many of these settings afford children the opportunity to interact with healthy, fit siblings and peers, as well as those at risk for health problems. Screening neonates, infants, children, and youth in these settings is an essential role of therapists practicing preventive care. A variety of screening tools are available that provide normative data for identifying children at risk or children with health impairments requiring appropriate interventions.

Genetics, or "nature," plays a key role in a child's physical and psychological makeup; however, physical activity and other environmental influences can "nurture" a child, greatly influencing a child's healthy growth, proper development, increasing fitness, and emergent wellness. Combinations of genetic and environmental factors, including stressors the mother may be encountering, play key roles in these maturational processes. Certain aspects of growth are more strongly influenced by genetic factors, including dental development, the sequence of bone ossification, and sexual differentiation during puberty. Other aspects of growth and development are more strongly influenced by maternal lifestyle habits. Chapter 8 provides suggestions for promoting prenatal wellness through healthy lifestyle habits during pregnancy.

Thompson CR.
Prevention Practice and Health Promotion: A Health Care Professional's Guide to Health, Fitness, and Wellness, Second Edition (pp 95-110).

Early Childhood Screenings

Newborns are generally screened by obstetricians using the APGAR test, a screening tool describing the infant's *activity/muscle tone (A), pulse (P)* or heart rate, *grimace/infantile reflex response (G), appearance (A)* in terms of normal skin color, and *respiration (R) rate.*[1] These key indicators provide a quick screening of the newborn's body functions at 1 minute and 5 minutes after birth. Each of the 5 indicators is scored up to 2 points for optimal function. A score of 7 to 10 is considered normal, whereas 4 to 6 may require some immediate medical assistance. Infants with scores below 4 require immediate medical attention and are at increased risk for problems during infancy, including significant neurological dysfunction.[1] If a newborn is suspected of having problems prior to or during birth, the infant is generally referred to an early intervention program for further assessment. In some cases, these infants do not receive follow-up care and may need to be identified through additional screening opportunities. Health care professionals are commonly trained in performing the Denver II Developmental Screening Test (Denver II), a screening tool designed to detect problems in young children.[2] The Denver II, an updated version of the original Denver Developmental Screening Test, is a simple, sensitive, and convenient test developed to screen children from birth to age 6 years. This test battery includes screening of *personal-social skills* (getting along with others and taking care of self), *fine motor-adaptive skills* (eye-hand coordination and hand skills such as drawing and coloring), *language skills* (hearing, following directions, and speaking), and *gross motor skills* (total body movements such as sitting, walking, and jumping.) Any suspected delays in function should be reported to the child's physician for further examination. When performing any developmental screening test, it is helpful to make additional observations of structural and functional aspects of the child indicating potential problems. It is helpful to ask the parents, guardians, and/or teachers about the child's nutritional habits, developmental milestones, physical development, psychosocial interactions, communication skills, medical history of illness or injury, environmental hazards, and impairments, such as hearing loss or visual deficits.[3] Other considerations include observations for signs of child abuse and information about the safety and enrichment of the child's home environment. If there are any concerns, the family physician should be contacted for collaborative strategies to address the child's needs.

The child's height and weight should be measured and compared with normative data for age and sex to detect delayed or disproportionate growth of the body. According to the Centers for Disease Control and Prevention (CDC), being overweight is having a body mass index (BMI) above the 95th percentile for the child's age, whereas a BMI above the 85th percentile puts the child at risk of becoming overweight.[4] Some children who are very athletic may have a large muscle mass contributing to a high BMI, but the vast majority of children with high BMI scores are overweight and need help with weight management. A child with a BMI below the 5th percentile is considered underweight.[4] Again, if the child is developing normally, has a healthy diet, and is extremely active and energetic, this BMI may be normal. If the child has been ill with diarrhea and vomiting, has a poor appetite, or has a low energy level, the child should be thoroughly examined to determine the cause of the problem.

Recent research indicates that there are racial differences in the timing of sexual maturation that can have a significant effect on growth assessment in the use of the growth charts. Within age and sex groups, children who are sexually more mature tend to be taller and weigh more than less mature children.[5] Rapidly maturing children tend to have larger BMI values than those who are maturing slowly.[5]

Factors Influencing Growth and Development in Early Childhood

Genetics play a key role in a child's appearance and in some behavioral aspects of development yet are not solely responsible for normal growth. More important are the environmental factors that facilitate, inhibit, and age tissue growth, such as gravitational forces, compression and traction forces, and other biomechanical forces that combine with healthy nutrition, adequate rest, and a healthy psychosocial environment. During the first 6 months of life, the body systems undergo dramatic changes to accommodate the dynamic physical changes of an infant. On average, babies grow 10 in (25 cm) in height while tripling birth weight by their first birthday.[6] After age 1, a baby's growth in length slows considerably, and by 2 years, growth in height usually continues at a fairly steady rate of approximately 2.5 in (6 cm) per year until adolescence. Children generally have a prepubescent growth spurt that begins at age 8 in girls and age 10 in boys. Throughout puberty, the growth spurt is accompanied by the development of secondary sex characteristics and the onset of menstruation for girls. By age 18, most youths have reached physical maturity.[5] Additional factors that should be considered when screening a child for health, fitness, and wellness include considerations of the child's physical health, including proper nutrition, sleep, exercise, arousal and alertness, reflexes, and satiation of needs, including eating, drinking, eliminating, and safety.

One area of great concern is the lack of physical activity by children. Nearly half of young people aged 12 to 21 years do not regularly engage in vigorous physical activity. This lack of activity leads to obesity and other significant complications, including increased risks for insulin resistance and type 2 diabetes mellitus; joint problems and musculoskeletal discomfort; risk for asthma and sleep apnea; high blood pressure and high cholesterol; fatty liver disease; gallstones; gastroesophageal reflux (ie, heartburn); fertility problems; and psychosocial consequences in the form of a negative self-image, poor self-esteem, social discrimination, emotional and behavioral problems, and depression.[7,8] Many prevention programs are aimed at increasing physical activity, monitoring nutrition habits, and dealing with psychosocial issues.[9]

Common Health Problems of Infants and Young Children

Common childhood problems include acute health problems, chronic illness, and developmental or behavioral problems. Acute health problems may present as excessive crying, sleep disorders, skin problems, ear infections, fever, and trauma. More chronic problems include allergies, asthma, chronic pain, problems with urination and constipation, and seizures. Developmental problems include developmental delays, attention-deficit/hyperactivity disorders, or other behavioral problems. In addition, structural problems related to the body systems can be observed when screening the child for normal growth and development.

Excessive Crying

Crying is an infant's means of communicating boredom or loneliness; discomfort from a dirty diaper; excessive gas; teething; or feeling cold, hungry, or thirsty. Excessive crying in an infant younger than 6 months of age may indicate that the infant has colic, suggesting possible acute abdominal pain, illness, infection, or other problem.[10] If the crying persists, a referral should be made to the child's physician for examination to determine whether the child has a pathology or dietary intolerance that needs to be addressed.[10]

Sleep Disorders

Sleep disorders, such as difficulty falling asleep or problems staying awake, are generally noted when the child reaches school age, when 9 hours of sleep is recommended for elementary schoolchildren. A sizeable proportion of elementary schoolchildren sleep less than the recommended 9 hours.[11] Although few pathologies are associated with pediatric sleep disorders, behavioral strategies may be recommended to help the parents deal with their child's sleeping problems. These sleep disorders are generally acute, but they can become chronic if they are not properly addressed. A referral to a child psychologist or the child's physician can provide the parents with additional resources for resolving these problems.

Fevers

Fevers are common in children and should be addressed by the child's pediatrician. However, fevers do not always necessitate a doctor visit. According to Bergman,[12] criteria for an office visit include (1) any feverish child under the age of 3 months, (2) fever accompanied by significant localized pain (headache, chest, throat, or abdominal pain) or dysfunction (persistent vomiting, bloody diarrhea, limping, or altered state of consciousness), (3) fever lasting more than 4 days unexplained by other illness, or (4) a child who does not meet the above criteria but whose parents are concerned.

Otitis Media

Otitis media, an infection that leads to inflammation behind the eardrum, is the second most common disease of childhood and the most common cause for childhood visits to a physician's office.[13] Over 33% of children have 6 or more episodes of acute otitis media by the age of 7 years.[13] A child with otitis media may be irritable, cry or whine, have a reduced appetite, and have some difficulty sleeping. Fever is not always necessary for the diagnosis. Whereas an older child may complain that the ear hurts, an infant may simply rub or tug at the auricle or dig a finger into the auditory meatus as an indication of discomfort. In older children, chronic otitis media may lead to hearing loss; complaints of ear stuffiness may be an indicator of the infection.[14] Pain referred to the temporomandibular joint could also be an indicator of otitis media in the older child.[14] Children with these symptoms should be referred to a pediatrician for a definitive medical diagnosis.

Urinary Tract Infections

Urinary tract infections are common in children, often accompanied by fever in infants 0 to 23 months of age. Clinical manifestations of urinary tract infections include vomiting, diarrhea, irritability, and poor feeding. In addition, the urine may smell foul. Children with these signs and symptoms should see their doctor for urinalysis to confirm the diagnosis.[15]

Skin Pathology

Skin problems may be noted during visual inspection of an infant or child. *Dermatitis* (inflammation of the skin) may be caused by irritants, such as diapers or infection; however, certain types are caused by a combination of genetic and environmental factors.[16] Often, this skin condition presents with edematous patches and plaques on the face, the trunk, and extremities. Similarly, *impetigo* (characterized by small infectious vesicles on the skin's surface) presents with redness and skin irregularities.[16,17] *Hemangiomas* (tumors that may be superficial or deep) are similarly red but are generally singular and are often raised from the skin's surface. Approximately 50% of these lesions resolve by age 9.[16,17] Warts are generally yellowish to brownish and are commonly seen on the hands. *Tinea capitis* (a scalp infection) appears as round or irregular patches of broken hairs on the scalp. Finally, *tinea corporis* (an infection on the body) presents as scaly, reddened patches with raised borders. Because many of these skin problems are infectious and all are treatable, immediate referral should be made to the physician for proper management.

Trauma (Accidental and Intentional)

Trauma during childhood can result from a variety of accidents, from minor falls and burns to near drownings or motor vehicle injuries. It is important to know whether injuries are from accidents or are intentionally inflicted. Caregiver risk factors suggesting abuse include the following[18]:

- The explanation of the injury is not plausible.
- The explanations are inconsistent or change.
- The seriousness of the child's condition is understated.
- There is a delay in obtaining treatment.
- The caregiver cannot be located.
- The male caregiver is not the child's father.
- There is a history of domestic abuse.
- There is a history of substance abuse.

If the clinician suspects any of these risk factors, contact must be made with the local child protection services.

The most common manifestation of abuse is bruises that are not on prominent surfaces over bones. Also, nonmobile infants rarely inflict wounds on themselves. Most suspect fractures are caused by twisting or pulling an extremity, causing damage to the *metaphysis* (the growing part of the long bone).[18] Perhaps the most difficult type of abuse to understand is *Munchausen by proxy syndrome (MBPS)*, a situation in which the parent, usually the mother, fabricates information about the child's health and intentionally makes the child ill. This psychological disturbance of the parent can prove lethal. Victims of MBPS need immediate medical attention because these children are at an increased risk of death or dangerous injury.[19] Clinicians should collect information about witnesses to any traumatic event, any history of previous injuries, and past medical records. Suspected child abuse must be reported to the local authorities. A helpful website listing contact information is the Childhelp USA National Child Abuse Hotline at http://www.childhelpusa.org/.

Allergies

It is estimated that over 20% of children have seasonal allergies that present with nasal congestion, sneezing, and *rhinorrhea* (a discharge from the nasal mucous membrane).[20] Chronic congestion can lead to mouth breathing. Another common sign is constant rubbing of the nose in an upward direction. Finally, edematous or swollen eyes lead to suspicion that the child is having an allergic reaction to a seasonal *allergen* (agent causing the allergic reaction). These allergic reactions are commonly caused by the pollen from nonflowering, wind-pollinated plants.[20]

Food allergies are more common in younger children and often decrease in prevalence once children reach the age of 4 (Table 6-1). In children, common allergy-provoking foods include cow's milk protein, hen's egg white, wheat, soybean or soybean products, codfish, peanuts, seafood, citrus fruit, and chocolate.[20] The oral allergy syndrome response is characterized by a red, itchy mouth and throat after eating the food. More generalized responses following the consumption of a large serving include rashes, flushing, abdominal pain, vomiting, diarrhea, and heart palpitations.[20] Although an antihistamine is the most effective treatment for suspected allergic reactions, the physician should be contacted whenever allergic reactions are a concern. It is important that the parent record a description of the child's symptoms; the amount of time elapsed between ingestion and the initiation of symptoms; the type, quantity, and processing of food eaten (cooked,

Table 6-1. Common Food Allergies of Children	
• Cow's milk protein • Hen's egg white • Wheat • Soybean or soybean products • Codfish	• Peanuts • Seafood (fish/shellfish/mollusks/crustaceans) • Citrus fruit • Chocolate

raw, processed with other foods); and the frequency of the allergic reaction. Because exercise may induce this allergic reaction, this should also be noted.[21]

Asthma

Asthma is a common pediatric condition that limits sports participation, causes sleep problems, leads to absences from school due to health care issues, and potentially reduces growth and development.[22,23] Asthma further affects the child's family in terms of recreational opportunities, as well as economic costs of dealing with this chronic illness. Whenever asthma is suspected, an immediate medical referral should be made to confirm the diagnosis. Once the diagnosis is established, caretakers should eliminate asthma triggers, including airborne allergens; upper respiratory tract infections; smoke and other lung irritants; cold, dry air; and various types of medications (aspirin and other nonsteroidal anti-inflammatory drugs and beta-blockers) while encouraging "normal" breathing and normal physical activity.[21-24] Swimming improves cardiorespiratory fitness in children with asthma and is asthmogenic (less likely to induce asthma) than other forms of exercise.[25] Exercise training has health-related benefits and improves the quality of life of children with asthma.

Chronic Pain

Chronic pain can be a potent stressor to children and family members. Certain pains are expected, such as teething pain accompanying tooth eruption in early childhood. "Growing pains" are generally experienced in the legs of young children during growth spurts, often between the ages of 3 and 10 years.[26] The complaints of pain are generally in the evening, and both legs are affected, although pains rarely awaken the child during sleep and are often resolved by morning. Massaging the affected area can effectively reduce the pain. Recurrent abdominal pain affects up to 11% of children and may be caused by a variety of factors.[27] Although food allergies are often suspected, recurrent abdominal pain may be caused by irritable bowel syndrome, gastroesophageal reflux, or infection.[27] In some instances, abdominal pain is associated with psychological distress. Because pain is a subjective sensation, it is important to tell parents that the pain should not be overemphasized. Also, parents should encourage the child's normal engagement in daily activities if no organic cause is determined.

Headaches

Headaches can be a concern if they are recurrent. Although recurrent headaches could suggest intracranial disease, migraine headaches can occur in childhood and can be treated with over-the-counter medications. Fatigue, exercise, or long periods in the sun can trigger headaches, as can nuts, caffeine (including cola drinks), and spiced meats.[28] Because there are many etiologies of headaches, it is important to have recurrent headaches examined by a physician. According to recent research, relaxation training and thermal biofeedback may be effective treatments for pediatric headache, reducing both the severity and frequency of headaches.[28] Chest pain is less common and can generally be attributed to a musculoskeletal problem, such as overuse from coughing or novel physical activity. Heartburn or esophageal pain can also occur in children and may be related to digestive problems. If it persists, a medical referral is appropriate.

Enuresis and Constipation

Approximately 15% to 20% of first graders have nocturnal *enuresis* (urinary incontinence)[29] and up to 2% have *encopresis* (involuntary defecation),[30] causing considerable concern to parents. Nearly 90% of these cases resolve over time; however, if these problems are not dealt with in a timely manner, they may cause subsequent maladaptive behaviors. A variety of medical and behavioral programs offer parents and their children considerable relief.[29,30]

Seizures

Seizures accompany high fevers in 2% to 5% of all young children. Approximately 50% of these infants younger than 12 months have a second seizure, indicative of epilepsy.[31,32] Seizures may present in a variety of ways but often last less than 5 minutes and cease on their own. Any seizure-like activity, such as a loss of consciousness, involuntary movements, or total body convulsions, should be reported to the child's physician. Questions that can help with the child's diagnosis include[32]:

- Was any warning noted before the spell? If so, what kind of warning occurred?
- What did the child do before, during, and after the spell?
- How long did the spell last?
- Was this the first spell? If not, how frequently do the spells occur?
- Did anything precede or precipitate the spells?

Developmental Delays

Health care professionals play a key role in the detection of children with developmental delays. Approximately 13% of children between birth and 21 years of age receive special educational services for developmental disabilities, ranging from cognitive delays to physical impairments.[33] Causes of developmental delay include emotional disturbance, specific learning disabilities, health impairments, visual impairments, traumatic brain injury, mental retardation, speech or language impairment, physical impairment, autism, hearing impairment, and/or delays in 2 or more areas of physical development, cognitive development, communication development, social or emotional development, or adaptive development.[33] A thorough examination by the physical therapist is important to help establish the degree of impairment limiting function. Pervasive developmental disorders (PDDs) are becoming more prevalent in the United States.[34] PDDs include *autism* (a condition associated with problems with social interaction, pretend play, and communication), *Asperger's syndrome* (a condition presenting with difficulties in social interaction and communication, but typically with average or above average intelligence), *childhood disintegrative disorder* (a condition that presents between ages 2 and 10 years and results in deteriorating functional abilities over time), *Rett's syndrome* (a genetic condition affecting development and motor function), and *pervasive developmental disorder not otherwise specified* (sometimes referred to as a milder form of autism).[34] According to the National Center on Birth Defects and Developmental Disabilities, an average of 1 in 110 children have autism.[35] PDDs are characterized by severe or pervasive impairment in social interaction skills, communication skills, or the presence of stereotyped behavior, interests, and activities generally presenting by age 3 years.[34] Children presenting with signs and symptoms indicating any of these disorders should have a complete examination by a psychologist to determine causality and diagnosis.

Attention-Deficit/Hyperactivity Disorder

According to the National Institute of Mental Health, up to 5% of all American children have attention-deficit/hyperactivity disorder (ADHD). This disorder presents with features of inattention, hyperactivity (or the inability to sit still), and impulsivity or uncontrolled interruptions of others.[36] Specific *Diagnostic and Statistical Manual of Mental Disorders, Fifth Edition* criteria for ADHD are listed at the following website: http://www.cdc.gov/ncbddd/adhd/diagnosis.html. These characteristics label people with a persistent pattern of inattention and/or hyperactivity-impulsivity that interferes with functioning or development as having ADHD if these behaviors present before age 12, persists across different environments (eg, school and home), and is not associated with another mental condition, such as anxiety disorder or schizophrenia.

Other Behavioral Problems

Other problems influencing a child's growth and development include a poor appetite, shyness or aggression, and spoiled behavior. These behaviors may be transitory but need to be recognized and discussed with parents. Pediatricians and psychologists are best trained to deal with these issues and can provide guidance as needed.

Obesity in Childhood

BMI should decrease during the preschool years, then increase into adulthood.[37] Recently, however, BMI has been increasing throughout childhood for individuals living in the United States. The percentage of children and adolescents who are defined as overweight has more than doubled since the early 1970s, with approximately 15% of children and adolescents being overweight.[37] Obese children and adolescents are more likely to become obese adults. Experts agree that weight management requires a combined approach of a sensible diet and regular exercise for weight loss. Before initiating a weight loss program for children with obesity, it is essential to contact the child's physician and a nutritionist to ensure a safe and enduring program for lifestyle changes that will safely manage the child's weight problem.[37] According to researchers at the Center for Human Nutrition, Johns Hopkins Bloomberg School of Public Health[38]:

> Most prevention programs include at least one of the following components: dietary changes, physical activity, behavior and social modifications, and family participation. School-based prevention programs may also include elements related to the school environment and personnel. Primary prevention programs cannot usually restrict caloric intake but may effectively reduce the energy intake by reducing the energy density of foods, increasing offering of fresh fruits and vegetables, using low-calorie versions of products, and reducing offering of energy-dense food items. Physical activity interventions have recently focused more on reducing inactive time, particularly sedentary behaviors such as computer use and television viewing.

Health care professionals should work collaboratively with others in the community to ensure that physical activity is integrated into all prevention programs for childhood obesity. The Centers for Disease Control and Prevention provides valuable resources for family education and evidence-based strategies for helping health care professionals manage childhood obesity at http://www.cdc.gov/obesity/childhood/solutions.html.

Anorexia and Bulimia

Other weight problems, particularly during adolescence, include *anorexia* and *bulimia*. Individuals with anorexia starve themselves because they suffer from a distorted self-image of being overweight when they may be grossly underweight. Likewise, individuals who engage in binge eating following by self-induced vomiting (referred to as bulimia) are equally at risk for poor health from lack of proper nutrition. Up to 7% of American females suffer from either disorder at some time during their lives.[39] Characteristics of these disorders include the following[39]:

- Binge eating repeatedly with a feeling that they cannot stop or control their eating, at least twice a week for the past 3 months
- Compensating for the overeating by using laxatives, fasting, exercising to exhaustion, or making themselves vomit at least twice a week for the last 3 months
- Critically judging their weight and body shape

Chemical imbalances from anorexia and bulimia can lead to heart arrhythmias and protein deficiencies.[39] If either of these 2 conditions is suspected, a physician or psychological referral should be made.

Factors Influencing Growth and Development in Children Aged 7 to 21 Years

During preadolescent and adolescent years, lifestyle behaviors, including limited physical activity, poor nutrition, poor stress management, exposure to infective agents, sun exposure, substance abuse, delinquency, psychological disorders, sports-related injuries, sexually transmitted diseases (STDs), and even homicide, pose significant health risks. Many of the leading causes of morbidity and mortality are interrelated, according to the Youth Risk Behavior Surveillance System (YRBSS),[40] which monitors priority health-risk behaviors contributing to unintentional injuries and violence, substance abuse, unintended pregnancy, STDs, and obesity. Additional risks are related to riding with a driver who had been drinking alcohol. Nearly one-third of students do not participate in sufficient vigorous physical activity. Similarly, one-third of students in this age group watch television more than 3 hours per day on an average school day, providing evidence of sedentary behavior contributing to health risks. Although excess body fat is a problem for certain students, taking laxatives and vomiting contributed to weight loss or was used as a strategy to prevent weight gain. Other health risks include significant underage alcohol use, cocaine use, desire to commit suicide, and cigarette use. Those engaged in physical activity are at increased risk of injuries if they are not wearing the appropriate protective gear. Chapter 12 offers preventive care for common sports injuries in this population.

Special Considerations for Screening Children and Youth

Screening preadolescents and adolescents may involve parents or may be performed in the absence of other adults. It is important to ask the youth about possible risk behaviors (sexual activity, substance abuse, psychological concerns, and physical inactivity) as well as growth pains that may accompany rapid growth spurts. Preadolescents and adolescents are particularly concerned about their body image and self-concept. Questions should address potential eating disorders, depression, or suicidal thinking. Using indirect statements, such as citing statistics related to risk

Table 6-2. Activity Profile for Children and Youth

Child's name: ____________ Grade: ____________ School: ____________

Please answer these questions based on behavior during a typical week:

1. How many hours each day do you watch television?
   - 0 minutes per day; I don't watch TV ____
   - 30 minutes to 1 hour per day (1 to 2 TV shows) ____
   - 1 to 2 hours per day (3 to 4 TV shows) ____
   - More than 2 hours per day ____
2. How much time do you spend exercising outdoors at school and at home?
   - 0 minutes per day ____
   - 30 minutes to 1 hour per day ____
   - 1 to 2 hours per day ____
   - More than 2 hours per day ____
3. How much time do you spend reading books, newspapers, or magazines at school and at home?
   - 0 minutes per day; I don't read at home ____
   - 30 minutes to 1 hour per day ____
   - 1 to 2 hours per day ____
   - More than 2 hours per day ____
4. How many servings of each food group do you eat on a typical day? Circle the answer.

Bread and cereal	1	2	3	4	5	6
Milk and cheese	1	2	3	4	5	6
Fruit and vegetables	1	2	3	4	5	6
Meat, chicken, fish, beans	1	2	3	4	5	6

WHAT ARE YOUR FAVORITE PHYSICAL ACTIVITIES? ____________

____

____

behaviors, may help the youth share more confidential information. Open questions could include the following: "How would you describe your extracurricular activities?" "How would you describe your general health?" "Have you had any loss of interest in favorite activities?" "What are your eating habits?" "What are your exercise habits?" and "Do you have a tendency to be worried or anxious?" The Activity Profile for Children and Youth is a short survey that can identify levels of physical activity, nutritional habits, and sedentary behaviors (Table 6-2).

A more comprehensive screening tool includes information about the teenager's medical history (childhood infections and illnesses; prior hospitalizations and surgery; significant injuries; disabilities; medications, including prescription medications, over-the-counter medications, complementary or alternative medications, vitamins, and nutritional supplements; allergies; immunization history; prior developmental history, and mental health history), family history, health status and age of family members, school information, job/career information, family, significant physical or mental illnesses in the family, and a review of systems.

An interview should focus on specific areas of concern for appropriate referral, as needed.[40] It is helpful to link high-risk behaviors related to physical health concerns, family dysfunction, sexual problems, substance abuse, emotional dysfunction, school, and social dysfunction. Early identification of potential problems provides an opportunity to help the youth make healthier lifestyle choices with support and knowledge. For positive findings in any areas of concern, clinicians should refer to the appropriate health care professional.

Fitness During Childhood

The average American child watches 1480 minutes of television per week, and studies have proven that parents rather than children choose television for a leisure time activity.[41] Reasons given by parents for using the television as a planned activity include:

- Providing the parent freedom from entertaining the child
- Preventing the child from becoming bored
- Socializing in regard to popular television shows
- Watching television is not considered harmful

The drawbacks of watching so much television are self-evident. The child develops a sedentary lifestyle that can lead to obesity. Furthermore, watching television has been shown to slow the development of cognitive skills, especially imagination, and can lead to violent and aggressive behavior. Research shows that children 5 years and younger who watch television "spend less time in creative play and less time interacting with parents or siblings."[42] Television watching should be avoided for children under the age of 2 years and restricted for older children, allowing time for alternative games and activities, especially physical exercise.[43]

Assessing Fitness in Children

Before recommending specific physical activities for children, a physical therapist should assess levels of fitness. The President's Challenge: Physical Activity and Fitness Program is a comprehensive program for children aged 6 to 17 years that incorporates activities designed to improve physical activity and physical fitness.[44] Tests used by this program to determine baseline levels of fitness include curl-ups or partial curl-ups, an endurance run for cardiorespiratory endurance, pull-ups and push-ups for upper-body strength, a sit-and-reach test for flexibility, and BMI for body composition. Many educational settings use The President's Challenge: Physical Activity and Fitness Program to address fitness needs of children and adults; nonetheless, children and youth are still prone to obesity and other health risks due to a predominantly sedentary lifestyle. The website for the President's Challenge (https://www.presidentschallenge.org/tools-resources/index.shtml) offers a wide range of tools and resources for encouraging fitness, healthy nutrition, and adaptive activities for all ages and ability levels.

Exercise for Children and Youth

Physical activity produces overall physical, psychological, and social benefits for children and youth. Inactive children are likely to become inactive adults, so physical therapists need to encourage physical activity in children and youth as physiological buffers to illness. As with adults, physical activity can improve fitness in children and youth by controlling weight, reducing blood pressure, raising high-density lipoprotein (HDL; "good") cholesterol, reducing the risk of diabetes and some kinds of cancer, and improving in many areas of psychological well-being, including gaining more self-confidence and higher self-esteem.[45]

The American Heart Association recommends that all children aged 2 years and older should participate in at least 60 minutes of enjoyable, moderate-to-vigorous physical activity every day.[45] Sufficient exercise for children with reduced endurance can be achieved by providing two 15-minute periods or three 10-minute periods in which they can engage in vigorous activities appropriate to their age, sex, and stage of physical and emotional development. Health care professionals need to play a significant role in the development and implementation of educational and physical activity programs that promote physical activity and behavior-change skills that reduce health risks posed by inactivity. Strategies for implementing the policies, programs, and initiatives for promoting physical activities in communities are outlined at the Let's Move website at http://www.letsmove.gov/.

Before any vigorous physical activity program is initiated, ask the physician to conduct a comprehensive physical to ensure that the child is not at increased risk for cardiopulmonary, neuromuscular, musculoskeletal, or other impairments from engaging in increased physical activity. Physical therapists are trained to modify exercise prescription based on potential pathological conditions and can decrease the intensity, duration, or frequency of exercises to meet the individual needs of the child or youth. Chapter 17 goes into greater detail about developing health and fitness programs that best suit the needs of children with developmental disabilities. This chapter will focus on children without physical impairments restricting normal physical activity.

Suggested Physical Activities for Children and Youth

Certain physical activities can be suggested for each age group based on the normal physical and psychosocial development of children as they mature. Although individual differences might warrant exploring other options, it is important to offer a variety of activities that are age appropriate.

Physical Activities for Children Aged 2 to 3 Years

Young children are just learning to run, jump, and catch a ball, so competitive sports are inappropriate at this level. Physical activity offering variety and minimal structure will afford young children an opportunity to explore their bodies and their environment. Children tend to be more egocentric at this age and may not understand the concept of performing as part of a team. Activities that will most likely provide the appropriate physical activity include unstructured playtime with other children, running and walking in a yard or playground, swinging or sliding on a child-sized playground set, water play, toddler gymnastics classes, and tumbling. At this age, all physical activity should be closely supervised and provided on soft play surfaces.

Physical Activities for Children Aged 4 to 6 Years

As children mature to elementary school age, they are capable of higher-level balance and coordination activities. They also are capable of sharing toys, such as a ball, and engaging in social activities with other children. Children aged 4 to 6 years enjoy dancing, playing games like hopscotch or tag, jumping rope, playing catch with a lightweight ball, and riding a tricycle or a bike with training wheels.

Physical Activities for Children Aged 7 to 10 Years

Children who are 7 years and older are capable of understanding the concepts of team sports and are more cautious about safety issues. Sports activities popular with children in this age group include baseball, gymnastics, soccer, swimming, and tennis.

Physical Activities for Children Aged 10 Years and Older

As children reach adolescence and mature into adult-sized physiques, more demanding physical activity is allowable; however, precautions are needed to avoid overstressing developing musculoskeletal structures. Popular physical activities for children and youth who are 10 years and older include biking, aerobic exercise and strength training, hiking, organized team sports, rowing, running and track and field events, and softball.

Older children may be interested in prescribed exercise programs to increase health-related fitness and sports-related fitness. Special precautions should be applied to exercise prescriptions designed for children. Children and youth may experience a higher incidence of overuse injuries or damage to the epiphyseal growth plates of bones if exercise is too strenuous.[45] Children must be careful when participating in activities that involve sudden, forceful external rotation of the ankle and foot. This kind of movement, especially in preadolescent children, can result in rotational injuries of the distal tibial growth plate.[45] Injury to the anterior cruciate ligament is one of the most common sports-related injuries of the knee, as are forearm fractures.[45] Children and youth should be advised to wear protective athletic gear and to avoid overuse injuries when participating in any types of sports activities. In addition, preparticipation physical examinations (PPPEs) should include comprehensive screenings of all body systems to reveal potential risks related to the musculoskeletal and cardiopulmonary systems. In one study at the Mayo Clinic, 2739 high-school athletes who had PPPEs performed at the clinic most commonly failed due muscle and bone problems.[46] Poorly healed injuries and joints unprepared for certain types of movement usually caused such disqualifications. Heart and vision problems were the next most common causes of disqualification.[46]

Exercise Prescription for Children

When prescribing exercise for children and youth, it is important to recognize that children do not have the same anaerobic capacity as adults. The ability to perform anaerobic or high-intensity exercise for a short duration increases with age.[47] Likewise, blood lactate levels at maximal exercise also increase with age, possibly secondary to increases in energy stores, muscle mass, and improved neuromuscular coordination.[47] One study demonstrated a 10% to 15% increase in anaerobic power in 10- and 11-year-old boys engaged in a 9-week interval training program.[47] Training children requires knowledge of exercise physiology, as well as familiarity with the fitness training principles, including the principles of individuality, overload, periodization, reversibility, progression, adaptation, and recovery. According to the American Academy of Sports Medicine, "All youth strength training programs must be closely supervised by knowledgeable instructors who understand the uniqueness of children and have a sound comprehension of strength training principles and safety guidelines (eg, proper spotting procedures)."[48]

Appropriate exercise prescription for children and youth requires minor modifications to standard exercise regimens to ensure that the growing child is not overstressed. Motor control, including balance and postural skills, enables children to begin strength training by 7 years of age, depending on the child's health status.[49]

Strength training offers many benefits for children and youth, including decreasing the risk of osteoporosis, strengthening ligaments and tendons, preparing soft tissues for flexibility and force production, and improving motor fitness skills, such as jumping and sprinting, which are often required in sports performance. However, it is important to distinguish strength training from weight lifting and power lifting. Strength training refers to a systematic and progressive program of exercises designed to increase an individual's ability to exert or resist force. Professional organizations have published position standards on prepubescent strength training and offer the following guidelines and principles[50]:

- The program should include at least one exercise for all major muscle groups.
- The child should learn movements without weight first.
- The program should be done on nonconsecutive days.
- The child should perform 1 to 3 sets of each exercise. Each set should include 6 to 15 repetitions.
- Weights for each child should be set within developmentally appropriate boundaries.
- Once a child has mastered an exercise with weight, additional weight can be added in 5% increments (typically 1 to 5 pounds) every 7 to 10 days.

> Strength training should be one part of a well-rounded fitness program that also includes endurance, flexibility, and agility exercises. Properly designed and competently supervised youth strength training programs may not only increase the muscular strength of children and adolescents, but may also enhance motor fitness skills and sports performance. Preliminary evidence suggests that youth strength training may also decrease the incidence of some sports injuries by increasing the strength of tendons, ligaments, and bone. During adolescence, training-induced strength gains may be associated with increases in muscle size, but this is unlikely to happen in prepubescent children, who lack adequate levels of muscle-building hormones. Although the issue of childhood obesity is complex, youth strength training programs may also play an important role in effective weight-loss strategies.[50]

Flexibility Exercises for Young Athletes

Although maintaining general fitness can be accomplished through a regular exercise program, most children and youth engage in sports activity to maintain fitness. To ensure that young athletes optimally benefit from sports activities, flexibility exercise can be helpful in preventing injury during competition. "Athletes must do each one of the exercises carefully; speed is not important."[51] Once the exercise routine is learned, the entire program should take no longer than 10 minutes. It also is important to warm up before doing any of these exercises. Good examples of warm-up activities are slowly running in place and walking for a few minutes.

Summary

Health care professionals play a key role in the health, fitness, and wellness of children with impairments, functional limitations, and disabilities but must recognize how important it is to reach out to children and youth who are at risk for illness and potentially life-threatening injury. As part of the health care team, each professional must communicate effectively with the obstetrician and gynecologist of pregnant women; the pediatrician or family physician regarding risk factors for children and youth; other professionals who support health, fitness, and wellness; and, most importantly, the family. Collaboration on all fronts offers the best opportunity for managing potential problems that threaten the health, fitness, and wellness of infants, children, and youth.

References

1. APGAR. National Institutes of Health. http://www.nlm.nih.gov/medlineplus/ency/article/003402.htm. Accessed May 30, 2013.
2. Frankenburg WK, Dobbs JB. *Denver Developmental Screening Test II-Screening Manual.* Denver, CO: Denver Developmental Materials; 1990.
3. Brachlow A, Jordan AE, Tervo R. Developmental screenings in rural settings: a comparison of the child development review and the Denver II Developmental Screening Test. *J Rural Health.* 2001;17(3):156-159.
4. Body mass index. Centers for Disease Control and Prevention. http://www.cdc.gov/nccdphp/dnpa/bmi/bmi-for-age.htm. Accessed May 30, 2013.
5. Tanner JM. Normal growth and techniques of growth assessment. *Clin Endocrinol Metab.* 1986;15(3):411-451.
6. Odegard RA, Vatten LJ, Nilsen ST, Salvesen KA, Austgulen R. Preeclampsia and fetal growth. *Obstet Gynecol.* 2000;96(6):950-955.
7. Renders CM, Seidell JC, van Mechelen W, Hirasing RA. Overweight and obesity in children and adolescents and preventative measures. *Ned Tijdschr Geneeskd.* 2004;48(42):2066-2670.
8. Basics about childhood obesity. Centers for Disease Control and Prevention. http://www.cdc.gov/obesity/childhood/basics.html. Accessed May 30, 2013.
9. Caballero B. Obesity prevention in children: opportunities and challenges. *Int J Obes Relat Metab Disord.* 2004;28 Suppl 3:S90-S95.
10. Crying–excessive (0-6 months). MedlinePlus. http://www.nlm.nih.gov/medlineplus/ency/article/003023.htm. Accessed May 30, 2013.
11. Spilsbury JC, Storfer-Isser A, Drotar D, et al. Sleep behavior in an urban US sample of school-aged children. *Arch Pediatr Adolesc Med.* 2004;158(10):988-994.
12. Bergman A. *Twenty Common Problems in Pediatrics.* St. Louis, MO: McGraw-Hill; 1990.
13. Otitis media. Medscape. http://emedicine.medscape.com/article/994656-overview. Accessed May 30, 2013.
14. Ear infections in children. National Institute on Deafness and Other Communication Disorders. https://www.nidcd.nih.gov/health/hearing/Pages/earinfections.aspx. Accessed May 30, 2013.
15. Chang SL, Shortliffe LD. Pediatric urinary tract infections. *Pediatr Clin North Am.* 2006;53(3):379-400.
16. Sidbury R. What's new in pediatric dermatology: update for the pediatrician. *Curr Opin Pediatr.* 2004;16(4):410-414.
17. Dermatology and skin. Johns Hopkins Children's Center. http://www.hopkinschildrens.org/pediatric-skin-disorders.aspx. Accepted May 30, 2013.
18. Oral R, Blum KL, Johnson C. Fractures in young children: are physicians in the emergency department and orthopedic clinics adequately screening for possible abuse? *Pediatr Emerg Care.* 2003;19(3):148-153.
19. Munchausen syndrome by proxy. MedlinePlus. http://www.nlm.nih.gov/medlineplus/ency/article/001555.htm. Accessed May 20, 2014.
20. Spergel JM, Beausoleil JL, Fiedler JM, et al. Correlation of initial food reactions to observed reactions on challenges. *Ann Allergy Asthma Immunol.* 2004;92(2):217-224.
21. Cabana MD, Slish KK, Lewis TC, et al. Parental management of asthma triggers within a child's environment. *J Allergy Clin Immunol.* 2004;114(2):352-357.
22. Satta A. Exercise training in asthma. *J Sports Med Phys Fitness.* 2000;40(4):277-283.
23. Mellon M, Parasuraman B. Pediatric asthma: improving management to reduce cost of care. *JMCP.* 2004;10(2):130-141.
24. Asthma. Medscape. http://www.emedicine.com/ped/topic152.htm. Accessed May 30, 2013.
25. Rosimini C. Benefits of swim training for children and adolescents with asthma. *J Am Assoc Nurse Pract.* 2003;15(6):247-252.
26. Evans AM, Scutter SD. Prevalence of "growing pains" in young children. *J Pediatr.* 2004;145(2):255-258.
27. Nygaard EA, Stordal K, Bentsen BS. Recurrent abdominal pain in children revisited: irritable bowel syndrome and psychosomatic aspects: a prospective study. *Scand J Gastroenterol.* 2004;39(10):938-940.
28. Powers SW, Mitchell MJ, Byars KC, et al. A pilot study of one-session biofeedback training in pediatric headache. *Neurology.* 2001;56:133.
29. Skoog S. How to evaluate and treat pediatric enuresis: behavioral modification, drug therapy are keys to controlling daytime, nighttime wetting. *Urology Times.* http://www.urologytimes.com/urologytimes/article/articleDetail.jsp?id=92007&&pageID=2. Accessed May 30, 2013.
30. Von Gontard A, Hollmann E. Comorbidity of functional urinary incontinence and encopresis: somatic and behavioral associations. *J Urol.* 2004;171(6 Pt 2):2644-2647.
31. Febrile seizures fact sheet. National Institute of Neurological Disorders and Stroke. http://www.ninds.nih.gov/disorders/febrile_seizures/detail_febrile_seizures.htm. Accessed May 20, 2014.
32. Yamashiroya VK. Febrile seizures. Case Based Pediatrics for Medical Students and Residents. Department of Pediatrics, University of Hawaii John A. Burns School of Medicine. http://www.hawaii.edu/medicine/pediatrics/pedtext/s18c03.html. Accessed May 20, 2014.

33. Students with disabilities. National Center for Education Statistics. http://nces.ed.gov/fastfacts/display.asp?id=64. Accessed May 30, 2013.
34. Pervasive developmental disorders. WebMD. http://www.webmd.com/brain/autism/development-disorder. Accessed May 30, 2013.
35. How many children have autism? Centers for Disease Control and Prevention. http://www.cdc.gov/ncbddd/features/counting-autism.html. Accessed May 30, 2013.
36. Attention Deficit Hyperactivity Disorder (ADHD). National Institutes of Mental Health. http://www.nimh.nih.gov/health/publications/attention-deficit-hyperactivity-disorder/what-is-attention-deficit-hyperactivity-disorder.shtml. Accessed May 30, 2013.
37. Prevention and treatment of childhood overweight and obesity. American Academy of Pediatrics. http://www2.aap.org/obesity/about.html. Accessed May 30, 2013.
38. Perspectives on childhood obesity prevention: recommendations from Public Health Research and Practice. Bloomberg School of Public Health. http://www.jhsph.edu/research/centers-and-institutes/johns-hopkins-center-for-a-livable-future/_pdf/research/clf_reports/childhoodobesity.pdf. Accessed May 30, 2013.
39. Norqvist C. What is anorexia nervosa? What is bulimia nervosa? Medical News Today. http://www.medicalnewstoday.com/articles/105102.php. Accessed May 30, 2013.
40. Youth Risk Behavior Surveillance System (YRBSS). Centers for Disease Control and Prevention. http://www.cdc.gov/healthyyouth/yrbs/. Accessed May 30, 2013.
41. Television watching statistics. Statistics Brain. http://www.statisticbrain.com/television-watching-statistics/. Accessed May 30, 2013.
42. Vandewater EA, Bickham DS, Lee JH. Time well spent? Relating television use to children's free-time activities. *Pediatrics*. 2006;117(2):e181-e191.
43. Media use by children younger than 2 years. American Academy of Pediatrics. *Pediatrics*. 2011;128(5)1040-1045.
44. President's Challenge: Physical Activity and Fitness Program. http://www.presidentschallenge.org/. Accessed May 30, 2013.
45. Ippolito E, Postacchini F, Scola E. Skeletal growth in normal and pathological conditions. *Ital J Orthop Traumatol*. 1983;9(1):115-127.
46. Smith J, Laskowski ER. The pre-participation physical examination: Mayo Clinic experience with 2,739 examinations. *Mayo Clin Proc*. 1998;73(5):419-429.
47. Rotstein A, Dotan R, Bar-Or O, Tenenbaum G. Effect of training on anaerobic threshold, maximal aerobic power and anaerobic performance of preadolescent boys. *Int J Sports Med*. 1986;7(5):281-286.
48. ACSM current statement: youth strength training. American College of Sports Medicine. http://www.acsm.org/docs/current-comments/youthstrengthtraining.pdf. Accessed May 30, 2013.
49. American Academy of Pediatrics. Strength training by children and adolescents. *Pediatrics*. 2008;121(4):835-840.
50. Ashmore A. Strength training guidelines for children–CEU Corner. *American Fitness*. Sept-Oct 2003.
51. Flexibility exercises for young athletes. American Academy of Orthopaedic Surgeons. http://orthoinfo.aaos.org/topic.cfm?topic=A00038. Accessed May 20, 2014.

7

Health, Fitness, and Wellness Issues During Adulthood

Catherine Rush Thompson, PT, PhD, MS

"Every human being is the author of his own health."—Swami Sivananda, *Bliss Divine*

Unique Challenges During Adulthood

The term *adult* suggests both physical maturation and psychosocial transition, from being dependent on others to becoming more self-reliant and responsible for personal behaviors. Although the body is physically mature between ages 21 and 25, the adult's psychosocial dimensions continually develop. Key life skills developing throughout adulthood enable the individual to function independently in the home, in the community, and in the world at large, yet many of the psychosocial skills that enable the individual to function independently in varying contexts are taught early in life. Recognizing these foundational psychosocial skills, health care professionals need a broad perspective for managing the adult client. Independent function in the home, in the workplace, and in leisure activities are all key to physical and mental health; however, interactions with others, including expanding friends and family, play an essential role in wellness.

During adulthood, there are many common characteristics between men and women; however, priorities vary as men and women move from early to late adulthood. The main life tasks that engage men and women are health or physical vigor, relationships with others (a spouse or partner, parents, and/or children), and financial security (property or income). Earlier in life, children dominate priorities, but income and property needed for financial stability and retirement become more important in later life. These priorities suggest key issues for preventive care: health, relationships, and income/property. Health care providers should promote the health of the individual while recognizing the importance of significant relationships and financial stability.

Whereas children and youth deal with adapting to ever-changing physiques, psychologists suggest that individuals progressing through adulthood seek 2 basic needs: (1) intimacy in human relationships (affiliation, social acceptance, or love and belonging) and (2) competence (achievement, generativity, or productivity). Freud felt that the healthy adult has the ability to both love and work.[1] Erikson described the 2 crises of early adulthood in terms of intimacy vs isolation, followed

Thompson CR.
Prevention Practice and Health Promotion: A Health Care Professional's Guide to Health, Fitness, and Wellness, Second Edition (pp 111-126).

by generativity vs stagnation.[2] Psychological health and happiness in adult years depend on how the individual envisions the future and what that individual does to bring about the desired vision. Generativity orients the individual toward the long-term goals in life and the future.

The key tasks of early adulthood include separating from parents, making choices in relationships, and achieving in the realms of education, career, community, and parenthood while accommodating to social demands. As individuals progress into adulthood, they become more conscious of their professional and personal goals, including issues associated with childbearing, career goals, social relationships, and mentoring others in life. Individuals with lower socioeconomic status often must leave school to begin work; they marry and, often, become parents at a younger age than other adults with more financial resources.[3] These additional responsibilities earlier in life can cause additional stresses that make people of low socioeconomic status more vulnerable to stress and illness.[3] Minority populations with certain genetic backgrounds are put at an even greater risk for pathology when living in poverty.

Relationships with close friends or sexual partners serve as buffers against stress or as sources of stress for many individuals. Many intimate relationships in adulthood do not survive adulthood challenges, as evidenced by the divorce rate. The average divorce and annulment rate in 2011 was 3.6 per 1000 total population, according to the Centers for Disease Control and Prevention.[4] "Divorced adults, particularly divorced men, experience early health problems to a much greater extent than married individuals. Premature death rates for divorced men from such causes as cardiovascular disease, hypertension, and strokes double that of married men. The premature death rate from pneumonia is seven times larger for divorced men than for married men...The suicide rate for divorced white men was four times higher than for their married counterparts."[5] The importance of healthy adult relationships cannot be overstated.

Work during adulthood is often a key aspect of an individual's identity. For many people, work is central to their lives for more than economic reasons. Workers who have been laid off or disabled often feel lost, depressed, and empty. According to one study, the indirect cost of illness due to lost wages exceeds the cost of medical services by a large margin.[6] Social characteristics of persons with physical impairments are more important than the medical condition characteristics in predicting whether disability will lead to work loss.[6] Physical therapists can help adult clients reach their full potential by providing needed resources for physical, mental, and psychosocial health through education, fitness programs, and appropriate referrals to needed services, including psychologists and social workers.

The health, fitness, and wellness needs of adults vary between men and women. Both sexes seek intimacy and generativity, but social roles, as well as genetics, lead to substantially different health risks.

Adult Health and Wellness Risks

Adults face health risks that affect all major body systems, including the integumentary, cardiovascular, neuromuscular, and musculoskeletal systems, commonly treated in physical therapy. In addition, risks for developing diabetes, cancer, chronic pain, substance abuse, gastrointestinal problems, migraine headaches, accidents, infections, and sleep disorders increase during the adult years. Many of these conditions are covered in the chapters discussing musculoskeletal, neuromuscular, cardiopulmonary, and other chronic conditions. The health care professional should be familiar with these risk factors to alert individuals to potential threats to health and to inform physicians of controllable factors potentially contributing to chronic illness.

Skin Conditions

Screening for skin conditions often occurs during a comprehensive examination but can be performed by asking questions related to common integumentary problems that arise in adulthood. Although warts, acne, impetigo, and tinea pedis are more common in youths and adolescents, adults often present with chronic skin problems such as dermatitis and psoriasis.[7]

Dermatitis (eczema) is commonly seen as skin inflammation, generalized redness, edema or swelling, and possible oozing, crusting, and scaling when long term.[7] *Contact dermatitis* is often produced by substances contacting the skin and causing toxic or allergic reactions. *Atopic dermatitis* has a genetic component that predisposes the individual to environmental agents or factors that precipitate skin inflammation. Although elimination of precipitating factors alleviates contact dermatitis, it does not ameliorate atopic dermatitis.[7] *Psoriasis* is a common chronic, recurrent skin disease that is characterized by dry, well-circumscribed, silvery, scaling papules and plaques of various sizes.[7] This skin condition often presents in a characteristic pattern on extensor surfaces of elbows and knees, scalp, back, anogenital region, and nails but may also appear on flexor surfaces, the tip of the penis, or the palms.[7] Examiners can ask about possible skin conditions or note skin rashes or irregularities during a physical examination. If an individual reports skin inflammation, itchiness, redness, soreness, or open wounds that fail to heal, medical attention is needed. All suspected skin conditions should be referred to a physician for a medical diagnosis and proper medical treatment.

To prevent skin problems, individuals need proper hydration. According to the Merck Manual,[8] water can be therapeutic as a cleanser and hydrating agent. When the environment has 60% humidity, the skin remains soft and smooth, but when water evaporates and humidity falls below 15% to 20%, the skin can become dry. With less humidity, the stratum corneum (the outermost layer of skin or epidermis) shrinks and cracks, breaking the epidermal barrier and allowing irritants to enter the skin and induce an inflammatory response. Replacement of water will correct this condition if evaporation is prevented. Therefore, dry and scaly skin is treated by soaking the skin in water for 5 minutes and then adding a barrier to evaporation. Oils and ointments prevent evaporation for 8 to 12 hours, so they must be applied once or twice per day. In areas already occluded (axilla), ointments or oils will merely increase retention of water and should not be used.[8]

Maceration (overhydration) can also occur. If sweat is prevented from evaporating (eg, in the axilla or groin), local humidity and hydration of the skin are increased. If humidity increases to 90% to 100%, the number of water molecules absorbed by the stratum corneum increases.[8] The tight lipid junctions between the cells of the stratum corneum are gradually replaced by weak hydrogen bonds; the cells eventually become widely separated, and the epidermal barrier falls apart. This occurs in immersion of the foot, axilla, and the like. The solution is to enhance evaporation of water in these areas by air drying.[8] When health care professionals are working in environments that are especially dry or humid, they can prevent skin problems by keeping the skin optimally hydrated. In addition, offering their clients water frequently, as well as having moisturizing lotions on hand, can help alleviate skin problems associated with reduced hydration.

Skin Cancer

Skin cancer should always be considered as a threat to all adults, especially fair-skinned individuals. Skin cancers, which are usually curable, are the most common type of cancer; most arise in sun-exposed areas of skin. According to the National Cancer Institute, there are more than 76,000 new cases of malignant melanoma (a fatal tumor affecting the skin, mucous membranes, eyes, and the central nervous system) yearly in the United States, causing more than 9000 deaths.[9] More information about skin screening and protection is provided in Chapter 16.

Type 2 Diabetes

Diabetes affects 8.3% of the population in the United States.[10] In 2007, the direct medical costs of diabetes were $116 billion, and the total costs were $174 billion. People with diabetes had average medical expenditures 2.3 times those of people without diabetes.[10] Diabetes is a chronic disease that has no cure but may be preventable. Advanced diabetes is a leading cause of blindness, kidney disease, nontraumatic lower limb amputations, and severe nerve damage.[11] Reported rates of gestational diabetes range from 3% to 10% of pregnancies.[11] Overall, the risk for death among people with diabetes is approximately twice that of people of similar age but without diabetes. Type 2 diabetes is most commonly diagnosed in individuals over the age of 30 years, but it also occurs in children and adolescents. Diabetes has diverse presentations, but both type 1 and type 2 diabetes generally present with *hyperglycemia* (high blood glucose). Symptoms of hyperglycemia include *polyuria* (frequent urination), followed by *polydipsia* (excessive thirst) and weight loss from dehydration. Other clinical manifestations of hyperglycemia include blurred vision, fatigue, and nausea, as well as susceptibility to fungal and bacterial infections.[11] Type 2 diabetes is commonly associated with obesity, especially of the upper body (visceral/abdominal), and often presents after a period of weight gain. Most patients are treated with diet, exercise, and oral drugs, with some patients requiring insulin to control symptomatic hyperglycemia. Type 2 diabetes patients with visceral/abdominal obesity may have normal glucose levels after losing weight.[11]

According to the American Diabetes Association, "people with pre-diabetes can prevent the development of type 2 diabetes by making changes in their diet and increasing their level of physical activity. They may even be able to return their blood glucose levels to the normal range. While some medications may delay the development of diabetes, diet and exercise worked better. Just 30 minutes a day of moderate physical activity, coupled with a 5% to 10% reduction in body weight, produced a 58% reduction in diabetes."[12] The American Diabetes Association has extensive, up-to-date information about diabetes prevention, including diet and nutrition recommendations.

Cancer or Uncontrolled Cellular Proliferation

Cancer or uncontrolled cellular proliferation is malignant by definition but not necessarily fatal. Most cancers are curable if detected in their early stages, and patients can help recognize early signs of possible malignancies. All individuals should be encouraged to perform self-examinations, including skin cancer and breast cancer (both men and women are vulnerable) and have appropriate diagnostic testing to screen for cancers that affect specific populations, such as cervical cancer in adult women and prostate cancer in adult men. Health care professionals should be on the alert for common symptoms that are associated with cancer, including a change in usual bowel habits (constipation, diarrhea, or both); stools that are narrower than usual; blood in or on the stool; general stomach discomfort, such as bloating, fullness, and/or cramps; frequent gas pains; a feeling of incomplete bowel emptying; weight loss with no known reason; and constant fatigue.[13] The most current recommendations for cancer screening by the American Cancer Society can be found at their website: http://www.cancer.gov/cancertopics/screening. This site describes the various types of screening tests and lists those recommended for specific types of cancer. This site also links to additional information about cancer and its management.

Obesity

According to the American Medical Association, obesity is the fastest-growing health problem in the United States. Currently, the US obesity rate is projected to reach 50% by 2030.[14] However, there are great disparities in the prevalence of obesity, with minority populations typically having higher rates of obesity. In general, women and men from lower-income families experience a greater prevalence of obesity than those from higher-income families.[14]

Table 7-1. Preventive Care for Obesity
1. Advocate lifestyles to promote a healthy weight.
2. Alert individuals to the risks of inappropriate weight gain and the benefits of weight loss.
3. Take baseline measures of weight, height, body mass index, waist circumference, and blood pressure to monitor the individual's progress.
4. Assess the current levels of physical activity, eating habits, and readiness to make long-term lifestyle changes.
5. Guide individuals toward weight management programs under the supervision of their physician.
6. Provide ongoing support and encouragement for individuals in weight treatment programs.
7. Recognize behavioral and environmental factors the may contribute to overweight and obesity.
8. Identify health professionals in the community who are critical to the treatment of adults who are obese, including registered dieticians, bariatric surgeons, and mental health professionals.
9. Provide relevant health education materials.
10. Become aware of and share community resources that can assist in the management of overweight and obesity problems.

Health risks associated with obesity include premature death, type 2 diabetes, hyperlipidemia, hypertension, coronary artery disease, stroke, certain types of cancer gastroesophageal reflux disease, gallstones and gall bladder disease, gout, nonalcoholic fatty liver disease, pregnancy complications, menstrual irregularities, bladder control problems, osteoarthritis, obstructive sleep apnea, infertility, and psychological disorders, such as depression, eating disorders, problems with body image, and low self-esteem.[14] The American Medical Association suggests that health professionals recognize the significant consequences of obesity. The total indirect and direct cost of obesity in the United States was $147 billion in 2008.[15]

The Harvard School of Public Health provides recommendations for managing obesity through obesity prevention policy and environmental change efforts at its website: http://www.hsph.harvard.edu/obesity-prevention-source/obesity-prevention/.

As health care professionals, we need to engage in all efforts to reduce this epidemic. Measures to decrease obesity are listed in Table 7-1.

Metabolic Syndrome

As many as 22% of American adults may have a sinister-sounding disorder called *syndrome X* or *metabolic syndrome*, a condition significantly increasing a person's risk of developing life-threatening chronic diseases.[16] According to the American Heart Association, risk factors associated with metabolic syndrome include the following[16]:

- Abdominal or "central" obesity (waist size greater than 40 inches in men and greater than 35 inches in women)
- High levels of fasting blood triglycerides (fats; greater than 150 mg/dL)

- Low levels of blood high-density lipoprotein (HDL) cholesterol (men less than 40 mg/dL and women less than 50 mg/dL)
- High blood pressure (greater than 130/85 mm/Hg)
- High levels of glucose (greater than 110 mg/dL as measured by a fasting glucose test)
- Insulin resistance

When metabolic syndrome is diagnosed early in its development, it can be slowed and, in some cases, even reversed.[16] Changes in diet and exercise can help significantly reduce the risk of developing this pathology. If an individual presents with risk factors for metabolic syndrome, the physician should be contacted for appropriate medical management. With obesity as a primary risk factor, physical activity under a qualified health care professional is advisable.

Insomnia

Insomnia is an individual's perception that sleep quality is inadequate or nonrestorative, despite having the opportunity to sleep. Insomnia includes difficulty falling asleep, sleeping too lightly, being easily disrupted with multiple spontaneous awakenings, or early morning awakenings with an inability to fall back asleep.[17] Insomnia is considered a disorder when it disrupts or impairs daily functioning. If an individual reports any difficulty with sleeping, the health care professional should note the duration of the symptom. Transient insomnia lasts less than 1 week; short-term insomnia lasts 1 to 6 months and is usually associated with persistent, stressful situations (such as death or illness of a loved one or environmental factors, such as loud environmental noises); and chronic insomnia lasts more than 6 months.[17] Insomnia can lead to depression and anxiety, abnormalities in metabolism, daytime sleepiness, and memory problems. Insomnia may be a problem of hyperarousal rather than mere sleep deprivation associated with stress. Individuals with insomnia should be referred to a physician for a more comprehensive examination and possible medical management.[17]

Sexually Transmitted Diseases

Sexually transmitted diseases (STDs) have serious and sometimes fatal complications. Sexually active teens and young adults are at highest risk, but STDs can affect all age groups. Those who are at increased risk of infection include the following[18]:

- People who have had multiple sex partners, especially those who have exchanged sex for money or drugs
- Males who have sex with males
- Injection drug users and their sex partners
- Individuals with exposure to HIV/AIDS, gonorrhea, syphilis, chlamydia, genital herpes, and genital warts

Approximately 40 million people are currently living with HIV infection, and an estimated 25 million have died from this disease.[19] Health care professionals need to be aware of the signs and symptoms of HIV infection, as listed below.[20]

Acute Retroviral Syndrome/HIV Infection

Presentation of acute retroviral syndrome/HIV infection occurs from 2 to 4 weeks up to 3 months after exposure to HIV. (Note: During primary HIV infection, there are higher levels of virus circulating in the blood, making it more easily transmitted to others.)

Symptoms can include the following:

- Fever
- Chills

- Rash
- Night sweats
- Muscle aches
- Sore throat
- Fatigue
- Swollen lymph nodes
- Ulcers in the mouth

Chronic phase or latency occurs after the initial infection and up to 10 years or longer. Symptoms may not be evident.

AIDS

Many of the signs and symptoms of AIDS come from opportunistic infections that occur in patients with a damaged immune system. They include the following:

- Chronic dry, scratchy cough; shortness of breath; tightness or pressure in the chest
- Rapid weight loss
- Profuse night sweats
- Continuous unexplained fatigue
- Diarrhea longer than 1 week (found in both early and late stages of HIV)
- Swollen lymph glands (lymphatic nodes in the neck, armpits, and groin)
- Sores, white spots, or blemishes in the mouth and on the gums and tongue
- Burning sensation and an altered sense of taste
- Pneumonia
- Shingles
- Excessive bruising and bleeding
- Herpes simplex affecting the rectal, genital, and esophageal regions of the body
- Loss of appetite
- Red, pink, brown, or purplish blotches on and/or under the skin
- Pain or difficulty swallowing
- Constant headaches
- Confusion or forgetfulness
- Unexplained change in vision
- Chronic yeast infections (women)
- Pelvic inflammatory disease (women)
- Cervical abnormalities (women)
- Skin conditions such as rash, hives, lumps, lesion, sores, spots, or abnormal growths
- Chronic mononucleosis-like illness
- Receding gums
- Constant fevers

Health care professionals can help educate the public about the continued risk of HIV infection and the need to practice safe sex with all partners.

Health Risks for Adult Males

"Men die at higher rates than women for all of the top 10 causes of death."[21] In the United States, the top 5 health risks for men are heart disease (leading cause of death), stroke, cancer, depression, and suicide.[21]

Heart Disease

Heart disease is the greatest health threat to men in the United States today. According to the American Heart Association, men have a greater risk of heart disease and have heart attacks much earlier in life than women.[21] Every man needs to take this disease seriously and understand that this number one killer can often be prevented. Physical and mental health problems can arise with the increasing family and work responsibilities that adult men face.

"Average annual rates of the first heart disease complication rise from 7 per 1,000 men at ages 35 to 44, to 68 per 1,000 men at ages 85 to 94. For women, similar rates occur, but they happen about 10 years later in life. The average age of a person having a first heart attack is 65.8 for men and 70.4 for women."[21] Risk factors contributing to heart disease include increasing age, male sex, family history and race (those with a family history, including African Americans, Mexican Americans, Native Americans, Native Hawaiians, and some Asian Americans), smoking, high blood cholesterol, high blood pressure, physical inactivity, obesity and overweight, and diabetes.[21]

Cancer

The most common cause of cancer death for men is lung cancer, and 90% of these deaths are linked to cigarette smoking.[21] Other risk factors for lung cancer include exposure to secondhand smoke, exposure to asbestos or radon, personal history, and air pollution.[21] Smoking cessation programs have been reducing the fatality associated with smoking.[21]

Men older than 50 years are also at risk for an enlarged prostate caused by a noncancerous condition called *benign prostatic hyperplasia* (BPH) or by cancer. Prostate cancer is the second-leading cause of cancer death among men. The American Cancer Society recommends an annual digital rectal examination and a prostate-specific antigen (PSA) test for healthy men aged 50 years or older. Men who have family history of prostate cancer or who are Black may want to ask their doctor about earlier testing. According to the American Cancer Society, other risk factors include increasing age, nationality (North America and northwestern Europe), and a high-fat diet (abundance of red meat and high-fat dairy products and insufficient fruits and vegetables).[21] "Thirty percent of prostate cancers occur in men under age 65. The younger a man is, the more aggressive the tumor is," says Stephen F. Sener, MD, American Cancer Society president.[21] Overall, about one-third of all cancer deaths are related to nutrition or other controllable lifestyle factors.

Stroke

Stroke is a leading cause of death in the United States and the third leading cause of death for men.[21] Stroke is one of the leading causes of disability as well. Risk factors for stroke include increasing age, sex (more common in men until age 75), race (African American men are at greatest risk), a personal history of stroke or a transient ischemic attack (mini-stroke), diabetes, high cholesterol, heart disease, smoking (including secondhand smoke), physical inactivity, and obesity.[21] Modifiable risk factors need to be incorporated in preventive care.

Depression and Suicide

William Pollack, PhD, Assistant Clinical Professor of Psychiatry at Harvard Medical School, stated, "Men are more prone to suicide because they're less likely to openly show depression and have somebody else recognize it early enough to treat it, or to have themselves recognize that they're in trouble."[21] Men are more likely to commit suicide compared with women, in part due to underdiagnosed depression in men. Signs of depression may include anger, aggression, work burnout, risk-taking behaviors, midlife crisis, and alcohol and substance abuse.[21]

One helpful measure that can be used to identify suicide risk factors is called the SAD PERSONS scale, which includes the following criteria:

- *S*ex (male)
- *A*ge younger than 19 or older than 45 years
- *D*epression (severe enough to be considered clinically significant)
- *P*revious suicide attempt or received mental health services of any kind
- *E*xcessive alcohol or other drug use
- *R*ational thinking lost
- *S*eparated, divorced, or widowed (or ending of significant relationship)
- *O*rganized suicide plan or serious attempt
- *N*o or little social support
- *S*ickness or chronic medical illness

The risk assessment for suicidal thoughts and behaviors should be performed by qualified mental health professionals. If depression is suspected, a referral for mental health services is critical.

Health care professionals need to be mindful of disease risks of the general population and of increased risk factors for men. Professionals can ask questions related to lifestyle behaviors contributing to illness (eg, sedentary behavior, poor diet, smoking, use of alcohol or other substances), and specific medical tests can screen for pathophysiological changes that clearly identify pathology. The government website http://womenshealth.gov/screening-tests-and-vaccines/screening-tests-for-men/ offers current screening guidelines, tests, and immunizations for adult men and is recommended by the US Preventive Services Task Force. Health care professionals should be familiar with these guidelines and encourage their male clients to follow these recommendations.

Screening Tests

Prostate Cancer Screening Test

The PSA test is a blood test that measures the amount of a protein secreted by the prostate gland and is used to screen for possible prostate cancer. According to the American Cancer Society,[22] both the PSA blood test and digital rectal examination should be offered annually, beginning at age 50, to men who have a risk for prostate cancer or who have recommendations for the screening from primary physicians. Men at high risk (Black men and men with a strong family history of one or more first-degree relatives [eg, father, brothers] diagnosed at an early age) should begin testing at age 45. Men at even higher risk due to multiple first-degree relatives affected at an early age could begin testing earlier. Depending on the results of this initial test, no further testing might be needed until age 45.[23] Symptoms of prostate cancer include the following:

- A need to urinate frequently, especially at night
- Difficulty starting urination or holding back urine
- Inability to urinate

- Weak or interrupted flow of urine
- Painful or burning urination
- Painful ejaculation
- Blood in urine or semen
- Frequent pain or stiffness in the lower back, hips, or upper thighs

Any man presenting with these problems should be referred for medical care.

Testicular Examination

A testicular self-examination can be performed to note any masses in the testicles or any change in size, shape, or consistency of the testes. Testicular cancer is the most common malignancy in American men between the ages of 15 and 35 years.[24] Common symptoms associated with testicular cancer include the following:

- A lump in either testicle
- An enlargement of a testicle
- A feeling of heaviness in the scrotum
- A dull ache in the lower abdomen or the groin
- A sudden collection of fluid in the scrotum
- Pain or discomfort in a testicle or in the scrotum
- Enlargement or tenderness of the breasts

These symptoms should be further examined by a medical professional for medical diagnosis.

Dental Checkup

Bruxinism is a behavior that is commonly seen as a reaction to stress or as a result of temporomandibular joint dysfunction. Regular dental examinations should be encouraged to monitor the teeth, gums, lips, and soft tissue, as well as the alignment of the jaws for a proper bite. A more thorough examination should be performed when oral motor dysfunction or temporomandibular joint impairment is suspected.

Screening Guidelines for Men and Women

In addition to performing a standard screening of adult clients, health care professionals need to remind adults of regular medical screening tests that are important for early detection of other common pathologies. Health care professionals should be familiar with the following common medical tests used to screen individuals for pathological changes in their body systems.

Blood Cholesterol

The level of blood cholesterol is a significant risk factor for heart disease, particularly coronary artery disease. A lipid panel should be routinely performed that measures total cholesterol, low-density lipoprotein (LDL) cholesterol (the "bad" cholesterol), HDL cholesterol (the "good" cholesterol), and triglycerides. The desired values in most healthy adults follow[25]:

- LDL cholesterol lower than 100 mg/dL is considered ideal (100 to 129 is near optimal; 130 to 159 is borderline high; 160 to 189 is high; and ≥ 190 is very high)
- HDL cholesterol greater than 40 to 60 mg/dL (<40 is low and >60 is high; higher numbers are desired)

- Total cholesterol less than 200 mg/dL is desirable (lower numbers are desired; 200 to 239 is borderline high and > 240 is high)
- Triglycerides 10 to 150 mg/dL (lower numbers are desired)

Electrocardiogram

An electrocardiogram can detect abnormalities such as heart damage after a heart attack, an irregular heart rhythm, or an enlarged heart.

Chest Radiographs

A chest radiograph images the size and shape of the heart and provides information regarding the lungs' condition. A chest radiograph is typically ordered when a patient has symptoms of lung pathology, including a persistent cough, a chest injury, chest pain, coughing up blood, or difficulty breathing.

Blood Chemistry Test

An adult's blood chemistry reveals the functional status of the liver, kidney, and pancreas, measuring sodium, potassium, calcium, phosphorus, and blood sugar, as well as liver enzymes, bilirubin, and creatinine. Normal results for a comprehensive metabolic panel may vary slightly depending on the laboratory processing the blood and changes with aging. Typical values for an adult are as follows:

- Albumin: 3.9 to 5.0 g/dL
- Alkaline phosphatase: 44 to 147 IU/L
- Alanine aminotransferase (ALT): 8 to 37 IU/L
- Aspartate aminotransferase (AST): 10 to 34 IU/L
- Blood urea nitrogen (BUN): 7 to 20 mg/dL
- Calcium: 8.5 to 10.9 mg/dL
- Chloride: 96 to 106 mmol/L
- Carbon dioxide (CO_2): 20 to 29 mmol/L
- Creatinine: 0.8 to 1.4 mg/dL
- Glucose test: 100 mg/dL
- Potassium test: 3.7 to 5.2 mEq/L
- Sodium: 136 to 144 mEq/L
- Total bilirubin: 0.2 to 1.9 mg/dL
- Total protein: 6.3 to 7.9 g/dL

Adults who have used certain medications are at increased risk for liver, muscle, and kidney damage. The American Diabetes Association recommends that pregnant women and adults 45 or older should have regular screening of their blood glucose, also referred to as the blood sugar, fasting blood sugar (FBS), fasting blood glucose (FBG), fasting plasma glucose (FPG), blood glucose, oral glucose tolerance test (OGTT or GTT), or urine glucose.[26]

Complete Blood Count With Differential

The complete blood count (CBC) is used to identify cardiovascular and hematological problems. The CBC measures *hemoglobin* (an indication of the blood's oxygen-carrying capacity), *hematocrit* (the percentage of red blood cells in total blood volume), *leukocytes* (the number and types of white blood cells in the blood), and the number of *platelets* (an indicator of blood coagulability). Blood counts may vary with altitude. In general, normal CBC results are as follows:

- Red blood cell (RBC) count: men, 4.7 to 6.1 million cells/µL; women, 4.2 to 5.4 million cells/µL
- White blood cell (WBC) count: 4500 to 10,500 cells/µL (segmented neutrophils, 34% to 75%; band neutrophils, 0% to 8%; lymphocytes, 12% to 50%; monocytes, 2% to 9%; eosinophils, 0% to 5%; basophils, 0% to 3%)
- Hematocrit: men, 42% to 50%; women, 36% to 45%
- Hemoglobin: men, 12.7 to 13.7 gm/dL; women, 11.5 to 12.2 gm/dL
- Red blood cell indices: mean corpuscular volume (MCV), 86 to 98 fL; mean corpuscular hemoglobin (MCH), 33.4 to 35.5 gm/dL; and mean corpuscular hemoglobin concentration (MCHC), 32 to 36 gm/dL. A CBC can help detect the presence of many conditions, including anemia, infections, and leukemia.[27]

Thyroid-Stimulating Hormone Test

This blood test identifies levels of thyroid stimulating hormone (TSH), a pituitary gland hormone used to produce the hormone thyroxine. TSH level should be between 0.4 and 4.0 mIU/L (milli-international units per liter), depending on the laboratory processing the test. This test is used to detect too little thyroxine (an indication of low thyroid activity or *hypothyroidism*) or too much thyroxine (an indication of increased thyroid activity or *hyperthyroidism*).[28]

Transferrin Saturation Test

This blood test measures the amount of iron bound to transferrin, an iron-carrying protein in the bloodstream, and is used to detect *hemochromatosis*, a condition of iron overload in the blood.[29] Transferrin saturation values higher than 45% are considered too high. Hemochromatosis, a treatable hereditary disease, can lead to diabetes, arthritis, heart disease, or liver disease. Because this condition is often underrecognized, the physical therapist should encourage individuals to have their blood tested regularly during medical visits.

Urinalysis

A urinalysis is helpful for detecting levels of glucose excreted from the body and the presence of red blood cells (signaling internal problems, including possible tumors in the gastrointestinal tract), white blood cells (indicating infection), and elevated bilirubin (suggesting liver disease).

The American College of Physicians lists additional preventive interventions for anemia, breast cancer, chronic kidney disease, chronic obstructive pulmonary disease, dementia, depression, diabetes, erectile dysfunction, low back pain, obstructive sleep apnea, osteoporosis, heart disease, and vascular disease at its website: http://www.acponline.org/clinical_information/guidelines/guidelines/.

Health care professionals should review these guidelines for individuals presenting with risk factors associated with these common medical conditions.

Oral Health

Oral health is essential during adulthood. Healthy dentition is critical for eating a variety of textured foods and for the pronunciation of certain words. All clients should be counseled to stop the use of all forms of tobacco and to limit consumption of alcohol to reduce the risk of oral cancer as well as cardiovascular pathology. Although clients generally have regular oral examinations by their dentists, health care professionals should be aware of the following potential indicators of disease[30]:

- Sore in the mouth that does not heal
- Lump or thickening in the cheek
- White or red patch on the gums, tongue, or lining of the mouth
- Soreness or a feeling that something is caught in the throat
- Difficulty chewing or swallowing
- Difficulty moving the jaw or tongue
- Numbness of the tongue or other area of the mouth
- Swelling of the jaw, causing dentures to fit poorly or become uncomfortable

Any of these signs or symptoms commonly associated with cancer should be immediately reported to the physician.

Fitness

Just as children and youth must complete a preparticipation examination, adults should be thoroughly screened prior to initiating a fitness program. Screening should provide the individual's personal medical information, information about any current medical information, medications (over-the-counter and prescription medications), a family history of medical conditions, as well as lifestyle behaviors (nutritional habits, exercise habits, stress, smoking, alcohol consumption). Any contraindications indicate the need for a referral to appropriate health professional.

Individuals at risk for exercise are those with unstable medical conditions (cardiopulmonary or metabolic disease processes) or conditions exacerbated by exercise. These individuals have what are considered high-risk factors, according to the American College of Sports Medicine. Additionally, those with special testing or exercise needs need a more thorough examination before initiating any program of physical activity. In these cases, the risks of exercise or physical activity may outweigh the benefits.[31] Individuals at moderate risk for exercise include men who are 45 years and older, women who are 55 years and older, and individuals of either sex with 2 or more risk factors for coronary artery disease.[31] The low-risk group includes men younger than 45 years, women younger than 55 years, and individuals with no more than one cardiovascular risk factor. Cardiovascular risk factors include smoking; high blood cholesterol and other lipids; diabetes mellitus; hypertension (systolic greater than 135 mm Hg and diastolic greater than 90 mm Hg); a family history of myocardial infarction, coronary revascularization, or sudden death before 55 years in a father or first-degree relative; hypercholesterolemia (total serum cholesterol greater than 200 mg/dL, HDL cholesterol less than 35 mg/dL, or LDL greater than 130 mg/dL); obesity (body mass index of 30 kg/m^2 or greater); a sedentary lifestyle (not participating in regular exercise); or impaired glucose fasting (fasting blood glucose of 110 mg/dL or greater).[32]

A more comprehensive fitness assessment includes information about the individual's knowledge of health-related fitness, the individual's current exercise program, and motivation for exercise. Although the risks of death or myocardial infarction are relatively small (less than 0.04%[33,34]), this information should be shared with individuals undergoing submaximal exercise testing.

Suggested Adult Physical Activities

A variety of adult-oriented activities are effective for burning calories and promoting general cardiopulmonary fitness. The following list provides the number of calories generally burned by an adult when performing each activity[35,36]:

Activity	Calories burned per hour
Bicycling 6 mph	240
Bicycling 12 mph	410
Jogging 5.5 mph	740
Jogging 7 mph	920
Jumping rope	750
Running in place	650
Running 10 mph	1280
Skiing (cross-country)	700
Swimming 25 yds/min	275
Swimming 50 yds/min	500
Tennis (singles)	400
Walking 2 mph	240
Walking 4 mph	440

A well-rounded exercise program should address all areas of health-related fitness, including muscular strength and endurance. A generic outline for a comprehensive exercise program, addressing all areas of health-related fitness includes flexibility, strengthening, muscular endurance, cardiopulmonary endurance, and postural exercises.

Weekend Warriors

Those who try to compress their exercise into their free time, usually the weekend, are referred to as *weekend warriors*. Do weekend warriors achieve the recommended amount of exercise? In the Harvard Alumni Health Study,[37] 8421 men (mean age, 66 years) without major chronic diseases provided survey responses to questions about their levels of physical activity in 1988 and 1993. Men were classified as sedentary (expending < 500 kcal/week), insufficiently active (500 to 999 kcal/week), weekend warriors (≥ 1000 kcal/week from sports/recreation 1 to 2 times/week), or regularly active (all others expending ≥ 1000 kcal/week). At baseline, 8421 men were classified as follows: 17% as sedentary, 13% as insufficiently active, 7% as weekend warriors, and 62% as regularly active. The study showed many weekenders reaching their calorie expenditure by playing tennis, golf, or gardening. Among the weekend warriors, over 75% exercised on 2 days per week, rather than 1. Between 1988 and 1997, 1234 men died. The study found that among men without major risk factors, weekend warriors had a lower risk of dying, compared with sedentary men (relative risk = 0.41; ie, less than half as likely to die) as compared with men with at least one major risk factor (relative risk = 1.02). The researchers concluded that regular physical activity generating 1000 kcal/week or more should be recommended for lowering mortality rates; however, among those with no major risk factors, even 1 to 2 episodes/week generating 1000 kcal/week or more can postpone mortality. There was no such advantage for the high-risk weekend warriors. "At the end of the study, sedentary men (500 calories or less energy expended through exercise per week) were found to be at highest risk of death from any cause, and regularly active men (1000 calories or more energy expended through exercise per week) were at lowest risk. The risk of death in insufficiently active men (500 to 1000 calories of energy expended through exercise per week) and weekend warriors (1000 calories or more energy expended through exercise per week, concentrated in 1 or 2 sessions) were slightly lower than that of sedentary men, but these differences did not reach statistical significance.[37] Further analysis revealed that weekend warriors who were not overweight, did not smoke, and did not have high blood pressure or high cholesterol levels had a risk of death similar to regularly exercising men. Interestingly, the presence of risk factors did not inhibit exercise benefits in men who exercised regularly, but weekend warriors who had any one of these risk factors had a risk of death similar to that of sedentary men."[37]

Authors examining the risk of mortality as it relates to energy expenditure per week recommended that: "Men who want to engage in weekend warrior exercise practices should consult a health care provider, because those who are overweight or smokers, or who have high blood pressure or high cholesterol levels are not likely to benefit from this type of exercise. Men with any of these risk factors should be encouraged to exercise regularly rather than sporadically. Weekend warriors should also be aware that the risk of sprains, strains, and muscle injuries, which was not evaluated in this study, could be higher for sporadic exercisers than for men who exercise frequently. The effects of various exercise patterns on the long-term health of women should also be examined in future studies."[37]

Although the Harvard study was conducted with only male participants, it is likely that women who are weekend warriors may have similar risks of injury and needs for appropriate exercise prescription based on their risk factors for cardiopulmonary disease. The 8 most common injuries sustained by weekend warriors included rotator cuff problems, elbow tendinitis, knee arthritis, hip arthritis, knee cartilage tear, anterior cruciate ligament tear, Achilles tendonitis, and lower back pain. Preventing these injuries involves protection, acute care of inflammation, and reduced intensity, in many cases.

Summary

For adult clients, it is important to recognize priorities that enable individuals to maintain a healthy lifestyle, manage stress, and sustain financial security while continuing healthy relationships at home and at work. Health care professionals can identify pathological risk factors, reduce stressors, address lifestyle habits that impair health, and recommend appropriate exercise programs to optimize limited time. A holistic approach to health care for adults includes an awareness of multiple responsibilities and needs affecting priorities and lifestyle habits. Chapter 8 offers additional suggestions to promote the health and well-being of women.

References

1. To love and to work: Adlerian thoughts on an anecdote about Freud. Bulletin of the Menninger Clinic. 1981;45(5):439-441.
2. Marcia J. Identity and psychosocial development in adulthood. *IIJTR*. 2002;2(1):7-28.
3. McAdams DP, St. Aubin ED, Logan RL. Generativity among young, midlife, and older adults. *Psychol Aging*. 1993;8(2):221-230.
4. Marriage and divorce. Centers for Disease Control and Prevention. http://www.cdc.gov/nchs/fastats/divorce.htm. Accessed May 30, 2013.
5. Larson S, Larson D. Divorce: a hazard to your health? *Physician*. 1990;(May/June):14.
6. Yelin E, Nevitt M, Epstein W. Toward an epidemiology of work disability. *Milbank Mem Fund Q Health Soc*. 1980;58(3):386-415.
7. Dermatology A-Z. American Academy of Dermatology. http://www.aad.org/dermatology-a-to-z/dermatology-a-to-z. Accessed May 30, 2013.
8. Dermatologic disorders. The Merck Manual for Health Care Professionals. http://www.merckmanuals.com/professional/dermatologic_disorders.html. Accessed May 30, 2013.
9. Melanoma. National Cancer Institute. http://www.cancer.gov/cancertopics/types/melanoma. Accessed May 30, 2013.
10. Diabetes statistics. American Diabetes Association. http://www.diabetes.org/diabetes-basics/diabetes-statistics/. Accessed May 30, 2013.

11. Khardori R. Type 2 diabetes mellitis. Medscape. http://emedicine.medscape.com/article/117853-overview#showall. Accessed May 30, 2013.
12. American Diabetes Association. Clinical practice recommendations. *Diabetes Care.* 1998;21(Suppl 1):S1-S70.
13. American Cancer Society. *Cancer Prevention & Early Detection Facts & Figures 2012.* Atlanta, GA: American Cancer Society; 2012.
14. Overweight and obesity: adult obesity facts. Centers for Disease Control and Prevention. http://www.cdc.gov/obesity/data/adult.html. Accessed May 30, 2013.
15. Overweight and obesity: causes and consequences. Centers for Disease Control and Prevention. http://www.cdc.gov/obesity/adult/causes/index.html. Accessed May 30, 2013.
16. Metabolic syndrome. American Heart Association. http://www.heart.org/HEARTORG/Conditions/More/MetabolicSyndrome/Metabolic-Syndrome_UCM_002080_SubHomePage.jsp. Accessed May 30, 2013.
17. Erman MK. Insomnia. In: Poceta JS, Mitler MM, eds. *Sleep Disorders: Diagnosis and Treatment.* Totowa, NJ: Humana Press;1998:21-51.
18. Sexually transmitted diseases (STDs). eMedicineHealth. http://www.emedicinehealth.com/sexually_transmitted_diseases/article_em.htm. Accessed May 30, 2013.
19. HIV/AIDS. eMedicineHealth. http://www.emedicinehealth.com/hivaids/article_em.htm#hivaids_overview. Accessed May 30, 2013.
20. HIV/AIDS symptoms and signs. The HIV/AIDS Network. http://www.hivaidssearch.com/facts/hiv_aids_common_symptoms.htm. Accessed January 28, 2006.
21. Men's top 5 health concerns. MedicineNet.com. http://www.medicinenet.com/script/main/art.asp?articlekey=46826. Accessed May 30, 2013.
22. Screening tests and immunizations guidelines for men. Office on Women's Health. http://www.womenshealth.gov/screening-tests-and-vaccines/screening-tests-for-men/. Accessed May 30, 2013.
23. Prostate cancer prevention: ways to reduce your risk. Mayo Clinic. http://www.mayoclinic.com/health/prostate-cancer-prevention/MC00027. Accessed May 8, 2013.
24. Testicular cancer. Mayo Clinic. http://www.mayoclinic.com/health/testicular-cancer/DS00046. Accessed May 8, 2013.
25. Third report of the National Cholesterol Education Program (NCEP) Expert Panel on detection, evaluation, and treatment of high blood cholesterol in adults (Adult Treatment Panel III). National Institutes of Health. http://www.nhlbi.nih.gov/guidelines/cholesterol/atp3xsum.pdf. Accessed May 8, 2013.
26. Diabetes basics. American Diabetes Association. http://www.diabetes.org/diabetes. Accessed May 8, 2013.
27. Beers M. Blood disorders. The Merck Manual of Medical Information. http://www.merckmanuals.com/home/blood_disorders/symptoms_and_diagnosis_of_blood_disorders/diagnosis_of_blood_disorders.html?qt=CBC&alt=sh#Laboratory%20Blood%20Tests. Accessed May 8, 2013.
28. Beers M. Thyroid disorders. The Merck Manual of Medical Information. http://www.merckmanuals.com/professional/endocrine_and_metabolic_disorders/thyroid_disorders/overview_of_thyroid_function.html. accessed May 8, 2013.
29. Beers M. Iron overload. The Merck Manual of Medical Information. http://www.merckmanuals.com/professional/hematology_and_oncology/iron_overload/overview_of_iron_overload.html?qt=Iron%20Overload&alt=sh. Accessed May 8, 2013.
30. Oral health. Indiana State Department of Health. http://www.in.gov/isdh/programs/oral/s-tobacco.html. Accessed January 28, 2006.
31. Thompson P, Buchner D, Piña I, et al. Scientific statement: eercise and physical activity in the prevention and treatment of atherosclerotic cardiovascular disease. *Circulation.* 2003;107:3109.
32. Heart disease and stroke statistics–2009 update. American Heart Association. http://www.nanocorthx.com/Articles/HeartDiseaseStrokeStatistics.pdf. Accessed May 8, 2013.
33. Pate RR, Pratt M, Blair SN, et al. Physical activity and public health: a recommendation from the Centers for Disease Control and Prevention and the American College of Sports Medicine. *JAMA.* 1995;273:402-407.
34. National Heart, Lung, and Blood Institute/American Heart Association. *Exercise and Your Heart: A Guide to Physical Activity.* DHHS, PHS, NIH Publication No. 93-1677.
35. Calories burned during physical activities. US Department of Veterans Affairs. http://www.move.va.gov/download/NewHandouts/PhysicalActivity/P03_CaloriesBurnedDuringPhysicalActivities.pdf. Accessed May 8, 2013.
36. Physical activity for a healthy weight. Centers for Disease Control and Prevention. http://www.cdc.gov/healthyweight/physical_activity/. Accessed May 8, 2013.
37. Sesso HD, Paffenbarger RS Jr, Lee IM. Physical activity and coronary heart disease in men: the Harvard Alumni Health Study. *Circulation.* 2000;102:975-980.

8

Women's Health Issues
Focus on Pregnancy

Shannon DeSalvo, PT and Catherine Rush Thompson, PT, PhD, MS

"For American women, being healthy is far more than getting a good checkup or being disease-free. Being healthy means both physical and emotional wellness and having a healthy family."
—National Women's Health Resource Center

Women's Health

The scope of health promotion for women's health encompasses care for problems seen most commonly in women, although men may have some similar issues. Common health concerns for women include unhealthy lifestyle habits, incontinence, pelvic/vaginal pain, prenatal and postpartum care, osteoporosis, and breast cancer. Although women's health issues often center on reproductive health, the top 5 medical conditions affecting adult women are heart disease, breast cancer, osteoporosis, depression, and autoimmune diseases.[1] These health problems span multiple body systems and may limit activities, affecting women's personal and professional roles in life. Using the World Health Organization model, health care professionals can identify common health concerns, determine activity limitations, explore environmental and personal factors contributing to these health issues, and determine appropriate resources for their management.

This chapter focuses on common women's health conditions, with an emphasis on their prevention, screening, and management. Specific topics include issues facing the female athlete, pregnancy, and changes occurring during perimenopause, menopause, and postmenopause.

Screening for Women's Health Issues

Health care professionals need to explore each individual's medical history and familiarity with preventive care, comparing results with national data for respective ethnic populations. Cultural, psychosocial, and environmental factors vary across groups and can guide appropriate

Thompson CR.
Prevention Practice and Health Promotion: A Health Care Professional's Guide to Health, Fitness, and Wellness, Second Edition (pp 127-140).

interventions. As mentioned in Chapter 5, a thorough interview can yield significant information baseline information. Questions on an intake form or by interview can elicit additional information, including the following:

- Do you have any concerns about pregnancy or the use of contraceptives?
- Do you have any concerns related to your risk for breast, uterine, or cervical cancer? Health care professionals should be mindful that women with a family history of cancer, particularly women over the age of 60, are at increased risk.[2]
- Do you experience bowel/bladder leakage, urgency or pain? Vaginal/rectal pain? Pain with intercourse? Pregnancy and childbirth often contribute to pelvic floor issues such as incontinence, prolapse of organs, or pain with intercourse. According to the National Association for Incontinence, "Urinary incontinence affects 30% to 50% of childbearing women by age 40. Up to 63% of stress-incontinent women report their problem began during or after pregnancy."[3]
- How would you characterize your health behavior, including exercise, nutritional intake, mental health, and use of cigarettes, alcohol, or other substances?
- Do you have any significant stressors in your life that may be affecting your health (including domestic problems, issues related to children, work-related stressors, or uncontrollable events causing stress)? Women play multiple roles in their personal and professional lives, leading to a variety of stressful situations. Stress management resources should be made readily available to women of all ages. Helpful information can be found at the Women's Health Section of the American Physical Therapy Association, the National Incontinence Society, the National Vulvodynia Association, the International Society of Vulvovaginal Diseases, and the American College of Obstetricians and Gynecologists (ACOG).
- Are you feeling overly fatigued or experiencing any unusual pain?
- Are you familiar with controllable risk factors for cancer, osteoporosis, and heart disease? Women's hormones contribute to the delay in heart disease up to 15 years.[4]
- Are you having regular health screenings for risk reduction performed by your physician or other health care professional? Women should be reminded of the following screening guidelines recommended for maintaining and monitoring health status:
    - The *breast self-examination* includes feeling for lumps and looking at the breasts carefully to detect any changes in shape or size, any dimpling or puckering, or any changes in the color of the skin or in the nipple. Breast cancer is the most common cancer in women. Risk factors for breast cancer include the following[1]:
        - Increasing age
        - Genetics (most commonly the BRCA1 and BRCA2 genes)
        - Family history of the disease
        - Personal history of the disease
        - Race
        - Earlier abnormal breast biopsy
        - Earlier chest radiation
        - Early onset of menstruation (before age 12) or menopause after age 55
        - Not having children
        - Medication use, such as diethylstilbestrol
        - Alcohol abuse
        - Obesity

- Health care professionals should be alert to the following symptoms of breast cancer[1]:
  - A lump or thickening in the breast or armpit
  - A change in the breast's size or shape
  - A change in the color of the breast or the areola (area around the nipple)
  - Any dimpling or puckering of the skin or change in the color or texture of the skin
  - An abnormal discharge from the nipple
  - Scaling of the nipple or nipple retraction
- *A Pap smear test* is used to identify precancer cells lining the cervix. A sample of cells is collected from the cervix and upper vagina and smeared onto a glass slide, then examined in the laboratory for abnormal changes. Pap tests should be taken as soon as a woman begins having vaginal intercourse (or at age 21) and performed routinely every 3 years to age 65. If the screen is negative, Pap tests can be done every 5 years. Risk factors for cervical cancer include diethylstilbestrol exposure before birth, HIV infection, or a weakened immune system due to organ transplant, chemotherapy, or chronic steroid use. Symptoms of cervical cancer that require a medical referral for more extensive testing include abnormal vaginal bleeding or discharge, bleeding after intercourse, or painful intercourse.[5]
- *Human papillomavirus test.* "Since infection with human papillomavirus (HPV) is the most important risk factor for cervical cancer and precancers, it is important to avoid genital HPV infection. This may mean delaying sex, limiting the number of sex partners, and avoiding a sex partner who has had several other partners. Condoms are important to prevent the spread of sexually transmitted diseases, but they can't give full protection against HPV since there may be skin-to-skin contact of exposed areas which can transmit the virus."[6] According to the US Preventive Services Task Force, the HPV test in combination with the Pap test can safely extend the interval between cervical cancer screenings from 3 years to 5 years in many women between the ages of 30 and 65.[6]
- *The cervix, uterus, ovaries, fallopian tubes, and rectum.* A speculum is inserted into the vagina so that the doctor can see the upper part of the vagina and cervix for possible abnormalities.[7]
- *Vagina and pelvic floor muscles.* If a woman has any concerns about weakness, pain, or incontinence, she should have her pelvic floor muscles examined. This can be done by her health care provider or a physical therapist who specializes in pelvic rehabilitation.

Exercise and Lifestyle for Women

Exercise and healthy lifestyle habits offer many benefits to women but must be monitored because cyclic hormonal changes affect women from puberty to postmenopause. Customized exercises for those with health concerns are best prescribed by a physical therapist with expertise in women's health.

Premenstrual syndrome (PMS) is a constellation of physical and psychological symptoms seen among women of reproductive age. Monthly symptoms are both psychological and physical, including irritability, anxiety or depression, diminished self-esteem, difficulty concentrating, sleep problems, appetite changes, low energy, bloating, headache, and breast swelling and tenderness.[7] Although the type and intensity of symptoms may vary between women, all can be distressing. Management of PMS includes lifestyle and stress management, dietary restrictions (salt or carbohydrate), diuretics, prostaglandin inhibitors, progesterone (hormone treatment), ovulation inhibitors, vitamins, lithium, and antidepressants.[7] Aerobic exercise may reduce stress associated with premenstrual syndrome and improve mood[8]; however, health habits during PMS may attenuate the symptoms commonly limiting engagement in regular exercise. The following suggestions may reduce the effect of PMS on women engaged in regular physical activity[9]:

- Eat smaller meals or snacks throughout the day. Snack suggestions include plain yogurt; unsalted nuts; unsalted sunflower seeds; unsalted popcorn; whole wheat bread with peanut butter; pumpkin, zucchini, or banana bread; graham crackers; unsalted whole grain crackers; bran or oatmeal muffin; raw vegetables; apple slices; celery with peanut butter; applesauce; raisins; dates; dried apricots or prunes; grapes; banana; grapefruit; or orange slices.
- Eliminate or reduce caffeine. Coffee, tea, colas, and chocolate all contain varying amounts of caffeine. Caffeine can make breast symptoms (ie, swelling and tenderness) and headaches symptoms worse.
- Reduce salt. Excess salt intake may worsen water retention symptoms.
- Reduce alcohol intake.
- Perform relaxation techniques. Relaxation exercises reduce the mood symptoms of PMS and are particularly helpful for women who are able to identify their stressors.[7]

The Female Athlete Triad

Women should exercise to maintain general health-related fitness, including preventing changes in body function secondary to hormonal changes across the lifespan. Although weight-bearing exercise is heralded for reducing the risks of osteoporosis, increased physical activity, especially increased female participation in organized athletics, has revealed a triad of medical conditions resulting from the hormonal shifts and lifestyle habits altering female regulatory systems. The *female athlete triad* includes: (1) *anorexia nervosa* and *bulimia* (eating disorders/disordered eating behavior), (2) *amenorrhea/oligomenorrhea*, and (3) decreased bone mineral density (*osteoporosis and osteopenia*), and requires intervention by a multidisciplinary team, including prevention, assessment, and intervention by physical therapists.[10] Female athletes who must maintain a certain body type or weight class are at the highest risk of developing eating disorders. Young female gymnasts and dancers are classic examples of athletes whose bodies are ideally lean and muscular. To maintain this ideal body weight, girls and women will limit healthy eating or will binge on food, then purge the meal to avoid weight gain.

- *Anorexia nervosa* is an eating disorder involving limited eating and weighing at least 15% less than the ideal weight. *Bulimia nervosa* is an equally unhealthy eating disorder that involves binge eating (eating large quantities of food at one sitting), regardless of hunger, often followed by vomiting or purging the food. Disordered eating can result in decreased athletic performance, increased morbidity, and occasional mortality.[10] Interventions include psychological counseling, encouraging healthy lifestyle habits, and hormone replacement therapy as needed to manage or stop the condition.[10]
- *Amenorrhea* occurs when a woman of childbearing age fails to menstruate. There are 2 types of amenorrhea: primary amenorrhea and secondary amenorrhea. *Primary amenorrhea* is often associated with delayed puberty and commonly occurs in girls who are very thin or very athletic. The normal puberty-related rise in body fat responsible for triggering the initial onset of menstruation is absent.[11] In some cases, the lack of menstruation may have causes other than body fat. *Secondary amenorrhea* is a condition in which a previously menstruating woman fails to menstruate for 3 consecutive months.[11] Secondary amenorrhea is naturally caused by pregnancy, breastfeeding, and menopause (the normal age-related end of menstruation); however, other conditions related to genitourinary or endocrine system pathology may cause this condition. Other preventable causes include obesity, frequent strenuous exercise, rapid weight loss, or stress, either emotional or physical.[11] Amenorrhea affects 2% to 5% of all

women of childbearing age in the United States. The incidence of menstrual irregularities is much higher in activities where a thin body is required for better performance. Female athletes, especially young women, may be more likely to have amenorrhea.[11] Although exercise or physical activity itself does not cause amenorrhea, it is more likely to occur in women who exercise very intensely or who increase the intensity of exercise rapidly. Women who engage in sports associated with lower body weight, such as ballet or gymnastics, are more likely to develop amenorrhea than women in other sports.

- *Oligomenorrhea* is the term used to describe infrequent or very light menstruation in a woman with previously normal periods.[11] Oligomenorrhea can also be caused by emotional and physical stress, chronic illnesses, tumors that secrete estrogen, poor nutrition, and eating disorders such as anorexia nervosa. Female athletes often develop oligomenorrhea secondary to their restricted diets, the use of anabolic steroid drugs, and strenuous exercise.[11] Oligomenorrhea can be caused by a hormonal imbalance.[11] For both amenorrhea and oligomenorrhea, individuals should be encouraged to eat a healthy diet, exercise moderately, use healthy stress management resources, and balance their lifestyle to reduce unnecessary emotional stress.
- *Osteoporosis* may result when the bone-maintaining properties of estrogen are compromised whenever menstrual cycles are altered. Of particular concern in female athletes is the increased risk for stress fractures from repetitive forces transferred to the bone, either through muscle fatigue or from the tensile forces generated by forceful muscle contractions.[12] Female athletes experiencing amenorrhea and increased fracture risk may benefit from decreases in both the intensity and duration of training, as well as increases in calcium intake (1200 to 1500 mg/day) and reduced use of contraceptives. The dietary alterations could be accomplished by adding 3 glasses of skim milk per day to the diet.[12] A program of resistance training designed to increase both muscle strength and mass may improve the skeletal profile of these athletes, as well as protect against soft tissue injuries. Estrogen replacement therapy may be considered by those unwilling to make changes in their diet and exercise regimen.[12]
- Although stress incontinence is not considered part of the female athlete triad, it is a common issue faced by athletic females, including those in sports, dance, and physically demanding vocations. Stress incontinence is discussed later in this chapter.

Pelvic Pain

Women of all ages experience pelvic pain. Pelvic pain occurs mostly in the lower abdomen area and may range in intensity and severity from mild and infrequent to constant and extremely painful, leading to limitations in daily activities. If a person experiences pelvic pain, it is helpful to inquire about the pain characteristics (eg, specific location, type of pain, frequency, intensity, and duration), antecedents to pain (eg, physical activity or diet), pain mediators (eg, rest or pain medication), possible factors contributing to the pain (eg, menstruation, emotional changes, and lifestyle habits), and the effect that pelvic pain has on the individual's life (eg, ability to sleep, ability to participate fully in daily activities or sports, and ability to engage in sexual activity).[13] Although pelvic pain is more common in women, it can also occur in men. In women, it typically indicates a problem with the uterus, ovaries, fallopian tubes, cervix, or vagina, whereas in men the problem is commonly the prostate gland. It could also be a symptom of infection or other problem with the urinary tract, lower intestines, rectum, muscle, or bone.

A team approach may be needed, including physical therapy, medications, psychological counseling, hormonal therapy, and in some cases, surgery. If the problem is not resolved within 6 months, if can become chronic pelvic pain. According to the International Pelvic Pain Society, 25% of women with chronic pelvic pain may spend 2 to 3 days in bed each month,[14] significantly limiting that individual's ability to participate in life.

Stress Incontinence

Stress incontinence occurs when urine leaks under any kind of physical stress, including laughing, coughing, sneezing, or sexual or physical activity. Most commonly, this problem occurs due to problems with pelvic sphincter muscles or the detrusor muscle. Risk factors for stress incontinence include: female sex, childbirth, chronic coughing, obesity, and smoking. Clinical examinations help to differentiate possible causes and may be accompanied by electromyography (muscle electrical activity), a pad test (exercising wearing a pad to check for leakage), pelvic or abdominal ultrasound, measuring urine left after urination (post-void residual), urodynamic studies to measure pressure and urine flow, cystoscopy (scope of the bladder), urinalysis or urine culture (for potential infection), urinary stress test (coughing with a full bladder), or radiographs with contrast dye of the kidneys and bladder.[15] Preventive care and management of stress incontinence includes the following[15-17]:

- Lifestyle behavior changes (quitting smoking; drinking less alcohol and caffeine; losing weight; avoiding food and drinks that irritate the bladder, such as spicy foods, carbonated drinks, and citrus fruits; and keeping blood sugars well controlled)
- Pelvic muscle training exercises, which are discussed later in this chapter, accompanied by biofeedback or electrical stimulation
- Medications that can control the bladder (eg, anticholinergic, antimuscarinic, and alpha-adrenergic drugs)
- Surgery if conservative management is not possible.

A consensus statement was developed by a panel of experts in urology, urogynecology, nursing, and behavioral therapy in 2010 recommending the following for personal bladder health:

- Consume an adequate amount of fluid (25 to 30 mL/kg per day)
- Empty the bladder every 3 to 4 hours (based on adequate hydration)
- Moderately consume foods or beverages known to irritate the bladder
- Assume a relaxed position for urination and allow time for the bladder to empty
- Use self-management practices of pelvic floor muscle training, bladder training, and preemptive pelvic floor contraction to improve and maintain bladder health
- Avoid constipation
- Avoid obesity
- Do not smoke

Health care professionals should alert their clients to these essential health tips to prevent bladder problems. Suggestions for maintaining the strength of the pelvic floor muscles are discussed later in this chapter.

Osteoporosis

"Osteoporosis threatens 44 million Americans, of which 68% are women and it is largely preventable [when the body builds up bone mass before age 30]," reports the National Osteoporosis Foundation. Risk factors for osteoporosis include female sex; increasing age; small, thin-boned frame; ethnicity (White and Asian women have the greatest risk); family history; sex hormones (infrequent menstrual cycles and estrogen loss due to menopause may increase risk); anorexia; diet (low in calcium and vitamin D); medication use (especially glucocorticoids or some anticonvulsants); a sedentary lifestyle; smoking; and excessive alcohol.[1] Changes in lifestyle, including increasing weight-bearing activities, a healthy diet, and certain medications, may prevent osteoporosis and slow the progression of the condition.

Perimenopausal, Menopausal, and Postmenopausal Changes

Menopause marks the physiological aging process after which a woman no longer menstruates. Menopause, typically commencing when a women turns 50 years old, results from hormone alterations affecting not only reproductive capabilities but other body systems as well.[18] Symptoms of *perimenopause* (the period prior to menopause as the woman's body transitions into menopause) and menopause that woman may experience include the following[18]:

- Hot flashes and skin flushing
- Night sweats
- Insomnia
- Mood swings, including irritability, depression, and anxiety
- Irregular menstrual periods
- Spotting of blood in between periods
- Vaginal dryness and painful sexual intercourse
- Decreased sex drive
- Vaginal infections
- Urinary tract infections
- Incontinence

Of particular interest to health care professionals are bone loss and eventual osteoporosis, changes in cholesterol levels, and greater risk of heart disease. Factors that reduce the age of onset of menopause include smoking, hysterectomy, and living at high altitudes.[18]

Various studies indicate that exercise, proper diet, and, if advisable, hormone therapy can help prevent or minimize many of the problems associated with menopause.[18-20] Because both the quantity and the quality of bone decline during perimenopause, it is particularly important to address changes as early as possible. Furthermore, it is important to identify women at high risk for fracture *postmenopause* (after the onset of menopause) through bone scans[19] and encourage healthy lifestyle habits, including eating a diet with sufficient calcium and vitamin D, regular weight-bearing activities, measures to reduce fall risk, smoking cessation, and moderation of alcohol intake.[20] Certain pharmacologic agents containing biphosphates and selective estrogen receptor modulators may increase bone mass and reduce fracture risk.[21]

Changes With Pregnancy

The female body undergoes significant changes with pregnancy to accommodate the growth of the fetus and to prepare for childbirth. After birth, the body continues to change to prepare for nursing and return to reproductivity. Professionals with expertise in areas of care related to pregnancy can help guide women through a healthy pregnancy.

Anatomical and Physiological Effects of Pregnancy

From conception to birth, a pregnant woman's body undergoes significant changes. Each system within the body uniquely adapts to support and sustain the growing fetus and prepare for the childbirth process. Although these changes are vital for the process of pregnancy, often the woman will develop discomfort because of them. For example, to create more room for the enlarged uterus, the ribcage expands, allowing the diaphragm to elevate up to 4 cm.[22] As a result, there is increased stress where the ribs articulate with the thoracic spine, leading to potential back pain. Furthermore, the elevated hormone levels responsible for the increased laxity within her joints often do not return to baseline for several months after the baby is born.[22] These musculoskeletal changes create the need for physical therapy if body function is disturbed. Understanding how each body system specifically adapts during pregnancy will help therapists optimally treat these complaints and differentiate between various clinical diagnoses.

During pregnancy, the levels of estrogen, progesterone, and relaxin drastically change, causing increased softening of ligaments, growth of breast tissue, and retention of fluid.[23] Relaxin is responsible for much of the relaxation that occurs in the ligaments, symphyses, and fibrocartilage of the pelvis, as well as in peripheral joints.[23] Relaxin also begins to affect tissues right after conception, reaching its peak at approximately 3 months, and then either remaining at a constant level or dropping 20% to 50% for the remaining months of pregnancy.[24] Due to this laxity, the sacroiliac joints, in particular, can become hypermobile and lead to pain with activities such as bed mobility, transfers, gait, and stair negotiation. If a woman chooses to breastfeed her child, her hormone levels may continue to remain elevated well after delivery, a key consideration for the postpartum woman. Ligamentous laxity may continue after birth as long as the mother breastfeeds her baby. Maternal hormones often do not return to normal until she has finished or greatly decreased her frequency of breastfeeding.[25]

Altering hormonal levels are also responsible for the mood changes, periods of fatigue, increased metabolism, and decreased tolerance to heat that women develop, whether pregnant or menstruating, often contributing to the inability to adhere to an exercise program.[25]

The musculoskeletal system uniquely adapts to support the growth of a pregnant woman's uterus. Unfortunately, the changes that take place within the musculoskeletal system often contribute to various discomforts. Although these physiological changes are common with pregnancy, the discomfort or dysfunction that may result is not something to be ignored. Physical therapists are experts in the treatment of musculoskeletal impairments and can often provide the relief that many women need. Table 8-1 lists musculoskeletal changes associated with pregnancy.[25]

Many of these anatomical changes are a direct result of the weight gain that occurs with pregnancy. The ACOG recommends an average weight gain of 27.5 pounds, unless the woman was under- or overweight prior to becoming pregnant.[26] As the abdomen enlarges, her center of gravity shifts forward, causing an increased *lumbar lordosis* (swayback) and eventually a more pronounced *thoracic kyphosis* (humpback). The shift in gravity, in addition to the *diastasis recti* (separation of the rectus abdominus muscles), leads to decreased back stability and often pain.[25] An abdominal support binder often relieves this pain during functional activities. Due to the increase in breast tissue, added stress is placed on the thoracic spine. To prevent discomfort, women should wear supportive undergarments. Specific back stretches and stabilization exercises may help as well.[25] In addition to lumbar pain, pregnant women often develop *sacroiliac dysfunction*, which can lead to sciatica or pain directly in the low back. These symptoms usually flare up with activity, especially asymmetrical movements, such as bed mobility, transfers, and stair negotiation.[25] Wearing a sacroiliac belt can often bring symptom relief in combination with a back stabilization program. If these strategies completely alleviate the symptoms, the pregnant patient may benefit from manual techniques to improve the alignment of the joint itself.

Pubic symphysis separation occurs at approximately 2 to 32 weeks' gestation as the pubic symphysis widens to approximately 4 to 7 mm to prepare the pelvis for a vaginal delivery.[27] Because

Table 8-1. Musculoskeletal Issues Associated With Pregnancy
• Increased lumbar lordosis
• Posterior shift/increased kyphosis of the thoracic spine
• Rib cage expansion to accommodate growing
• Diastasis recti (thinning of the linea alba, causing separation of the rectus abdominus muscles)
• Rounded shoulders due to increasing weight of breasts
• Sacroiliac joint hypermobility
• Pubic symphysis separation (4 mm, nuliparas women; 4.5 to 8.0 mm, multiparas women)
• Round ligament pain
• Pelvic floor muscle weakness/incontinence
• Increased subtalar joint pronation
• Increased knee hyperextension
• Nerve compression (carpal or tarsal tunnel syndrome, thoracic outlet syndrome)
• Swelling or lymphedema issues

of the attachments of both the abdominal and pelvic floor muscles to this area, some women may develop pain as their muscles stretch. Others may develop a waddling gait because of the separation, potentially leading to back pain. Wearing a sacroiliac belt will help provide added stability during gait and transfers, and exercises that stress the adductor muscles should be avoided.

Round ligament pain results from the stretch of ligaments suspended from the lateral aspects of the uterus to the labia majora during pregnancy. Often, this considerable stretching causes sharp pain in the woman's groin and/or vagina. Commonly, pain is experienced after prolonged periods of standing or walking, although some women report sharp pains in this region when transferring out of a chair or bed. Limited weight-bearing activities, wearing an abdominal support binder, or taping techniques often relieve this pain with functional activities. Some women may even find relief from simply lifting their abdomen with their hands when they have one of these sharp pains.

Pelvic muscle weakness results from the added pressures on the pelvic floor muscles during pregnancy. Pelvic floor muscles, located at the base of the pelvis, have 3 major roles: sphincteric, supportive, and sexual (the "three S's").[28] These muscles connect the pubic bones to the sacrum by forming a sling. When at their optimal strength and length, pelvic floor muscles have the ability to perform the following 4 functions: (1) control the passing of urine, feces, or gas; (2) support the pelvic organs (bladder, bowel, and uterus); (3) facilitate enhanced sexual pleasure; and (4) provide stability of the pelvic girdle (pubic and sacroiliac joints).[28] As the uterus increases in size throughout pregnancy, added pressure is placed on the pelvic floor muscles, causing them to stretch and possibly weaken. If they are not strong enough to withstand this force, bladder and bowel control may be impaired, resulting in incontinence.[17,24]

When a woman's bladder becomes full, stretch receptors within the bladder send a message to the brain that it is time to find a bathroom. If the woman is not near a bathroom, a message is sent from the brain to the pelvic floor muscles to "hold it" or contract. The contraction of the pelvic floor muscles causes the smooth muscle lining of the bladder (the *detrusor muscle of the bladder*) to relax and continue to hold the urine. Once she is ready to void, she relaxes her pelvic floor muscles, causing the detrusor to contract and urine then flows out. If a woman's pelvic floor muscles are weak, they may not be able to sufficiently contract. This can lead to insufficient closure of the urethral sphincter, causing leakage of urine. There are 3 common types of incontinence associated with pregnancy: (1) *stress incontinence* (leakage of urine during an event of increased intra-abdominal pressure, such as sneezing, coughing, laughing, or lifting); (2) *urge incontinence* (leakage of urine due to an inability to delay a strong, sudden urge to urinate [ie, overactive bladder syndrome]); and (3) *mixed incontinence* (a combination of both stress and urge incontinence).[29] Due to these pelvic floor issues, it is crucial that physical therapists help educate woman about the importance of pelvic floor strengthening. This is a topic not only for the pregnant population but for all women. Age, hormonal changes, and the effects of gravity and certain physical activities all contribute to pelvic floor muscle weakness and the potential for incontinence, or even *pelvic organ prolapse* (the descent of an organ within the pelvic cavity).

A pregnant woman's feet take quite a toll during pregnancy. With more weight to support, the arches begin to fall and a resulting pronation occurs.[24] The equal and opposite ground reaction force is then altered, causing added stress on the knees, hips, and, once again, the low back. Due to these issues, it is important that pregnant women wear supportive shoes and try to avoid standing with their knees hyperextended.

By the end of pregnancy, most women retain an extra 3 liters of fluid.[24] With more time spent in weight-bearing positions, fluid tends to pool in the lower extremities, causing discomfort. Wearing supportive hose can often improve lower extremity circulation and help decrease this discomfort. This additional fluid within their connective tissues can also lead to various nerve compression syndromes. Due to the postural changes that pregnant women develop and the amount of fluid they retain, nerves can often become compressed. Some of the more common *nerve compression syndromes* are *carpal tunnel syndrome, tarsal tunnel syndrome, thoracic outlet syndrome, lateral femoral cutaneous nerve entrapment, iliolinguinal nerve compression, intercostal neuralgia, and peroneal nerve compression*.[24] Often splints, supportive garments, postural education, and instruction on various stretches and nerve mobilization can help women with these complaints.

The respiratory system goes through incredible changes to accommodate the demands of pregnancy. "Oxygen consumption alone increases by 14% (half going to the fetus and placenta and the other half going to the uterine muscle and breast tissue)."[30] Due to the increase in overall tidal volume, women may develop dyspnea or hyperventilation.[24] The women's hyperventilation helps with the diffusion of carbon dioxide from the fetus to maternal circulation.[30] As stated earlier, the diaphragm elevates up to accommodate the enlarged uterus. This diaphragmatic elevation causes the mother's breathing pattern to become more chest breathing than abdominal breathing. Due to all of these changes within the respiratory system, the overall pulmonary function of the mother is not impaired.[30]

Like each of the other body systems, the cardiovascular system uniquely adapts to meet the needs of the growing fetus. Blood volume increases by 40% to 50%, causing an eventual increase in overall cardiac output to 50% above nonpregnant values, leading to increases in stroke volume and heart rate.[30] It is important to note that a pregnant woman's resting heart rate will be higher than it was prepregnancy. Some say that being pregnant is exercise in and of itself because of this. However, overall blood pressure decreases throughout pregnancy. This decrease in blood pressure is primarily due to the smooth muscle relaxation taking place within the blood vessel walls with increasing levels of progesterone.[30]

Exercise During Pregnancy

Although each system of the female body uniquely adapts to the physiological demands of pregnancy, it is still important to be cautious when advising someone on prenatal exercise. Caution should be taken to not exceed the thresholds of the metabolic, respiratory, or cardiac thresholds.[30] The ACOG no longer suggests a specific heart rate for pregnant woman to stay under during exercise; rather, they advise exercise within 60% to 75% of maximal heart rate, which is approximately 140 bpm for most women.[30] Because factors such as age, fitness level, and overall health affect a pregnant woman's ability to exercise, it is always important to first consult with the involved physician before initiating an exercise program. Health care professionals should recommend that pregnant women seek out exercise classes designed specifically for pregnant women, especially in the latter trimesters. The benefits of exercise during pregnancy include the following[30]:

- Increased muscle tone
- Increased endurance/energy level
- Decreased tension/stress
- Decreased swelling
- Improved posture and body mechanics
- Improved circulation
- Improved pelvic floor muscle strength
- Decreased discomfort/pain
- Better sleep patterns
- Preparation for the intensity of labor and delivery
- Quicker return to prepregnancy shape
- Improved self-esteem
- Networking with other pregnant women

The pregnant woman should be educated about signs and symptoms to monitor while exercising. According to the ACOG, certain clinical manifestations suggest potential problems needing medical attention, such as pain, vaginal bleeding, persistent dizziness, numbness or tingling, faintness, shortness of breath, generalized edema, severe headache, or severe calf pain, swelling, or redness.[31] Women with heart disease, complicated births (placenta previa, premature labor, ruptured membrane), hypertension, lung disease, incompetent cervix, or risk for premature labor should not engage in exercise during pregnancy, according to the ACOG.[31] Specific recommendations for exercise during pregnancy and during the postpartum period are listed at http://bjsm.bmj.com/content/37/1/6. Signs and symptoms to stop exercise and contact a physician include dizziness, vaginal bleeding, chest pain, headache, calf pain, uterine contractions, decreased fetal movements, or vaginal leakage.[31] Information about exercise during pregnancy is available in a helpful fact sheet for women located at the ACOG website at http://www.acog.org/~/media/For%20Patients/faq119.pdf.

The health care professional should be familiar with the client's medical history and exercise tolerance, recognizing relative and absolute contraindications to exercise in pregnancy.

Exercises for pregnancy are designed to address the issues that are precipitated by the various anatomical and physiological changes that occur during the months preceding delivery. The most familiar exercises are the Kegel exercises, known to strengthen the pelvic floor muscles and prevent incontinence.

> The principle behind Kegel exercises is to strengthen the muscles of the pelvic floor, thereby improving the urethral and rectal sphincter function. The success of Kegel exercises depends on proper technique and adherence to a regular exercise program. Some people have difficulty identifying and isolating the muscles of the pelvic floor. Care must be taken to learn to contract the correct muscles. Typically, most people contract the abdominal or thigh muscles, while not even working the pelvic floor muscles. These incorrect contractions may even worsen pelvic floor tone and incontinence.[32]

Additional details about the history of Kegel exercises, how to perform these exercises, techniques to identify the correct muscles, and how biofeedback is used to facilitate muscle contractions can be found at http://www.nlm.nih.gov/medlineplus/ and in an encyclopedia.[32]

Prenatal Care

In addition to concern about her own body during pregnancy, a pregnant woman is also concerned about her unborn child's health. A health care professional can remind women to practice healthy lifestyle habits to promote their unborn child's good health at birth. Embryological and fetal development are generally predictable in terms of structures that develop from one month to the next; however, environmental factors, such as the mother's diet, smoking habits, use of alcohol, or other risky behaviors, can significantly affect the normal development and function of these structures. After the first 8 weeks following conception, the fetus' developing organs mature throughout the remainder of gestation for full function at birth yet are continually susceptible to the mother's lifestyle habits. Maternal factors that can negatively affect a developing embryo and fetus include exposure to infections (eg, rubella, syphilis, genital herpes, AIDS, cytomegalovirus); inadequate nutrition; high levels of stress; advanced age; use of drugs or alcohol; metabolic disorders; placental inadequacy; and preeclampsia.[33] One of the most feared toxic agents to the fetus in current times is radiation exposure.[34] Health care providers should obtain complete occupational and medical histories and discuss risk of exposure with pregnant clients.

Prenatal undernutrition had permanent effects on cardiovascular risk factors. Infants exposed to famine during gestation have an increased risk of coronary heart disease in later life. Either maternal or fetal metabolic disorders can alter normal growth patterns in the developing fetus. Phenoketonuria is a hereditary enzymatic defect that results in an accumulation of phenyalanine in the body and its conversion to abnormal metabolites.[35] If this condition continues unrecognized, the child may appear normal at birth, but within a year can develop progressive mental retardation.

Preeclampsia is another common condition that some women experience in the second half of pregnancy.[36] The condition is more common during the first pregnancy and in women who are older than age 40, teenage mothers, and mothers who are carrying multiple babies. Clinical manifestations of preeclampsia include high blood pressure and continuous swelling. Additional signs and symptoms include severe headaches; vomiting blood; excessive swelling of the face, feet and hands; decreased urine output; bloody urine; rapid heartbeat; excessive nausea; drowsiness; fever; double vision; and ringing in the ears.[36] Preeclampsia can prevent the placenta from providing sufficient blood to the fetus. This deprivation can cause low birth weight and other problems for the baby.

It is recommended that all pregnant women be screened for gestational diabetes, a carbohydrate intolerance that starts or is first recognized during pregnancy.[37] An oral glucose tolerance test between the 24th and 28th week of pregnancy is commonly used to detect this type of diabetes, and nearly 40% of women develop persistent diabetes up to 10 years following the initial diagnosis.[37] Risk factors for developing gestational diabetes include the following[37]:

- Race (Black or Hispanic)
- Overweight
- Atypical previous birth (baby weighing more than 9 pounds, unexplained death of fetus or newborn)
- Recurrent infections
- Older age

Maintaining blood glucose levels within normal limits for the duration of the pregnancy can improve the mother's health, as well as that of the fetus.[37]

If any prenatal health risks are suspected, the health care professional should advise the mother to seek medical attention to address maternal problems contributing to fetal injury. Prenatal care should be continually encouraged throughout the pregnancy.

Summary

Women have special health needs, particularly during pregnancy, that are commonly addressed by health care professionals. With the ever-increasing risk of heart disease, along with problems with osteoporosis, incontinence, pelvic or vaginal pain, and prenatal and postpartum musculoskeletal pain, health care providers play essential roles in preventive care. Physiological and anatomical changes during pregnancy and competition by female athletes warrant particular attention and should be carefully monitored by physical therapists with expertise in physical therapy. In addition, preventive care for an unborn child should be considered whenever working with women of childbearing age.

References

1. Women's health. WebMD. http://women.webmd.com/features/5-top-female-health-concern?page=2. Accessed May 8, 2013.
2. Breast cancer risk by age. Centers for Disease Control and Prevention. http://www.cdc.gov/cancer/breast/statistics/age.htm. Accessed May 8, 2013.
3. The many myths of bladder health. National Association for Incontinence. http://www.bladderhealthawareness.org/tag/incontinence/. Accessed May 8, 2013.
4. Epidemiology of cardiovascular disease. National Institutes of Health. http://www.ncbi.nlm.nih.gov/books/NBK45688/. Accessed May 8, 2013.
5. Women's health: pap smear. WebMD. http://women.webmd.com/guide/pap-smear. Accessed May 8, 2013.
6. Understanding cervical cancer–prevention. WebMD. http://www.webmd.com/cancer/cervical-cancer/understanding-cervical-cancer-prevention. Accessed May 8, 2013.
7. Bhatia SC, Bhatia SK. Diagnosis and treatment of premenstrual dysphoric disorder. *Am Fam Physician.* 2002;66(7):1239-1249.
8. Daly A. Exercise and premenstrual symptomatology: a comprehensive review. *J Women's Health.* 2009;18(6):895-899.
9. Goodale IL, Domar AD, Benson H. Alleviation of premenstrual syndrome symptoms with the relaxation response. *Obstet Gynecol.* 1990;75(4):649-655.
10. Birch K. The female athlete triad. *BMJ.* 2005;330:244-246.
11. Otis CL. Exercise-associated amenorrhea. *Clin Sports Med.* 1992;11:351-362.
12. Hobart U, Smucker D. The female athlete triad. *Am Fam Physician.* 2002;61:11-13.
13. Pelvic pain. MedlinePlus. http://www.nlm.nih.gov/medlineplus/pelvicpain.html. Accessed May 8, 2013.
14. Pelvic pain: diagnosis and management. International Pelvic Pain Society. http://www.pelvicpain.org/. Accessed May 8, 2013.
15. Gerber GS, Brendler CB. Evaluation of the urologic patient: history, physical examination, and urinalysis. In: Wein AJ, Kavoussi LR, Novick AC, Partin AW, Peters CA, eds. *Campbell-Walsh Urology.* 10th ed. Philadelphia, PA: Elsevier Saunders; 2011:18-21.
16. Deng DY. Urinary incontinence in women. *Med Clin North Am.* 2011;95:101-109.
17. Lukacz ES, Sampselle C, Gray M, et al. A healthy bladder: a consensus statement. *Int J Clin Pract.* 2011; 65(10):1026-1036.
18. Women's reproductive health: menopause. Centers for Disease Control and Prevention. http://www.cdc.gov/reproductivehealth/womensrh/. Accessed May 30, 2013.
19. Borer KT. Physical activity in the prevention and amelioration of osteoporosis in women: interaction of mechanical, hormonal and dietary factors. *Sports Med.* 2005;35(9):779-830.
20. Green JS, Stanforth PR, Rankinen T, et al. The effects of exercise training on abdominal visceral fat, body composition, and indicators of the metabolic syndrome in postmenopausal women with and without estrogen replacement therapy: the HERITAGE family study. *Metabolism.* 2004;53(9):1192-1196.
21. Keenan NL, Mark S, Fugh-Berman A, et al. Severity of menopausal symptoms and use of both conventional and complementary/alternative therapies. *Menopause.* 2003;10(6):507-515.
22. Hall C, Thein L. *Therapeutic Exercise: Moving Toward Function.* Philadelphia, PA: Lippincott Williams & Wilkins; 1999.
23. Novak J, Danielson LA, Kerchner LJ, et al. Relaxin is essential for renal vasodilation during pregnancy in conscious rats. *J Clin Invest.* 2001;107(11):1469-1475.
24. Stephenson R, O'Connor L. *Obstetric and Gynecologic Care in Physical Therapy.* 2nd ed. Thorofare, NJ: SLACK Incorporated; 2000.

25. Prather H, Hund D. Issues unique to the female runner. *Phys Med Rehabil Clin N Am.* 2005;16:691-670.
26. Stotland N, Haas J, Brawarsky P, Jackson R, Fuentes-Afflick E, Escobar G. Body mass index, provider advice, and target gestational weight gain. *Obstet Gynecol.* 2005;105(23):633-638.
27. Ritchie J. Orthopedic considerations during pregnancy. *Clin Obstet Gynecol.* 2003;46(2):456-466.
28. Nishimoto T. How fit is your pelvic floor? Denver Physical Therapy Women's Corner. 1998;4:1.
29. Bauman B, Frahm J, Hakeem F, McDonald G, Wallace K. *Incontinence: A Physical Therapist's Perspective.* Alexandria, VA: American Physical Therapy Association; 2005.
30. Wang T, Apgar B. Exercise during pregnancy. *Am Fam Physician.* 1998;57:8.
31. Exercise during pregnancy and the postpartum period. American College of Obstetricians and Gynecologists. http://www.acog.org/Resources%20And%20Publications/Committee%20Opinions/Committee%20on%20Obstetric%20Practice/Exercise%20During%20Pregnancy%20and%20the%20Postpartum%20Period.aspx. Accessed May 25, 2013.
32. Kegel exercises. MedlinePlus. http://www.nlm.nih.gov/medlineplus/ency/article/003975.htm. Accessed February 6, 2006.
33. Psychosocial and environmental pregnancy risks. Medscape. http://emedicine.medscape.com/article/259346-overview. Accessed May 8, 2013.
34. Hall C. The fetal and early life origins of adult disease. *Indian Pediatr.* 2003;40:480-502.
35. Anderson PJ, Wood SJ, Francis DE, et al. Neuropsychological functioning in children with early-treated phenylketonuria: Impact of white matter abnormalities. *Develop Med Child Neurol.* 2004;46(4):230-238.
36. Odegard RA, Vatten LJ, Nilsen ST, Salvesen KA, Austgulen R. Preeclampsia and fetal growth. *Obstetr Gynecol.* 2000;96(6):950-955.
37. Gestational diabetes. MedlinePlus. http://www.nlm.nih.gov/medlineplus/ency/article/000896.htm. Accessed February 6, 2006.

9

Prevention Practice for Older Adults

Ann Marie Decker, PT, MSA, GCS, CEEAA; Gail Regan, PhD, MS, PT; and Catherine Rush Thompson, PT, PhD, MS

"If I'd known how old I was going to be, I'd have taken better care of myself."—James Hubert (Eubie) Blake, *The Observer*, February 13, 1983

Older adults are our "national treasures"[1] and, as such, deserve considerable attention, particularly in the area of health and wellness. As they adjust to retirement, they shift from the stresses of maintaining a vocation to, in many cases, exploring a new avocation. This adjustment includes realigning their financial resources to manage their health and livelihood. Often, older adults can focus more of their energies on their personal relationships, allowing new opportunities to rediscover the unique qualities of their spouses and others.

Many maintain active lifestyles and remain engaged in various social roles in their community. According to Erikson,[2] the final stage of psychosocial development presents the challenge of accepting one's whole life and reflecting on it in a positive manner vs sensing despair, fearing death, and reflecting negatively on the final years of life. Choices of the older adult may reflect this relatively positive or negative view of the aging process. Health care professionals should recognize the unique value of each older adult and support continued engagement in the community to the fullest extent possible. Health care professionals are uniquely positioned to identify problems in the older adult that, over time, lead to decreased independent function, and to provide education to seniors, making them more aware and knowledgeable about maintaining their own health in their golden years.

Although aging is commonly associated with declines and changes in body systems, current evidence strongly suggests that genetic predisposition to illness and individual lifestyle behaviors significantly affect the aging process; the decline of the human body, once thought to be an inevitable consequence of aging, is as much related to the long-term consequences of lifestyle choices as to an individual's chronological age. It has been estimated that by the year 2030, the US population older than 65 years will number 70 million, with the fastest growing segment of the population being those 85 and older.[3] More women than men live well into old age, with almost half of women aged 65 and older being widowed.[3] Difference in life expectancy is not purely a sex difference, but

Thompson CR.
Prevention Practice and Health Promotion: A Health Care Professional's Guide to Health, Fitness, and Wellness, Second Edition (pp 141-157).

rather a sex-related combination of genetic, hormonal, and social influences. Extended lifespan is not only attributable to good health but is also related to technological advances in keeping people alive. In developed countries, there is an interest in slowing or reversing the aging process. Nutritional status and activity level, especially physical activity, are considered to be 2 important factors in influencing the rate and extent of physiological and cognitive changes in the aging process.[4]

People age in different ways and at different rates, although there is some consensus of opinion as to normal aging and what may be termed *successful aging*. On the simplest level, chronological age may determine whether an individual is classified as an older adult. Many sources categorize people as older adults, or senior citizens, if 65 years or older; some further distinguish between the *young-old* (those between 65 and 74 years), *old* (those between 75 and 84 years), and *old-old* (those 85 and older). The *frail elder* is described in the literature as the older adult with problems in multiple domains or who is vulnerable, fragile, and lacking resilience. The Fried definition of frailty includes 3 of the following 4 factors: (1) unintentional weight loss, (2) self-reported exhaustion, (3) slow walking speed, and (4) low physical activity.[5] Even 2 of these factors suggest intermediate frailty with increased risk of becoming frail in the next 3 to 4 years.[5]

Frail elders are generally older than 65 years and present with deficiencies in at least 2 of the following domains: physical, cognitive, nutritive, and sensory. The frail older adult has less physiologic reserve on which to draw and, therefore, is at increased risk of disability. It is important to note that frailty can result from the synergistic effects of aging, disease, malnutrition, disuse, and/or abuse.

What was once thought to be *normal aging* is now viewed as *typical aging*, and further study is helping elucidate *successful aging*. Although a segment of the population may escape most chronic disease and disability until later life, statistics suggest that it is much more common for individuals to experience a chronic illness or loss of function over time.[3] Typical aging results in highly variable changes in the function and overall health status of older adults. Exercise tolerance, strength, and balance frequently experience a decline with age, yet regular activity and exercise has been shown to preserve these functions over time and, in some cases, reverse the usual decline.

Anatomical and Physiological Changes With Aging

Muscle Strength

Muscle strength and postural alignment are critical to efficient and effective function in the older adult. Loss of isometric and dynamic strength has been documented in individuals as young as 50 to 59 years old.[6] Decline in muscle strength is closely associated with increased age, loss of type II muscle fibers, and loss of muscle mass. Normal changes in the aging musculoskeletal system, including reduced muscle mass and loss of bone density, can be compounded by physical inactivity. Generally, within 2 weeks of discontinuing resistance training, more than 5% of the benefits gained are greatly diminished.[6] Not only can physical inactivity accelerate the physiologic decline associated with aging, but it can also hamper the ability to cope with acute physiologic stressors. If older persons are forced by illness or injury to spend days or weeks exclusively on bed rest, muscle strength and aerobic capacity swiftly decline; muscle strength is lost at approximately twice the rate it takes to regain it. Decreased muscle mass leads to increased rate of disability.

The concept of threshold values for strength necessary for independent function is an interesting one. For example, there is a threshold value for quadriceps strength necessary to rise from a chair or toilet seat. At worst, when deterioration of function prevents an older adult from carrying out essential daily activities independently, professional assistance either in the home or a care center is warranted. On the other hand, a small strength gain may translate into considerable functional improvement. For example, an increase in muscle strength that allows one to transfer independently can make a substantial difference in quality of life and potential living possibilities. Numerous studies have suggested that loss of muscle strength may be slowed or reversed with progressive resistive exercise programs.[7] Although loss of muscle strength appears typical in older adults, regular strength training 3 times per week minimizes and, in some instances, reverses this loss. A range of health care professionals may be able to assist the older adult in maintaining his or her overall muscle strength. However, physical therapists are the best-equipped health care professionals to screen for loss of muscle strength in the older adult and make recommendations related to specific muscle strengthening exercise programs.

Bones and Joints

Age-related bone density differs from site to site. More peripheral sites, such as the radius, experience relative stability in density until menopause, whereas more central skeletal structures, such as the spine and the neck of the femur, show bone loss 5 to 10 years earlier.[8] Men and women aged 65 years and older can reverse bone loss and reduce fracture risk through the vitamin supplementation (500 mg of calcium and 700 IU of vitamin D). In addition, weight-bearing exercises minimize bone loss and, in some instances, diminish the decrease of bone density commonly seen with advancing age.[8]

Loss of joint fluid commonly associated with aging also adds to the wear and tear on the joint. Joint changes seem almost inevitable with advanced age; in fact, osteoarthritis is one of the conditions nearly all 100-year-olds experience.[8] Exercise and activity that promote optimal postural alignment and strength assist in reducing the occurrence of these changes until very late in life.

Changes associated with the spine are the primary reason behind the postural changes typically noted in the older adult. With aging, the intervertebral disks lose water, flatten, become porous, and undergo other deleterious changes at a cellular level.[8] These changes account for loss of disk height and compression of the spinal column—hence the inevitable height loss for all older adults. Spinal compression, combined with decrease in strength of intrascapular muscles and gradual wedging of the thoracic vertebrae, are contributing factors in increased thoracic spine *kyphosis* (rounding of the shoulders with a forward lean) commonly seen in elderly individuals.

Cardiopulmonary Function

Although aerobic capacity generally declines as one ages, the rate of decline can be diminished through physical activity.[8] *Maximum ventilatory uptake* (the maximum amount of oxygen the body inhales) usually drops between 5% and 10% per decade between the ages of 20 and 80.[9] Aerobic capacity, as measured by *maximal rate of oxygen consumption* (VO_2 max), declines in sedentary and active people with aging; however, the rate may be modulated by exercise training. Because cardiorespiratory capacity declines with age, it becomes less important to measure peak or maximal aerobic capacity unless monitoring the effectiveness of a particular cardiorespiratory intervention. Decline in VO_2 max can be attributed to a decrease in maximum heart rate with aging and to decreased muscle mass and decreased muscle demands, requiring less oxygen.[9] The metabolizing tissue contributing to VO_2 max measurement is almost exclusively muscle tissue, and, unless exercising to preserve muscle mass and strength, older adults experience a gradual loss of both. Improving the lung's functional capacity and functional reserve are keys to slowing the rate of decline of VO_2 max.[9] Older adults may increase functional capacity with aerobic exercise training. Individuals who report consistent physical activity over the course of their life have been found to maintain ventilatory oxygen uptake at a higher level than those who are inactive.[9]

Psychomotor and Psychological Functions

In general, there is a slowing in psychomotor performance in older adults, although differences in cognitive processing during the aging process are also subject to individual differences related to intelligence, health, and years of formal education.[10] Cerebrovascular disease and coronary heart disease can negatively affect cognition. Examples of some of the commonly observed changes in cognition with aging are (1) a decrease in *choice reaction time* (where a decision has to be made between tasks or in sequencing) and (2) an increase in *processing time for working memory* for complex tasks (such as involved mental arithmetic and lengthy sentence comprehension). *Fluid intelligence* (the ability to learn new information) is believed to decline with age, as opposed to *crystallized intelligence*, which reflects experiential learning.[10] Examples of crystallized abilities, which are generally understood to be maintained or improved over the lifespan, are verbal knowledge and comprehension.

Exercise over the long term has been found to be positively correlated with delaying the age-associated slowing of cognitive processing, specifically simple, discrimination, or choice reaction time.[10] Age-related cognitive decline is variable in both rate and onset, as evidenced by cross-sectional and longitudinal studies.[11-13] However, it has been observed that the reduction in cognitive efficiency seems to differentially affect knowledge-based and process-based abilities (also called *crystallized abilities* and *fluid abilities*, respectively).[10] Although the process-based abilities appear more vulnerable to decline, there is no single definitive mechanism to explain that observation. Sensory deficits, decreased attention, decreased processing speed, impaired neurotransmitter function, and impaired frontal lobe function are all possible contributing factors to the change in fluid abilities with age.[10]

Alzheimer's disease, stroke, and Parkinson's disease are the most prevalent brain pathologies with obvious cognitive impairments affecting older persons. Although physical activity may preserve functional independence to a point and promote oxygen delivery to the brain, claims cannot be made for it serving in a direct preventive manner against Alzheimer's disease and Parkinson's disease. These 2 health problems have more complicated etiologies than inactivity.

Physical activity can be used to reduce the risk of depressive disorders among adults and treat unpleasant symptoms of depression.[14] Exercise is a useful early intervention for mild to moderate depression, and chronic exercise has been associated with decreased depression. Unfortunately, only 34% of all adults with depressive symptoms are diagnosed and treated.[14] In light of depression's prevalence, the importance of healthy preventive tactics cannot be overstated. In most adults, effects of depression include lethargy, slowing of thought processes, moderate to severe sadness, possible confusion, memory loss (or difficulty retrieving memories), appetite loss, and, perhaps less commonly, restlessness and irritation.[14] Physical activity can help promote self-efficacy in the physical tasks of self-care and housekeeping.[14]

Mobility for Older Adults

Mobility is crucial to functional independence. There are several factors that contribute to a slowing of walking speed, primarily decrease in leg strength, lack of confidence in mobility or fear of falling, and an increased response time to environmental stimuli. The gait pattern of older adults often reflects a decreased stride length, a decrease in velocity, and concomitant higher cadence. Decreased joint flexibility can add to the slowing of walking speed because it encourages a decreased stride length and may also influence compromised balance. Walking should be encouraged for all older adults to maintain functional independence and stamina.

Successful Aging

Individuals who are at least 100 years of age, referred to as *centenarians*, are increasing in number, and many of these individuals live independently and participate in leisure and work activities. According to the New England Centenarian Study, individuals who live to be 100 years of age appear to escape some of the typical changes associated with aging; they have fewer instances of disease, hospitalization, and functional decline.[15] In the study, 8% had no incidence of life-threatening cancer, and 89% were living independently at age 92.[15] A survey of approximately 900 licensed physical therapists living into their ninth decade indicated that they experienced some declines in physical function and ambulation but less than those experienced by peers of the same age.[10] One might suspect that physical therapists possess the knowledge from their training about health and disease guiding their healthy lifestyle habits. Although a debate remains regarding how much genetics control longevity, current evidence suggests that engaging in regular exercise and maintaining a healthy weight contributes significantly to a longer and healthier life. The Harvard Alumni Health Study[16] followed a large group of men aged 45 to 84 beginning in 1977 through 1988 or until they reached the age of 90. The Harvard study strongly supports the physical exercise-longevity relationship. Essentially, it was found that the more active people were, the lower the risks of death from all causes between 1977 and 1988.[16]

Fitness and physical activity have been shown to positively influence cognitive functioning, working memory, risk and symptoms of depression, anxiety, positive self-concept, high self-esteem, mental well-being, and positive perceptions of health. There is a growing amount of evidence that the level of physical fitness, particularly cardiorespiratory fitness, is inversely related to the rate of cognitive decline.[17] The direct effects of physical activity include increased cerebral blood flow, increased glucose metabolism, neural efficiency, and increased production of neurotransmitters associated with memory storage and retrieval. Whereas typical aging seems to result in the development of chronic health conditions and loss of function, individuals who experience successful aging maintain a higher quality of life and overall health than other older adults.

Common Health Problems of Older Adults

Osteoarthritis

Osteoarthritis, also known as *degenerative arthritis,* is a form of arthritis occurring mainly in older persons that is characterized by chronic degeneration of the cartilage of the joints. Osteoarthritis is by far the most prevalent condition among older adults. Estimates for those affected by osteoarthritis range as high as 8%.[18] Traditionally, health professionals have advised older adults with osteoarthritis to refrain from many types of exercise for fear that exercise would lead to joint destruction, increased pain, and possible further injuries. Fortunately, the National Institutes of Health (NIH) and the American Geriatrics Society have both issued consensus statements supporting exercise in the prevention and treatment of osteoarthritis.[18] Regular exercise does not hasten disease progression but rather contributes to the reduction of pain, stiffness, and maintenance of range of motion in affected joints.[18] In addition to walking, more vigorous exercise, such as fairly high-intensity resistance training (60% to 80% of 1 repetition maximum weight) and stair climbing protect bone mass over time.[18] Not only does progressive resistance training assist in maintenance of bone mass, but it has been shown to lead to increases in muscle mass and strength, important contributors to fall prevention and overall functional independence.[18]

Although weight bearing is generally beneficial in terms of bone density, individuals prone to osteoarthritis may benefit from exercising at least 50% of the time in a nonweight-bearing or low-impact environment, such as aquatic exercise or bicycling. Exercise programs for persons who either have osteoarthritis or who are at high risk for osteoarthritis should be modified at the first mention of joint pain with exercise. Close attention to proper alignment and technique is also essential for safe completion of the recommended exercise program.

Cardiovascular Disease

Among the leading causes of death and disability of older adults are cardiovascular disease, stroke, and cancer.[19] Approximately 9% of adults aged 70 and older are affected by strokes every year. Incidence of stroke was followed as part of the Harvard Alumni Health Study, and all but light-intensity activities appeared protective of stroke for this group of approximately 11,000 men when data for stroke incidence were gathered in 1988 and 1990.[19]

Heart disease in older adults is commonly the culmination of lifelong lifestyle habits, including exercise, diet, and stress management. Additional information about cardiovascular disease can be found in Chapter 14.

Diabetes

Diabetes is a common chronic disease that causes mortality and complicates other health problems that older adults experience. Risk factors for type 2 diabetes include advancing age (older than age 45 years), obesity, family history, and a history of gestational diabetes. Research examining the effectiveness of the Diabetes Prevention Program found that intensive counseling on effective diet, exercise, and behavior modification reduced their risk of developing diabetes by 71% in adults older than age 60.[20] Additional information about the Diabetes Prevention Program and management of diabetes can be found at the National Diabetes Information Clearinghouse website: http://diabetes.niddk.nih.gov/dm/pubs/preventionprogram/.[20]

Chronic Obstructive Pulmonary Disease

Approximately 11% of older adults are affected by one form of *chronic obstructive pulmonary disease (COPD)*. Exercise benefits the physical functioning, the ability to breathe, and the mood of adults with this condition, but it also offers cognitive benefits to older adults. In a study of older adults with COPD (mean age, 67.8 ± 74 years), acute aerobic exercise for 20 minutes was associated with improved cognitive functioning, including improved verbal fluency and verbal processing.[21] This study further supports the benefits of physical activity to reduce pathology and improve mental health, particularly in the older adult population. Additional information about COPD is provided in Chapter 14.

Screening Older Adults for Health, Fitness, and Wellness

After screening the older adult for past medical conditions, prior treatment, use of medications, current complaints, and general health, more specific questions can address the areas that are often at risk in the older adult: mental, psychological, and physical function. Although an in-depth examination of these 3 areas of function is beyond the scope of this text, recognizing the comprehensive nature of screening is critical for identifying and addressing the health needs of the older adult.

Older adults who are isolated with minimal interaction have been shown to experience more depression and perceive that their life has a lower quality than individuals who report more regular interactions with family and friends. Increasing numbers of seniors are being identified as having problems associated with addiction to alcohol or drugs. Estimates of alcohol abuse range from 2% to 17%, with most experts agreeing the incidence will increase as the generation known as the baby boomers enter their seventh decade.[22]

The older adult dependent on family or health care organizations for any daily living activities is particularly vulnerable to abuse; the incidence of elder abuse varies widely, from 450,000 to 2 million.[23] Screening procedures by physical therapists should include information related to the signs and symptoms of elder abuse. Information about red flags for elder abuse and appropriate referrals are discussed in Chapter 12.

Recognizing signs and symptoms of abuse and taking appropriate steps to report the information is critical to promoting basic safety and security in older adult clients.

Nutrition Screening

Good nutrition is essential for physical function and is often overlooked during a health screening. Approximately 16% of elderly persons living in the community consume less than 1000 kcal per day, an amount that does not maintain adequate nutrition.[24] Individuals who are dehydrated or inadequately nourished can also experience dizzy spells contributing to falls.[24] The following nutrition screening tool can be used to identify older adults who may not be eating appropriate foods for optimal function:

- Does the individual appear dehydrated (dry lips, dry skin, parched mouth, difficulty speaking, frail skin)?
- Does the individual take any vitamin or mineral supplements?
- How many calories does the individual consume?

The Nutrition Screening Client Interview Form in Table 9-1 may prove useful in collecting additional information for a nutrition referral.[25]

Mental Health Function

Mental health function is often referred to as *psychological function*, or a person's mental and affective skills and abilities. Although the complete examination and treatment of mental and affective function is outside of a physical therapist's area of practice, recognizing problems within these functional areas and making appropriate referrals is critical for long-term health and wellness of the individual. Common tests used for screening older adults' mental function status include the Mini-Mental Status Examination (MMSE)[26] and the Geriatric Depression Scale (GDS). Another recent cognitive screening tool is the St. Louis University Mental Status (SLUMS) examination. This easy and freely available tool distinguishes between older adults with mild and more advanced dementia and also takes into consideration the level of secondary education completed. Similar to the MMSE, the SLUMS may identify problems with orientation, attention, immediate and short-term recall, language, and the ability to follow simple verbal and written commands.[27] The GDS is a short screening tool used to identify older adults who are at risk for depression or who are depressed when screened.[28] Individuals experiencing depression should be referred to the his or her primary physician or a psychologist for a more comprehensive examination of presenting signs and symptoms.

Physical Health Function

Because physiologic markers of fitness change as one ages, it becomes more important to measure physical fitness in elderly individuals in a way that does not use standards formulated with young persons. Relative improvements in oxygen uptake and use become more important with aging than absolute increases in maximal oxygen consumption. Physical mobility and gait are commonly measured with the same screening tools. Physical mobility may incorporate balance skills, transfer skills, and gait, as measured by the *Berg Balance Scale*, or may be focused on gait speed and the ability to stand up, as measured by the *Timed Up and Go Test*.[29] The *Tinetti Mobility Index* is another commonly used mobility scale that focuses primarily on balance and gait.[30]

Table 9-1. Nutrition Screening Client Interview Form

Client's name ______________ Date of screening: ______________

Introduce self and purpose of visit: (I would like to ask you some questions so that we can assess your nutritional status.)

1. Have you experienced any changes in your weight in the last 6 months?
   - Weight loss of ______________ lb
   - Weight gain of ______________ lb
   - No change in weight ______________
   - If weight loss, was it planned (were you trying to lose weight)? ______________
2. What is your usual weight? ______________ lb

   If weight loss calculate:

   % weight change = usual weight − current weight/usual weight × 100 =

   ____

   Evaluate significance of weight loss as follows:

TIME	SIGNIFICANT WEIGHT LOSS (% OF CHANGE)	SEVERE WEIGHT LOSS (% OF CHANGE)
1 week	1 to 2	> 2
1 month	5	> 5
3 months	7.5	> 7.5
6 months	10	> 10

   Calculate: % usual body weight: current weight/usual weight × 100 = ______________.

   Enter % of usual body weight on screening form: ______________

3. How would you describe your appetite? (circle one)

Excellent	Good	Fair	Poor*	No appetite*

4. Are you having any of the following problems? (check all that apply).

   _____ Difficulty chewing
   _____ Difficulty swallowing
   _____ Nausea
   _____ Vomiting
   _____ Constipation
   _____ Diarrhea
   _____ Mouth sores

5. Are there any foods that you are allergic to?
6. Do you have any food preference (likes or dislikes) you'd like to tell us about?
7. Have you been following any special diet at home? Are you currently taking any liquid supplements like Ensure or Sustacal? How often? Flavor preference?
8. Are you currently taking any vitamin, mineral, or herbal supplements? What kind?

Completed by: ______________ Date: ______________

*If patients are having any of these problems, refer to dietitian.

Adapted from Laporte M, Villalon L, Payette H. Development and validity of a single malnutrition screening tool adapted to adult and elderly populations in acute and long term care facilities [abstract]. *Can J Diet Pract Res*. 1998;59:160.

Social Function

Understanding the role of social function is critical to the health care professional. Healthy social function is a component of the healthy older adult. Attending to this area of function is critical for assuring the long-term health and wellness of the older individual. Questionnaires and surveys associated with frequency of interactions with family and friends, frequency of trips outside the home, and schedule of activities for volunteer or work purposes provide some insight into an individual's social function.

Comprehensive Screening Tools

Many of these surveys or questionnaires are incorporated into more comprehensive screening tools, such as the *Short Form (SF)-36*. The recently updated SF-36 (version 2) has proven useful in surveys of general and specific populations, comparing the relative burden of diseases and differentiating the health benefits produced by a wide range of different treatments.[31] As a measure of perceived health, the SF-36 v.2 has greater face validity than the single-question self-ratings of health described previously because it encompasses 8 health concepts using multi-item scales, plus 1 single item pertaining to change in perceived health during the past 12 months. General health perception (5 items) is 1 of the 8 scales of the SF-36 v.2.[31] The other 7 health concepts addressed by the multi-item scales are physical functioning (10 items), role limitations caused by physical health problems (4 items), role limitations caused by emotional problems (3 items), social functioning (2 items), emotional well-being (5 items), energy/fatigue (4 items), and pain (2 items).

The *World Health Organization Quality of Life (WHOQOL-BREF)* is another self-report questionnaire that can identify quality of life issues in older adults across multiple areas.[32] The 26-item questionnaire provides information in 4 domains: physical health, psychological health, social relationships, and environment. Used extensively in research, this questionnaire had been translated into 19 languages and serves as a useful tool for screening individuals from different cultures.[32]

Because older adults are at an increased risk for falls, many of the physical factors contributing to falls are screened using tools described in the multiple-dimension assessment of falls. Self-report questionnaires that combine measures of psychological, mental, and physical function are easily administered and provide valuable information. The *Health Survey* is a questionnaire updated to accommodate the special needs of older adults, providing a more consistent format and wording than earlier versions. The Health Survey is composed of 36 questions that address the physical components (physical function, physical role, bodily pain, and general health) and mental components (mental health, emotional role, social function, and vitality) of health.[33] This self-report tool yields an 8-scale profile of functional health and well-being scores, as well as psychometrically based physical and mental health summary measures and a preference-based health utility index.

Screening for Fall Risk

The Centers for Disease Control and Prevention (CDC) National Center for Health Statistics estimates that by 2020, the health care costs for fall injuries among people older than 65 will reach more than 30 billion dollars per year.[34] Falls are a result of multiple factors, both intrinsic and extrinsic. Intrinsic, individual factors to consider include decreased sensory system function, decreased postural control and balance, increased reactions to single and multiple medications, musculoskeletal impairments, and decreased cognition. Extrinsic factors that contribute to falls include the environment the individual resides in and equipment used for safety and mobility. Physical therapists are uniquely qualified to screen for both intrinsic and extrinsic factors that may place an individual at increased fall risk. Preventing or reducing falls in the elderly should be of primary importance to the physical therapist. Early identification of high-risk individuals allows for steps to be taken to decrease the chance for future falls. Evidence suggests that a prior fall places an individual at increased risk for future falls. Therefore, simple questionnaires requesting information related to fall frequency and the factors surrounding the fall should include, but not be limited to, the following: (1) location of fall, (2) activity prior to fall, (3) loss of consciousness, (4) use of walking aids (eg, cane, walker) and/or protective devices (eg, hip protectors, helmet), (5) environmental conditions (eg, snow, ice), and (6) injuries that resulted from the fall. The CDC recently published the STEADI (Stopping Elderly Accidents, Deaths and Injuries) guidelines, which include a questionnaire and physical tasks for the older adult to complete to better understand the person's risk for falls. Results from both the questionnaire and the physical tasks are best interpreted by a physical therapist to determine an individual's risk for falls and to make appropriate recommendations related to referrals and lifestyle changes that may decrease his or her fall risk. Educational material is also available through the STEADI program, which provides useful information on how to decrease fall risk.

Screening for Vital Signs

Basic physiological functioning, measured by vital signs at rest and during exercise, helps to identify problems with blood pressure, respiration, or other body functions that may be compromised by acute illness or injury. For example, individuals with untreated hypotension are at increased risk of falling as they transition from one position to another, often a result of *orthostatic hypotension* (dropping blood pressure when positioned antigravity).

Screening for Medications

In addition to questions related to fall history, a thorough history of current medications is needed when examining fall risk because certain medications can contribute to increased fall risk. It is particularly important to review current prescribed medications, over-the-counter medications, dietary supplements, and recreational drugs (including alcohol) the individual may be using. Common side effects of drugs include drowsiness, confusion, dizziness, lethargy, sedation, changes in bladder or bowel function, impaired balance and reaction time, and hypotension. The use of multiple drugs, or *polypharmacy*, may further compromise motor function and lead to increased fall risk. Drug side effects commonly impair postural control and balance. Generalized sedation, postural hypotension, and impaired psychomotor abilities are common associated drug reactions that older adults experience with medication use. Limited evidence suggests multiple medications, as well as some specific classifications of medications, such as benzodiazepines, result in side effects that diminish an individual's balance ability.[35] In addition, medications for cardiovascular problems cause *hypotension* (a reduction in blood pressure of 20 mm Hg 1 or 3 minutes after moving between supine and stand). Orthostatic hypotension may place a client at an increased risk for falls if he or she has a recent history of one or more falls. Table 9-2 summarizes the side effects associated with commonly prescribed medications.[36] A careful medication history is critical to understanding and identifying an individual's fall risk.

Screening of Sensory Systems

A visual screening may help identify those at increased risk for falling. Using a Snellen chart, the health care professional may determine visual acuity. Questions that are helpful for identifying visual problems include asking about current problems with poor visual acuity, problems related to a reduced visual field, impaired contrast sensitivity, and problems with depth perception. Note the date and results of most recent eye examination. All older adults should be advised to have regular visual screening tests performed by their regular physician or an ophthalmologist. Vestibular dysfunction is also more common in older adults. Generally, individuals will complain of dizziness,

Table 9-2. Side Effects of Geriatric Medications	
DRUGS AFFECTING MOBILITY	**ADVERSE DRUG REACTIONS**
Tricyclic antidepressants	May cause postural hypotension, tremor, cardiac arrhythmias, or sedation
Benzodiazepines and sedative hypnotics	May cause sedation, weakness, decreased coordination, or confusion
Narcotic analgesics	May cause sedation, decreased coordination, or confusion
Antipsychotics	May cause postural hypotension, sedation, or extrapyramidal effects
Antihypertensives	May cause postural hypotension
Beta-adrenergic blockers	May decrease ability to respond to workload

Adapted from Drugs associated with increased risk of falls in the elderly. Davis's Drug Guide. http://www.drugguide.com/ddo/ub/view/Davis-Drug-Guide/109640/all/Drugs_Associated_with_Increased_Risk_of_Falls_in_the_Elderly. Accessed May 20, 2014.

difficulties with balance, or decreased tolerance to standing for long periods of time. Likewise, pain can alter overall posture, leading to an increased risk for falls in older adults.

Screening Upright Control and Balance

Screening tools that examine upright control and balance tasks are recommended. Although strength and range of motion contribute to overall functional gait and balance, assessing fall risk requires the examiner to attend to functional tasks associated with upright postural control and balance. The Timed Up and Go Test, Functional Reach Test, and Berg Balance Scale have all been shown to have limited predictive value of future falls.[37]

Falls are a complicated issue and are almost always multifactorial in nature (ie, not purely the result of a single factor, such as poor balance). Used in combination, these screening tools and carefully crafted questionnaires and scales assist the physical therapist in identifying who would benefit from future follow-up from a physician, physical therapist, or other health care or social service provider. Older adults and their health care provider(s) should be provided with all information collected through the screening, including the physical therapist's recommendations. Physical therapists involved in identifying older adults at fall risk provide older adults, their families, and their communities with an important service. Even more importantly, this early identification gives the older adult an opportunity to modify fall risk through appropriate physical activity and exercise, environmental adjustment, and medical treatment. Recommendations for exercise to assist in prevention of falls usually include resistance training, aerobic exercise, dynamic weight-bearing exercise such as dance or t'ai chi, or sports such as tennis and water exercise.[38]

Environmental Assessment

An environmental assessment can often identify modifiable risk factors, such as rugs, floor mats, a lack of handrails in toilets, or clutter, that potentially cause falls in older adults. For individuals with poor vision, nonglare surfaces on walls, floors, and stairs improve the ability to see potential obstacles in their path. Also, glare-free lighting enables a better view for walking. Often wet floors or icy steps contribute to falls both inside and outside of the home. All individuals should be cautioned about venturing onto surfaces, such as freshly-cleaned floors, that lack traction for safe walking.

Fall Prevention Programs for Older Adults

After performing the screening for falls, the physical therapist must determine if the risk factors are modifiable or nonmodifiable. Health education about the modifiable risk factors should be discussed in detail with resources for future reference. The American Physical Therapy Association provides a helpful booklet entitled "What You Need to Know about Balance and Falls" that can be obtained through their website at http://www.apta.org.[39]

In addition, the National Institute on Aging offers advice for preventing falls and fractures because osteoporosis is one of the most common pathologies in older adults. The website (http://www.niapublications.org/engagepages/falls.asp) lists a number of suggestions for preventing falls and making the home safe.[40] The Home Safety Council, an organization whose mission is to educate and assist families in taking preventive action, lists similar information on its website at http://www.homesafetycouncil.org.[41] As mentioned previously, one of the most comprehensive, current resources specific to older adult safety was designed by the CDC and is available at http://www.cdc.gov/homeandrecreationalsafety/Falls/steadi/index.html.

Comprehensive fall prevention programs are the most effective efforts for reducing the risks of falls, so the physical therapist should work with a team of health care professionals to reduce risk factors for older adults. Interventions for fall prevention include the following:

- Identification of individual risk factors that contribute to falls
- Identification of the environmental factors that contribute to falls
- Determining factors associated with the movement by the individual (such as reaching, lifting, walking, or turning)
- Properly managing medications and other health supplements
- Improving physical mobility through exercise programs, balance, gait training, and appropriate use of walking aids
- Educating family members about risk factors
- Continence promotion and toileting programs
- Addressing any other factors that could potentially contribute to falls

The most successful fall prevention programs are individualized to the unique needs of the senior after careful consideration of the areas listed above.

Health education is a key component of reducing risks of falls. The National Center for Injury Prevention and Control (http://www.cdc.gov/ncipc) provides the following brochures free of charge: *Check for Safety: A Home Fall Prevention Checklist for Older Adults* (099-6156), *Check for Safety* (Spanish) (099-6590), and *What YOU Can Do to Prevent Falls* (Spanish) (099-6589).[42]

Assessment of Physical Activity

Physical therapists are uniquely qualified to assess the physical activity of older adults. Physical activity, a complex behavior with no single standard measurement, has been shown to increase the quality and longevity of life. Current techniques include behavioral observation and diaries, physiological markers, electronic monitors, and self-report instruments. No single instrument meets all criteria of being valid, reliable, and practical.

Over the course of one's life, physical activity may not always lead directly to favorable results as indicated by the customary markers of physical performance and fitness, such as VO_2 max and body composition. There are now instruments, such as pedometers (devices that measure walking distance) and accelerometers (devices that measure body movement in 3 planes), as well as laboratory methods such as *calorimetry* that confine a person to a closed space to measure calorie expenditure. However, the most frequently used tools are self-reports covering a range of frequencies (one day to decades). The *Minnesota Leisure-Time Physical Activity Questionnaire*,[43] the *Yale Physical Activity Survey for Older Adults*,[44] and the *Modified Baecke Questionnaire for Older Adults*[45] are 3 well-validated, easily administered activity assessments. *The Minnesota Leisure-Time Physical Activity Questionnaire* is an interviewer-administered tool that covers the past 12 months and is, in part, completed by an interviewer.

Before initiating an exercise program, the older adult should be screened for possible signs and symptoms that need medical attention. The following clinical manifestations warrant a visit to the physician before initiating a standard exercise program: chest pain or pressure, shortness of breath, heartbeat irregularities, blood clots, infections or fever, unplanned weight loss, foot or ankle sores that will not heal, a hernia, joint swelling, pain or trouble walking after a fall, a bleeding or detached retina, recent eye surgery or laser treatment, recent hip surgery, light-headedness or dizziness, difficulty with balance, or nausea. The fitness levels of older adults vary considerably based on the physical activity and general health of the older adult. To obtain a complete picture of the health-related fitness of the older adult, one needs to assess cardiorespiratory function, muscular strength, muscular endurance, flexibility, and body composition.

There are several ways to assess cardiorespiratory fitness or estimated VO_2 max. However, for some elderly individuals, these tests can taxing. The Rockport 1-Mile Walk Test, involving a 1-mile walk at the fastest pace possible, is commonly used.[46] The YMCA 3-Minute Step Test is another alternative for estimating VO_2 max from postexercise recovery heart rate; however, it is not feasible for extremely deconditioned individuals or those with visual perception or balance deficits. If conducted properly, a submaximal VO_2 test provides a valid measure of cardiorespiratory fitness; however, it does not measure physical fitness in a broader sense.

Functional fitness refers to "the physical capacity of the individual to meet ordinary and unexpected demands of daily life safely and effectively."[47] A functional fitness test provides health-related fitness information that can be used to determine independent living in the later years. The focus of functional fitness assessments is on assessment of the individual's capacity to perform skills for daily activities and evaluation of the individual's routine. For those at risk for functional dependence, functional fitness tests are more sensitive than traditional measures of cardiorespiratory fitness.[47] Besides being a more holistic approach to fitness than strictly VO_2 max, a functional fitness test has a second practical value of potentially challenging elderly participants without pushing them to exhaustion. Because physical mobility problems contribute the most to lost functional independence,[47] it is prudent to rely on a functional test that assesses several mobility-related fitness parameters. Functioning testing can also identify risk factors or developing problems missed on self-report questionnaires.

Functional measures have shown their usefulness in predicting outcomes, such as mortality or nursing center placement, as well as in assessing present mobility and independence in activities of daily living.[47] Another important consideration in the older adult population is that factors such as pain, visual deficits, and compromised balance may modify the association between strength and function. Conducting a functional fitness test enables the examiner to evaluate whether any of these aforementioned factors affect physical performance.

The *Continuous Scale Physical Functional Performance Test (CS-PFP)* examines upper body strength, lower body strength, flexibility, balance and coordination, and endurance and comprises several tasks quantified by time, distance, or weight.[48] An example of a CS-PFP item in the lower body strength domain is timed performance of 5 repetitions of sit-to-stand movements. A limitation of this examination tool is the significant amount of time needed to instruct and observe each test item; however, it can be helpful in demonstrating clinical improvements in specific health-related areas.[48]

The *physical performance test (PPT)* assesses multiple domains of function simulating activities of daily living: strength, mobility, and dexterity.[49] Meant to be administered in 10 minutes or less, there are 2 versions: one with 9 items and one with 7. The abbreviated version does not entail stair climbing. Tasks are varied, ranging from writing a sentence to walking 50 feet, enabling the examiner to identify limitations in separate domains of function.

AAHPERD Test Battery for Older Adults was developed for the American Alliance for Health, Physical Education, Recreation and Dance (AAHPERD) as a sound, practical measure of fitness; however, there are 2 features that limit its use.[50] The flexibility measure must be completed from a straight-leg position on the floor, and the test of aerobic endurance is challenging for many because it is a half-mile walk.

The *Senior Fitness Test* is a battery of performance tests designed to assess the physical parameters associated with functional mobility in older adults.[51] The motive behind the development of this functional test was to detect physical decline and address it because some physical decline during aging is preventable and, to some extent, reversible. The *6-Minute Walk*, a subtest of the Senior Fitness Test, has been used to effectively determine exercise capacity in older patients with congestive heart failure, and has convergent validity with self-rated health and physical functioning. Development trials for the senior fitness test show that lower extremity function subtests (the Chair Stand, the 8-Feet Up-and-Go, and the 6-Minute Walk) are strongly associated with walking, moving quickly when necessary, stair-climbing, dressing, and bathing. In older adults, if muscle weakness develops in the lower extremities, it may lead to the inability to perform fundamentally important activities, such as getting up from a seated position. The chair stand subtest is also helpful in identifying older adults who are more active.

It is important that functional fitness tests be administered by health professionals or professionals trained in exercise science, not only to insure safety of those participating in the test, but also because of the knowledge necessary to interpret the results. Baseline vital signs should be taken and closely monitored during and following more strenuous tests.

Fitness for Older Adults

The general recommendation of 30 minutes or more of moderate intensity exercise on most, and preferably all, days of the week applies to older adults who are not limited by serious health problems. One feature of this public health recommendation is the acknowledgment that intermittent, brief sessions of physical activity are appropriate for meeting the 30-minute total.[52] Some examples are walking 2 miles in 30 minutes, shoveling snow for 15 minutes, and raking leaves for 30 minutes. Swimming laps at a moderate pace for 30 minutes burns about twice as many calories. Barbara Ainsworth of the School of Public Health at the University of Minnesota, along with several exercise science colleagues, has developed a compendium of occupational, household, recreational, and sport physical activities.[52] The main impetus for development of this compendium was to develop comparable coding systems for physical activities across research studies. This resource lists activities by purpose and energy cost. There is a *metabolic equivalent unit (MET)* listed for each activity. Moderate-intensity physical activities are generally 3 to 5 MET. However, many older adult clients are more attuned to energy expenditure in terms of kilocalories or time spent on an activity.

In light of the expected growth of the older segment of the population, increasing the knowledge about the relationships between physical fitness, physical activity, and health in the senior citizen has the potential to positively influence overall health and wellness for this population. According to the CDC, 28% to 44% of adults over the age of 65 are inactive (ie, they participate in no leisure time physical activity).[52] Inactivity is more common in older people than in middle-aged men and women, and women were more likely than men to report no leisure time activity. Because successful aging is largely determined by individual lifestyle changes, this portion of the population is at the greatest risk of developing pathology secondary to a sedentary lifestyle. Women who are inactive and nonsmoking at the age of 65 have 12.7 years of active life expectancy compared with active, nonsmoking women, who have 18.4 years.[52] Estimates for 2000 indicated that only 13% of individuals between the ages of 65 and 74 reported engaging in vigorous physical activity for 20 minutes 3 or more days per week, and only 6% of those 75 and older reported such exercise.[52]

By 2030, the number of older adults in the United States is expected to reach 70 million, and the percentage of the total population aged 65 or older is expected to grow to 20%.[52] This growing population will place increasing demands on the public health system and on medical and social services. "Lack of physical activity and poor diet are the major causes of an epidemic of obesity that is affecting the elderly as well as middle-aged and younger populations. An estimated 18% of adults over age 65 in the United States are obese, and another 40% are overweight, putting them at substantially increased risk for diabetes, high blood pressure, heart disease, along with other chronic diseases."[52] Being inactive also affects balance as a result of losses in muscle strength and increased the risk of falls. Every year, fall-related injuries among older people cost the nation more than $20.2 billion. By 2020, the total annual cost of these injuries is expected to reach $32.4 billion.[52] Preventing chronic illness and injury in older adults should be cause enough to engage in regular physical activity. Older adults can benefit physically, cognitively, and psychosocially from physical activity performed on a regular basis. For this reason, increased physical activity in older adults should be promoted on a local, state, and national level.

Substantial health benefits occur with a moderate amount of activity (eg, at least 30 minutes of brisk walking) on 5 or more days of the week. Brief episodes of physical activity, such as 10 minutes at a time, can be beneficial if repeated. Sedentary persons can begin with brief episodes and gradually increase the duration or intensity of activity. One review of the literature revealed that programs to build muscle strength, improve balance, and promote walking significantly reduced falls in older persons. Experts recommend that older adults should participate at least 2 days a week in strength training activities that improve and maintain muscular strength and endurance.[52] Older adults are sensitive to the effects of physical activity, and even small amounts of activity are healthier than a sedentary lifestyle. Water exercises and low-impact exercises can be complemented by strength training exercises. Exercise programs that involve t'ai chi have been shown to help enhance balance, whereas yoga can improve flexibility.[52]

A recent study found that only half of all adults were asked about their exercise habits by their health care provider; older patients were asked less often than younger patients; and individuals who had been asked reported being more active than those who were never asked.[52] Collecting information from older clients about their activity level is a critical step all health care professionals should undertake in the overall management of the geriatric client. Physical therapists are best qualified to assist their older clients with chronic conditions in setting activity and fitness goals and recommend individually tailored physical activity regimens All health care professionals need to have knowledge of community resources of benefit to the older adult interested in improving overall health, wellness, and fitness.

Summary

Older adults are a diverse population with significant needs in the areas of long-term health, wellness, and fitness. Various health care professionals can optimize older adults' lives by providing health education and making recommendations to assist the older adult in maintaining or improving overall health, fitness, and wellness. Perhaps more so than any other age group, older adults experience a wide variety of changes in their bodies and abilities due to their unique genetic make-up, lifestyle, and environment. Assessing body systems for needed therapeutic activity, viewing environments where daily activities take place, and screening for falls offer primary prevention. Promoting healthy lifestyle habits that incorporate physical activity, healthy nutrition, mental fitness, and social engagement may reduce the risks of common chronic conditions, such as depression, diabetes, osteoporosis, and cardiovascular disease.

REFERENCES

1. Celebrate long-term living during Older Americans Month. Kentucky Cabinet for Health and Human Services. http://chfs.ky.gov/news/Older+Americans+Month+1.htm. Accessed June 1, 2013.
2. Erickson E. *Erikson on Development in Adulthood: New Insights From the Unpublished Papers*. London, UK: Oxford University Press Inc; 2002.
3. Centers for Disease Control and Prevention. Unrealized prevention opportunities reducing the health and economic burden of chronic disease. Atlanta, GA: CDC National Center for Chronic Disease Prevention and Health Promotion; 1997.
4. Fried LP, Tangen CM, Walston J, et al. Frailty in older adults: evidence for a phenotype. *J Gerontol A Biol Sci Med Sci*. 2001;56(3):M146-M156.
5. Rosenberg IH, Miller JW. Nutritional factors in physical and cognitive functions of elderly people. *Am J Clin Nutr*. 2000;55:1237S-1243S.
6. Nelson ME, Fiatarone MA, Morganti CM, Trice I, Greenberg RA, Evans WJ. Effects of high-intensity strength training on multiple risk factors for osteoporotic fractures: a randomized controlled trial. *JAMA*. 1994;272:1909-1914.
7. Slovik DM. Osteoporosis. In: Fronters WR, ed. *Exercise in Rehabilitation Medicine*. 3rd ed. Champaign, IL: Human Kinetics; 1999:313-348.
8. Turner CH, Robling AG. Designing exercise regimens to increase bone strength. *Exerc Sports Sci Rev*. 2003;31:45-50.
9. Spirduso WW. *Physical Dimensions of Aging*. Champaign, IL: Human Kinetics; 1995.
10. Gucionne A, ed. *Geriatric Physical Therapy*. 2nd ed. St. Louis, MO: Mosby; 2000.
11. Aartsen MJ, Smits CH, van Tilburg T, Knipscheer KC, Deeg DJ. Activity in older adults: cause or consequence of cognitive functioning? A longitudinal study on everyday activities and cognitive performance in older adults. *J Gerontol B Psychol Sci Soc Sci*. 2002;57(2):P153-P162.
12. Markowska AL, Savonenko AV. Protective effect of practice on cognition during aging: implications for predictive characteristics of performance and efficacy of practice. *Neurobiol Learn Mem*. 2002;78(2):294-320.
13. McArdle JJ, Ferrer-Caja E, Hamagami F, Woodcock RW. Comparative longitudinal structural analyses of growth and decline of multiple intellectual abilities over the life span. *Dev Psychol*. 2002;38(1):115-142.
14. Churchill JD, Galvez R, Colcombe S, Swain RA, Kramer AF, Greenough WT. Exercise, experience and the aging brain. *Neurobiol Aging*. 2002;23:941-955.
15. Dellara T, Wilcox M, McCormick M, Perls T. Cardiovascular disease delay in centenarian offspring. *J Gerontol Sci Med Sci*. 2004;59:M385-M389.
16. Lee IM, Hsieh CC, Paffenbarger RS. Exercise intensity and longevity in men. The Harvard Alumni Health Study. *JAMA*. 1995;273(15):1179-1184.
17. Colcombe S, Kramer AF. Fitness effects on the cognitive function of older adults: a meta-analytic study. *Psychol Sci*. 2003;14(2):125-130.
18. American Geriatrics Society Panel on Exercise and Osteoarthritis. Exercise prescription for older adults with osteoarthritis pain: consensus practice recommendations: a supplement to the AGS Clinical Practice Guidelines on the management of chronic pain in older adults. *J Am Geriatr Soc*. 2001;49(6):808-823.
19. American Heart Association. *Heart And Stroke Statistical Update*. Dallas, TX: American Heart Association; 2002.
20. The Diabetes Prevention Program and management of diabetes. National Diabetes Information Clearinghouse. http://diabetes.niddk.nih.gov/dm/pubs/preventionprogram/. Accessed June 1, 2013.
21. Berry MJ, Rejeski WJ, Adair NE, Ettinger HH Jr, Zaccaro DJ, Sevick MA. A randomized, controlled trial comparing long-term and short-term exercise in patients with chronic obstructive pulmonary disease. *J Cardiopulm Rehab*. 2003;23:60-68.
22. Williams GD, Stinson FS, Parker DA, Harford TC, Noble J. Demographic trends, alcohol abuse and alcoholism, 1985-1995 [epidemiologic bulletin no. 15]. *Alcohol Health & Research World*. 1987;11(3):80-83.
23. Reed R, Mooradian A. Treatment of diabetes in the elderly. *Am Fam Physician*. 1991;44(3):915-924.
24. Dietary targets for your senior years. PDR Health. http://www.pdrhealth.com/content/nutrition_health/chapters/fgnt20.shtml. Accessed February 12, 2006.
25. Laporte M, Villalon L, Payette H. Development and validity of a single malnutrition screening tool adapted to adult and elderly populations in acute and long term care facilities [abstract]. *Can J Diet Practice Res*. 1998;59:160.
26. Folstein MF, Folstein, SE, McHugh PR. Mini-mental state: a practical method for grading the state of patients for the clinician. *J Psychiatr Res*. 1975;12:189-198.
27. VAMC SLUM exam. Department of Veterans Affairs. http://medschool.slu.edu/agingsuccessfully/pdfsurveys/slumsexam_05.pdf. Accessed December 20, 2013.
28. Brink TL, Yesavage JA, Lum O, Heersema P, Adey MB, Rose TL. Screening tests for geriatric depression. *Clin Gerontol*. 1982;1:37-44.

29. Steffen TM, Hacker TA, Mollinger L. Age- and gender-related test performance in community-dwelling elderly people: Six-Minute Walk Test, Berg Balance Scale, Timed Up & Go Test, and gait speeds. *Phys Ther.* 2002;82(2):128-137.
30. Tinetti ME, Williams TF, Mayewski R. Fall risk index for elderly patients based on number of chronic disabilities. *Am J Med.* 1986;80(3):429-434.
31. Friedman B, Heisel M, Delavan R. Validity of the SF-36 five-item Mental Health Index for major depression in functionally impaired, community-dwelling elderly patients. *J Am Geriatr Soc.* 2005;53(11):1978-1985.
32. World Health Organization. Study protocol for the World Health Organization project to develop a Quality of Life assessment instrument (WHOQOL). *Qual Life Res.* 1993;2(2):153-159.
33. 36-Item Short Form Survey from the RAND Medical Outcomes Study. Rand Health. http://www.rand.org/health/surveys_tools/mos/mos_core_36item.html. Accessed May 30, 2013.
34. Falls and hip fractures among older adults. National Center for Injury Prevention and Control. http://www.cdc.gov/ncipc/factsheets/falls.htm. Accessed June 1, 2013.
35. Allain H, Bentue-Ferrer D, Polard E, Akwa Y, Patat A. Postural instability and consequent falls and hip fractures associated with use of hypnotics in the elderly: a comparative review. *Drugs Aging.* 2005;22(9):749-65.
36. Drugs associated with increased risk of falls in the elderly. Davis's Drug Guide. http://www.drugguide.com/ddo/ub/view/Davis-Drug-Guide/109640/all/Drugs_Associated_with_Increased_Risk_of_Falls_in_the_Elderly. Accessed May 20, 2014.
37. Thapa PB, Gideon P, Brockman KG, Fought RL, Ray WA. Clinical and biomechanical measures of balance as fall predictors in ambulatory nursing home residents. *J Gerontol A Biol Sci Med Sci.* 1996;51(5):M239-M246.
38. Li F, Harmer P, Fisher KJ, et al. Tai chi and fall reductions in older adults: a randomized controlled trial. *J Gerontol.* 2005;60A(2):187-194.
39. Physical therapist's guide to falls. American Physical Therapy Association. http://www.moveforwardpt.com/symptomsconditionsdetail.aspx?cid=85726fb6-14c4-4c16-9a4c-3736dceac9f0#.U3vPnCgngTI. Accessed May 20, 2014.
40. Preventing falls and fractures. National Institute of Aging. http://www.niapublications.org/engagepages/falls.asp. Accessed February 12, 2006.
41. Home Safety Council. http://www.homesafetycouncil.org. Accessed May 30, 2013.
42. Check for safety: a home fall prevention checklist for older adults (099-6156). The National Center for Injury Prevention and Control. http://www.cdc.gov/ncipc. Accessed February 12, 2006.
43. Folsom AR, Jacobs DR Jr, Caspersen CJ, Gomez-Marin O, Knudsen J. Test-retest reliability of the Minnesota Leisure Time Physical Activity Questionnaire. *J Chronic Dis.* 1986;39(7):505-511.
44. Dipietro L, Caspersen CJ, Ostfeld AM, Nadel ER. A survey for assessing physical activity among older adults. *Med Sci Sports Exerc.* 1993;25(5):628-642.
45. Buchheit M, Simon C, Viola AU, Doutreleau S, Piquard F, Brandenberger G. Heart rate variability in sportive elderly: Relationship with daily physical activity. *Med Sci Sports Exerc.* 2004;36(4):601-605.
46. Pober DM, Freedson PS, Kline GM, McInnis KJ, Rippe JM. Development and validation of a one-mile treadmill walk test to predict peak oxygen uptake in healthy adults ages 40 to 79 years. *Can J Appl Physiol.* 2002;27(6):575-589.
47. Blair SN, Cheng Y, Holder JS. Is physical activity or physical fitness more important in defining health benefits? *Med Sci SportsExerc.* 2001;33(6 Suppl):S379-S399.
48. Cress ME, Buchner DM, Questad KA, Esselman PC, deLateur BJ, Schwartz RS. Continuous-scale physical functional performance in healthy older adults: a validation study. *Arch Phys Med Rehabil.* 1996;77(12):1243-1250.
49. Falconer J, Hughes SL, Naughton BJ, Singer R, Chang RW, Sinacore JM. Self report and performance-based hand function tests as correlates of dependency in the elderly. *J Am Geriatr Soc.* 1991;39(7):695-699.
50. Clark BC. Test for fitness in older adults, AAHPERD fitness task force. *Journal of Physical Education, Recreation and Dance.* 1989;60(3):66-71.
51. Reuben DB, Valle LA, Hays RD, Siu AL. Measuring physical function in community-dwelling older persons: a comparison of self-administered, interviewer-administered, and performance-based measures. *J Am Geriatr Soc.* 1995;43(1):17-23.
52. Ainsworth BE, Haskell WL, Leon AS, et al. Compendium of physical activities: classification of energy costs of human physical activities. *Med Sci Sports Exerc.* 1993;25(1):71-80.

10

Stress Management

Martha Highfield, PhD, RN and
Catherine Rush Thompson, PT, PhD, MS

"The longer I live, the more I realize the impact of attitude on life. Attitude, to me, is more important than facts. It is more important than the past, than education, than money, than circumstances, than failure, than success, than what other people think or say or do. It is more important than appearances, giftedness or skill. It will make or break a company...a church...a home. The remarkable thing is we have choice every day regarding the attitude we will embrace for that day. We cannot change our past...or cannot change the inevitable. The only thing we can do is play on the one string we have, and that is our attitude...I am convinced that life is 10% what happens to me and 90% how I react to it. And so it is with you...we are in charge of our attitudes."—Charles Swindoll, *The Grace Awakening*

Stress

Stress is a description of how any individual reacts to physical, psychosocial, environmental, or other stressors or situations that are challenging and require action to restore balance.[1,2] Stress may be viewed as positive (*eustress*), neutral (*neustress*), or negative (*distress*), depending on how the individual perceives the stressor. Stresses may be created by situations desirable to the individual (eg, a job promotion), whereas other stressful situations could cause the person distress (eg, loss of a loved one or living with chronic illness). Everyone experiences at least one type of stress on a daily basis. Common sources of daily stress include work-related issues, financial problems, relationship issues, home and transportation concerns, health problems, and unexpected schedule conflicts. Whereas a certain situation may be stressful for one individual, another person may feel little, if any, stress at all. For example, a flat tire may not stress an auto mechanic working in a repair shop, but the same problem might prove distressing to a new graduate driving to her first job interview.

Acute (or short-term) stress is the immediate response to any challenging situation. Stress causes a physical reaction that involves a surge of hormones (primarily cortisol) in the body, resulting in a defensive "fight" response to confront the problems or a defeatist "flight" response

Thompson CR.
Prevention Practice and Health Promotion: A Health Care Professional's Guide to Health, Fitness, and Wellness, Second Edition (pp 159-174).

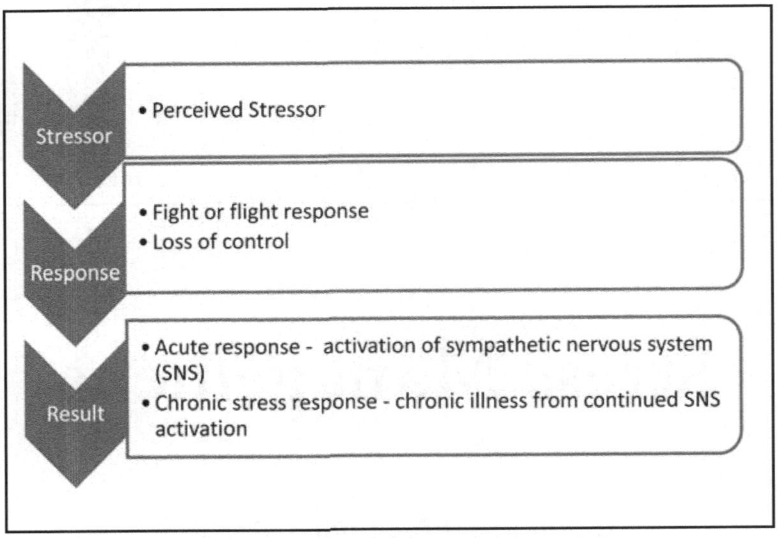

Figure 10-1. Stress response.

to give up control of the situation, as illustrated in Figure 10-1. Both responses are mediated by the sympathetic nervous system. Once the pressure or threat has passed, hormone levels usually return to normal, mediated by the parasympathetic nervous system. Although the body typically recovers rapidly from acute stress, it can precipitate or trigger health problems, such as a cardiac arrhythmia or a myocardial infarction (heart attack). Long-term stress is caused by persistent, unresolved situations, which, if left unmanaged, could lead to chronic pathology.

Chronic Pathology and Stress

Individuals experiencing chronic pathology and their caretakers are challenged by additional stresses associated with managing physical impairments and dealing with compromised functioning in activities of daily living. Generally, individuals with chronic health conditions have pain and lose strength, musculoskeletal flexibility, and cardiovascular endurance from decreased activity during acute illness. *Hypokinesia* (abnormally decreased motor function or activity)[3] is a major contributor to the chronic health problems leading to disability resulting from inactivity and deconditioning. Other health concerns associated with chronic illness include altered psychological status, changes in social interactions, altered sleep habits, unhealthy nutritional habits, changes with digestion and elimination, reduced balance and coordination, altered cognitive status (often secondary to medications), financial strain, and concurrent use of several drugs that may pose additional health risks.

Any chronic condition can trigger depression, but the risk increases with the severity of illness and the degree of life disruption it causes. Although depression alone can limit functional abilities, it can also aggravate signs and symptoms of pathology, including fatigue, lethargy, and pain, and lead to social withdrawal. Although the risk of becoming depressed is approximately 10% to 25% for women and 5% to 12% for men in the general population, the risk increases for individuals with chronic illness.[4] Examples of chronic illnesses leading to depression include heart disease, Parkinson's disease, multiple sclerosis, stroke, cancer, diabetes, and chronic pain syndrome. Behaviors associated with depression include poor health habits (drinking alcohol, smoking, lack of exercise, and poor eating habits) and poor adherence to interventions. The National Alliance for Mental Illness provides a helpful depression and chronic illness fact sheet for patients and health care professionals that outlines coping strategies recommended for individuals with chronic illness (http://www.nami.org).

Denial, anger, and frustration commonly accompany the realization that a chronic illness may be incurable. While coping with changes that diseases impose on lifestyle, those with chronic illness need to restore a sense of control in their lives. Providing information about pathological conditions, suggesting support groups, and directly addressing modifiable factors are all resources to help clients regain control of their lives. Emotional management of chronic illness includes regular exercise, maintaining daily activities, connecting with family and friends, as well as attending a support group on a regular basis, pursuing personal hobbies, maintaining a positive attitude, and seeking professional help from a psychologist when depression becomes evident.

Clients with chronic illness and their caretakers often have new, demanding schedules that incorporate regular medical visits, specific medical regimens, prescribed diets, and extra time required for self-care activities. These changes in lifestyle require time management skills to meet the multiple time demands of clients with chronic illness. Additionally, these clients must maintain some flexibility to best adapt to their new lifestyles and uncertain futures.

Recognizing the unique stresses caused by chronic illness, health care professionals can help clients and their caretakers focus on functional activities and time management skills to optimize time and effort required for daily activities. Routines can be established that help clients manage the healthy habits of grooming, exercising regularly, eating appropriate foods, tracking their health status, attending to proper administration of medications, maintaining the home, and managing finances. The physician should be contacted whenever progression of the pathology is apparent. The priority of health care is optimizing each individual's quality of life.

Job-Related Stress

Often, stress results from experiencing a loss or change for which the individual lacks needed resources to manage the problem, including problems at work. According to the National Institute for Occupational Safety and Health,[5] job stress is more strongly associated with health complaints than financial or family problems. According to the American Psychological Association (APA), job stress alone costs the nation $400 billion annually, including costs of absenteeism, lost productivity, and insurance claims.[4] Statistics compiled by the APA illustrate the importance of recognizing job-related stress and implementing preventive practice to reduce stress in the workplace[6]:

- 36% of employees report feeling tense or stressed out during their workday.
- 49% of employees said low salary is significantly affecting their stress level at work.
- 20% report that their average daily level of stress from work is an 8, 9, or 10 on a 10-point scale.
- 36% of employees report they are typically stressed out during the workday.
- The top 5 stressors at work are low salaries, lack of opportunity for growth and advancement, too heavy a workload, unrealistic job expectations, and long hours.

Because stressors are perceived differently between individuals, stress management should be tailored to the needs of the person experiencing stress. Customizing stress management to the needs of the individual requires awareness of stress symptoms as well as valid and reliable measures of stress.

Stress Assessment

Health care providers need to recognize the range of stress symptoms that may be evident in both their client population and the population at large. Symptoms of stress include emotional, physical, cognitive, and behavioral symptoms associated with stress that may warrant preventive measures and potential mental health referrals. Examples of emotional stress include moodiness, social withdrawal, low self-esteem, depression, difficulty relaxing, and loss of self-control. Physical symptoms include lethargy, pain (eg, headaches, chest pain, stomach pain), gastrointestinal problems (eg, dry mouth, difficulty swallowing, nausea, diarrhea, constipation), illness (eg, colds and infections), insomnia, loss of sexual appetite, muscle tension (eg, clenched jaw), and nervousness behaviors (eg, sweating palms). Behavioral symptoms are likely to manifest as poor lifestyle behaviors (eg, drinking, smoking, using alcohol or drugs, unhealthy eating, procrastinating, and avoiding responsibilities). Cognitive symptoms may not be readily apparent if individuals are unwilling to share their concerns, but the health care professional should explore these symptoms during the interview process if other symptoms are evident. Cognitive symptoms include constant worrying, racing thoughts, forgetfulness, disorganization, inability to focus, and poor judgment.

Two common self-administered surveys that appraise psychological stress include the *Social Readjustment Rating Scale*[7] for adults and the *Adolescent Life Change Event Scale*[8] for youth. Additionally, the *Perceived Stress Scale (PSS)* is one of the most widely used tests for measuring the perception of stress based on experiences in the past month.[9] This 10-question Likert scale includes questions such as, "In the last month, how often have you been upset because of something that happened unexpectedly?" The PSS provides the health care provider with a tool to explore perceived stress and to discern the need for referral.

A valid and reliable clinical measure for detecting anxiety and depression (commonly associated with stress) is the *Hamilton Anxiety Rating Scale (HAM-A)*,[10,11] a short psychological questionnaire used to rate the severity of an individual's anxiety. Table 10-1 lists the questions on the HAM-A, a test commonly used by mental health clinicians.

Electrocardiography (measurement of heart activity) and *galvanic skin tests* (measurement of the autonomic nervous system) are 2 psychophysiological measures that can be useful in detecting less dramatic bodily changes occurring with stress. Health care providers may detect increased blood pressure during rest due to emotional stress experience by clients in a clinical setting, commonly known as *white coat syndrome*.

If stress is not well managed, chronic stress can result in overstimulation of body organs, leading to possible organ failure. Chronic stress-related illnesses include migraine headaches, tension headaches, psoriasis, panic attacks, ulcers, colitis, gastritis, cancer, noncardiac chest pain, heart attacks, dizzy spells, low back pain, rheumatoid arthritis, and high blood pressure. Behavioral consequences of chronic stress include overeating or a loss of appetite, smoking, alcohol abuse, sleeping disorders, emotional outbursts, and violence and aggression. Whenever treating any of these chronic conditions, health care professionals should screen for possible stressors that could be mediated by stress management strategies that meet the individual's needs.

A person's general mental health can play a significant role in his or her perception and response to stress. "Normal individuals possess a powerful motive to survive, and therefore, behavior contrary to that motive, such as self-mutilation or suicide, is considered abnormal."[12] Other abnormal characteristics include unrealistic thoughts and perceptions, inappropriate emotions, and unpredictable behavior (as compared with the social norm). Clinical assessment of mental health may include affect and emotional tone, motor behavior (eg, unusual purposeless movements), inappropriate ideas or thinking, describing nonexistent sounds, difficulties recalling events or performing tasks of memory and concentration, or problems with a logical flow of thoughts and logical conclusions. Psychological issues should be addressed by mental health professionals with appropriate resources to address these clients' needs.

Stress Management

Individuals experiencing stress may need a variety of resources for its management. Resources for stress management range from learning how to schedule time more efficiently and effectively to relaxation training. One of the primary causes of work-related stress is when the job demands cannot be met by the worker's capabilities. Health care professionals should advocate for stress

TABLE 10-1. HAMILTON RATING SCALE FOR ANXIETY
Instructions: This checklist is to assist the health care provider in screening an individual for anxiety or a pathological condition. Rate each of the following based on the following scale:
NONE=0 MILD=1 MODERATE=2 SEVERE=3 SEVERE, GROSSLY DISABLING=4
1. Anxious—Worries, anticipation of the worst, fearful anticipation, irritability
2. Tension—Feelings of tension, fatigability, startle response, moved to tears easily, trembling, feelings of restlessness, inability to relax
3. Fears—Of dark, of strangers, of being left alone, of animals, of traffic, of crowds
4. Insomnia—Difficulty in falling asleep, broken sleep, unsatisfying sleep and fatigue on waking, dreams, nightmares, night terrors
5. Intellectual—Difficulty in concentration, poor memory (cognitive)
6. Depressed—Loss of interest, lack of pleasure in hobbies, depression, early waking, diurnal mood swing
7. Somatic—Pains and aches, twitching, stiffness, myoclonic jerks, grinding of teeth (muscular)
8. Somatic—Tinnitus, blurring of vision, hot and cold flushes, feelings of weakness (sensory), pricking sensation
9. Cardiovascular—Tachycardia, palpitations, pain in chest, throbbing of vessels, fainting feelings, missing beat
10. Respiratory—Pressure or constriction in chest, choking feelings, sighing, dyspnea
11. Gastrointestinal—Difficulty in swallowing, wind, abdominal pain, burning sensations, abdominal fullness, nausea, vomiting, borborygmi, looseness of bowels, loss of weight, constipation
12. Genitourinary—Frequency of micturition, urgency of micturition, amenorrhea, menorrhagia, development of frigidity, premature ejaculation, loss of libido, impotence
13. Autonomic—Dry mouth, flushing, pallor, tendency to sweat, giddiness, tension headache, raising of hair
14. Behavior—Fidgeting, restlessness or pacing, tremor of hands, furrowed brow, strained face, sighing or rapid respiration, facial pallor, swallowing, belching, brisk tendon jerks, dilated pupils, exophthalmos
Adapted from Hamilton M. The assessment of anxiety states by rating. *Br J Med Psychol.* 1959;32(1):50-55.

management education or additional job training to help workers develop needed skills to match job demands as one of many solutions to reduce stress in the workplace. Health care professionals need to work with each other and in the community to explore options to reduce stress in all sectors of society. Steps for managing stress include the following:

- Identifying stressors
- Using relaxation or coping strategies to relieve the stress
- Seeking solutions for avoiding or controlling the stress
- Being as fit and healthy as possible
- Changing a way of thinking, as needed

Healthy nutrition and adequate rest, using relaxation techniques, time management, a positive attitude, and physical activity have all been shown to effectively reduce stress. For all types of stress management programming, interventions should be targeted to the individual; they should be behaviorally based, and they should be integrated into lifestyle behaviors through practice and reinforcement. It is helpful for health care professionals to help stressed individuals to set goals to reduce stress. These easy steps can help guide stress management:

- Identify stressors and determine how the individual reacts to stressors. Journaling or recording stressful events and stress responses may offer a clue to a person's coping strategies.
- Write a long-term and a short-term goal to focus attention on the stressor and successful attempts to manage stress. Thinking about healthy options for managing a stressor before it happens may allow time for acquiring needed resources before the stressor recurs. Incorporating physical activity into the daily routine can also reduce stress and allow time for reflecting on important tasks and values. Time must be allowed to reconnect the heart, the mind, and the soul. For example, "I will spend 30 minutes walking at the end of each workday to reflect on my daily activities and gratitude for what I experienced that day."
- Plan for setbacks to avoid discouragement.
- Share goals with friends and family to gain reinforcement and encouragement for reaching goals. Refer the individual to counseling if additional support is needed.

The remainder of this chapter will offer various options for reducing or managing stress as well as resources for improving mental, spiritual, and emotional health and wellness.

Sleep

Individuals need adequate sleep to function normally and to manage stress. Sleep allows the body to repair and restore itself; over 70% of the body's daily dose of growth hormone is circulated during sleep.[13] Sleep is also an important time for the regeneration of the immune system, so missing sleep reduces the body's ability to resist and fight infection. Adequate sleep is essential for mental ability and concentration. The ability to undertake useful mental work declines by 25% every 24 hours without sleep; in shift work, this can lead to a much higher possibility of job-related accidents.[13] Studies suggest that sleep loss leads to lethargy during the day and contributes to more than 100,000 highway crashes, causing over 71,000 injuries and more than 1500 deaths each year in the United States alone.[13]

Nearly 12% of the US population experiences *insomnia* (difficulty falling asleep, sleeping too lightly, being easily disrupted with multiple spontaneous awakenings, or early morning awakenings with an inability to fall back asleep).[13] Approximately one-third of all Americans have sleep disorders at some point in their lives. Increasing age predisposes individuals to sleep disorders (5% in persons aged 30 to 50 years and 30% in those aged 50 years or older).[13] Older individuals commonly experience a decrease in total sleep time, with more frequent awakenings during the night. Often, older adults need to take medications on a regular schedule throughout the night, leading to sleep disruption.

Health care professionals should ask their clients about sleep difficulties and locate resources for sleep management. Medications may be useful in managing insomnia in most cases. Surgery may be indicated to correct some underlying medical conditions causing insomnia, such as palate surgery in some cases of sleep apnea. If sleep is a chronic problem, health care professionals may offer techniques to help reduce stress and induce relaxation.

Relaxation Techniques

Relaxation techniques have been widely used to reduce stress in a variety of populations, including patients with mental and physical health conditions. Herbert Benson coined the term *relaxation response*, referring to the body's natural response to restore homeostasis in the body:

> Each of us possesses a natural and innate protective mechanism against 'overstress,' which allows us to turn off harmful bodily effects to counter the effects of the fight-or-flight response. This response against 'overstress' brings on bodily changes that decrease heart rate, lower metabolism, decrease the rate of breathing, and bring the body back into what is probably a healthier balance.[14]

Various relaxation techniques enable individuals to self-manage stress. Relaxation techniques include the following:

- *Progressive muscle relaxation* is a technique commonly used to reduce symptoms of stress, anxiety, insomnia, and certain types of chronic pain. The technique of progressive muscle relaxation was described by Edmund Jacobson in the 1930s and involves simple isometric contractions of one muscle group at a time, followed by a release of the tension.[15] The muscle contraction and relaxation technique is performed on a succession of muscles progressing from the lower body toward the head, ending with contractions of facial muscles. The progressive relaxation may be facilitated by verbal directions, either in person or on audiotape: "Close your eyes (pause). Now tighten the muscles as hard as you can in your toes and hold for 5 seconds ...1...2...3...4...5... now relax." The technique may be performed when sitting comfortably on a supportive surface or when lying in a relaxed posture. Each muscle group is contracted for 5 to 8 seconds, then relaxed. After relaxing for approximately 30 seconds, the next set of muscles may be contracted and relaxed. Once all muscle groups have been contracted and relaxed, the individual may rest in this posture as long as possible to achieve complete relaxation. This technique may be augmented by visual imagery.
- *Visual imagery* is the practice of using one's imagination to create mental pictures in a way that promotes relaxation and helps relieve pain. A combination of relaxation and imagery is effective in improving the sleep of critically ill adults, but may be contraindicated for individuals with mental illness who may become agitated by visual images.[16] Health care professionals should screen their patients for good mental health prior to using visual imagery for relaxation purposes.
- *Meditation*, one of the most common mind-body interventions, is a conscious mental process that induces a set of integrated physiological changes that relaxes the body.[17] The 2 most popular forms of meditation in the United States include *transcendental meditation*, characterized by repeating a mantra (a single word or phrase), and *mindfulness meditation*, which is focusing one's attention on moment-by-moment thoughts and sensations. Meditation has been shown in one study to produce significant increases in left-sided anterior brain activity, associated with positive emotional states as well increased antibody titers to influenza vaccine. These findings suggest potential linkages among meditation, positive emotional states, localized brain responses, and improved immune function.[17] Meditation has not only a relaxing effect, but possibly the ability to augment the body's immune response.
- *Autogenic training* uses visual imagery and body awareness to elicit a relaxation response. The individual self-regulates the body by focusing on specific areas needing relaxation, including the limbs, lungs, heart, diaphragm, and head. The individual attempts to induce the following physiological responses through concentration: increased muscle relaxation, increased peripheral blood flow, lowered heart rate, lowered blood pressure, slower and deeper breathing, and reduced oxygen consumption. In separate meta-analyses examining the effects of autogenic

training, researchers revealed a significant reduction in patients' tension and migraine headaches, decreased blood pressure for clients with mild to moderate essential hypertension and coronary heart disease, reduced asthma symptoms, reduced symptoms associated with somatoform pain disorder (unspecified type), decreased symptoms of Raynaud's disease, reduced impairments from anxiety disorders, reduction of mild to moderate depression, and improvement in sleep for patients with functional sleep disorders.[17]

- *Biofeedback* is a technique using feedback from body functions to increase the person's awareness of internal body workings. Body function is measured with electrodes and displayed on a monitor that both the participant and his or her practitioner can see. The monitor thereby provides feedback to the participant about the internal workings of his or her body. Biofeedback is an effective therapy for many conditions, but it is commonly used to treat tension headaches, migraine headaches, and chronic pain.[17]
- *Massage* involves the manipulation of soft tissues for the purpose of reducing muscle tension or normalizing other soft tissue structures. There are various types of massage, including *relaxation massage* (to promote general relaxation, improve circulation, enable full range of movement, and relieve muscular tension), *therapeutic massage* (to restore function to injured soft tissue or move abnormal fluids from one body compartment to another), *sports massage* (to enhance sports performance and recuperation postinjury), *acupressure massage* (pressure at particular acupressure points associated with visceral structures), and *Oriental massage therapies*, such as acupressure and shiatsu (designed to treat points along the acupressure meridians, aiming to release discomfort).[12] Essentially, all types of massage can provide several benefits to the body, including increased blood flow, reduced muscle tension and neurological excitability, and increased well-being.[17] Massage techniques include *petrissage* (kneading or rubbing with force to manipulate tissues and muscles), *effleurage* (characterized by light or heavy stroking of the skin designed to improve flow to the circulatory and lymphatic systems), and *friction massage* or, more specifically, *deep transverse friction massage* (using firm finger pressure in soft tissue to treat muscles, tendons, ligaments, and joint capsules).
- *Fluid exercise*, such as t'ai chi and yoga, as discussed in Chapter 4, can also contribute to mental health and relaxation.

Self-Help

Education about a stressor can help individuals learn to cope effectively with unexpected problems. Braden's self-help model[18] has been used in multiple health care settings to help patients manage medical problems, including rheumatoid arthritis, chronic pain, breast cancer, heart failure, and HIV/AIDS. Braden defines self-help as "an informed process of facing definable, manageable adversities by maintaining control of everyday problems" as a healthier reaction than passively avoiding problems or remaining uninformed.[18]

"Self-help is part of the healthy self-management process necessary to facilitate chronic patient flexibility and to enable a greater number to adjust to their condition and to face life challenges ahead."[18] This self-help model supports the use of patient education for managing chronic stress and illness. One study reported that "self-help can enhance independence, reduce dependence on family and social resources, reduce health care costs, and increase mental and social well-being."[18] Nearly every type of medical condition has a support group or a website with information that can begin the educational process.

Time Management

Time management is a universal problem, and difficulties with prioritizing key tasks and procrastination contribute significantly to stress. Many people spend their days in a frenzy of activity, but they achieve little because they fail to concentrate on essential tasks. To concentrate on results, the individual must establish priorities and devise a plan to optimize strengths while downplaying weaknesses. The following process helps the individual determine strengths and weaknesses, identify goals to accomplish, and prioritize those goals for a concerted effort to accomplish each one.

Establish Priorities

An individual's highest priorities should center on that person's unique strengths and attributes. One way to determine an individual's strengths and weaknesses is to do a SWOT analysis, which asks the following questions[19]:

- Strengths: What advantages do you have? What do you do well? To which relevant resources do you have access? What do other people see as your strengths?
- Weaknesses: What could you improve? What do you do badly? What should you avoid? Do other people seem to perceive weaknesses that you do not see? Are others doing any better than you?
- Opportunities: Where are the good opportunities facing you? What are the interesting trends you are aware of? (Note: Useful opportunities can come from such things as changes in technology and markets, changes in government policy related to your field, changes in social patterns, population profiles, lifestyle changes, and local events.) Do personal strengths open up any opportunities? Alternatively, consider how opportunities increase by eliminating weaknesses.
- Threats: What obstacles are you facing? What is threatening you? Are the required specifications for a job, products, or services changing? Is changing technology threatening the position? Do you have bad debt or cash-flow problems? Could any of your weaknesses seriously threaten your roles in life?

This SWOT analysis can be helpful in pointing out what needs to be done and in putting problems into perspective. Overall, the SWOT analysis is a framework for analyzing strengths and weaknesses as well as the opportunities and threats the individual faces. This analysis helps the individual prioritize and focus on strengths, minimize weaknesses, and take advantage of opportunities while keeping in mind what could threaten the person's future.

Monitor Current Time Use

Track the schedule of time spent over the past 7 days (where can time be spent more and where can time be spent less). Highlight how much time is spent on priorities vs nonprioritized activities. Many computer programs offer electronic calendars for listing daily activities and tasks. In addition to listing tasks, the individual should note the times when fatigue, energy, or other emotions emerge throughout the day. Also, important health habits, such as eating well, having adequate sleep, and exercising on a regular basis, should be noted.

Analyze Current Time Use

The individual needs to analyze how time is spent and determine if the time spent matches personal priorities. Is the current schedule affording adequate time to accomplish desired goals? Does the current schedule allow time for healthy eating, sleeping, and exercise behaviors? Does the current schedule incorporate time for socializing with family and friends?

Make a Schedule

The next step is to develop a plan that lists activities based on priorities. The plan should also be based on what the individual desires for the long term, rather than what must be done from one moment to the next. What goals does the individual want to accomplish in the next 10 years? These goals need to be broken down into achievable tasks that can be accomplished within reasonable time frames. The plan should realistically incorporate activities that emphasize strengths while reducing time that relies on areas of weakness. A simple to-do list can be used to list the individual's tasks in order of priority and importance. Tackling the most important tasks will ensure that long-term goals are not overlooked.

Personal goals may be focused on particular areas; however, long-term goals probably address the multifaceted aspects of life, including artistic goals, attitudinal goals, career goals, educational goals, family goals, financial goals, physical or athletic goals, recreational goals, and public service goals. Once these goals are determined, they need to be prioritized and broken down into short-term, achievable goals.

Delegate Tasks

The final step is to determine what can be delegated to others and what can be most easily managed by the individual. It is logical to consider delegating those tasks that are areas of weakness or responsibilities that do not directly contribute to the long-range plan the individual envisions.

Overall, time management can be a useful stress management tool, as well as a means of accomplishing personal goals in a meaningful time frame. The individual should always allow some time for unexpected or uncontrollable events; this flexibility allows the plan to stand the test of time.

Coping

Coping means to constantly change cognitive and behavioral efforts to manage specific internal and/or external demands that are appraised as taxing. When experiencing stress, the individual needs to appraise the situation to determine whether the stressor justifies concern and, if so, what resources are available to manage the stress. Coping resources include exercise, self-talk skills, problem-solving skills, communication skills, social support, material resources, and community services.

The Schafer coping model[20] offers 3 options for coping with stress:

1. Altering the stressor (eg, pacing life's demands in a more realistic manner)
2. Avoiding the stressor (eg, making changes that reduce its presence)
3. Adapting to the stressor (eg, using self-talk to resolve conflict or alter perception of the stressor, using health buffers like exercise, nutrition, and sleep and controlling physical stress responses through relaxation and breathing)

Additional methods for adapting to a stressful situation include avoiding maladaptive health behaviors (eg, alcohol, smoking, overeating, overspending, blaming others, escapism, or unloading difficult issues on others). Seeking coping resources, including social support, money, community services, and a belief system, can provide a buffer to potential stressors. Finally, controlling one's personal actions can have a positive effect on adapting to stressors. Being assertive, using effective communication (especially listening), and sharing concerns with others can often deter further complications.

Locus of Control

Locus of control is the tendency to attribute success or difficulty to either internal factors (such as personal effort) or to external factors (such as fate or others' behaviors). An *internal locus of control* (ie, under one's own personal control) can be a mediating factor of actions taken to prevent health problems. Individuals with a perceived internal locus of control showed a reduced cortisol response (stress response) to an experimental stressor if they believed that they have some control over the stressor. Furthermore, studies have shown that *psychological hardiness* (a personality style consisting of commitment, control, and challenge)[21] can help buffer the negative effect of stressors and can enhance personal development. It is crucial that clients take control of their lives, recognizing healthy lifestyle behaviors and choices responsible for mitigating the effect of disease and injury.

Emotional Health

Many positive traits promise to improve quality of life and mitigate distress, ultimately preventing pathology. These traits include optimism, hope, wisdom, creativity, future-mindedness, courage, spirituality, responsibility, and perseverance. *Positive psychology*, a newer branch of psychology, examines how optimism and hope affect health. The ultimate goal of positive psychology is to make people happier by understanding and building positive emotion, gratification, and meaning.

According to Abraham Maslow's theory of development, individuals become self-actualized as they experience personal growth. When the individual takes responsibility and uses personal strengths, that person becomes more free, powerful, happy, and healthy. People with good emotional health are aware of their thoughts, feelings, and behaviors. They have learned healthy ways to cope with the stress and problems that are a normal part of life. They feel good about themselves and have healthy relationships. Those in emotional distress may not be in touch with their thoughts, feelings, and behaviors. The following are physical signs that an individual's emotional health may be out of balance: back pain, changes in appetite, chest pain, constipation or diarrhea, dry mouth, extreme tiredness, general aches and pains, headaches, high blood pressure, insomnia, lightheadedness, palpitations, sexual problems, shortness of breath, stiff neck, sweating, upset stomach, and weight gain or loss. If an individual presents with these physical health problems, emotional problems should not be ruled out. A referral to a psychologist is appropriate, especially if the individual expresses emotional distress or feeling depressed.

Maintaining a Balance Between Work and Play

Frequently, stress mounts when life is out of balance. Too often, work demands crowd out more leisurely or playful activities. Play is generally engaging in activity voluntarily, with the reward being intrinsic and a sense of freedom from life's demands.[21] To restore a sense of balance and wellness to one's life, play is essential. In particular, laughter and humor can play a key role in releasing stress.

Spirituality

Health care professionals are expected to recognize, respect, and respond to each individual with compassion and with sensitivity to individual and cultural differences,[22] including each individual's spirituality. *Spirituality* can be defined as a search for meaning and connectedness with others, nature, the self, and a greater power. All people experience this search as a longing and need for forgiveness, hope, life purpose, and giving and receiving love and support. To the extent that these longings and needs are met, the person moves toward wellness. Those whose spiritual needs are met will have a sense of peace, describe life as meaningful, and experience supportive, caring relationships. For these individuals, spiritual values provide a sense of hope and that life and health problems are manageable. To the extent that they are not met, the person moves away from wellness. These individuals may experience conflicting values, loss of purpose in life, few or no trusting relationships, anger, inner conflicts regarding beliefs and values, and a sense of emptiness. Health care professionals must be aware of similar or conflicting spiritual values to ensure that their clients are able to maximize their own health-promoting spiritual resources and possibly facilitate access to new resources. These efforts require ongoing self-assessment and developing competence.

Religion

Religion is complementary to and yet different from spirituality. It may be defined as those individual and community values, beliefs, and practices through which individuals meet their spiritual needs. Research suggests that religious involvement may be health promoting. Religious involvement has been associated with lower morbidity and mortality, shorter hospital stays, less depression, improved blood pressure, lower substance abuse, improved pain control, and other indicators of positive physical and psychosocial health. Additionally, religious organizations and churches often provide emotional and material support for their members, a phenomenon particularly recognized among some minority communities. Recent data suggest that most clients are religiously involved. In 2012, 77.3% of Americans told Gallup interviewers that they identified with a Christian religion (51.9% Protestant/other Christian, 23.3% Roman Catholic, and 2.1% Church of Jesus Christ of Latter-Day Saints [LDS]), 4.9% identified with a non-Christian religion, 15.6% said they had no religious identity at all, and another 2.2% did not respond.[22,23] They note that for the past 5 decades, at least 50% have reported having a religious faith. This poll also revealed that religiousness increases with age, women and Blacks are more religious than other populations, Mormons most value religion and religious attendance, and where an individual lives affects religiousness. The Southern states are the most religious, whereas the Northeast and Northwest are the least religious.[23]

Health care professionals should listen to how each client describes any involvement in religion, and then identify how that client's framework may facilitate health promotion. For clients who do not consider themselves religiously involved, other organizations may address their needs for support, hope, and meaning as the context for health promotion. Religious involvement can be unique to that individual or it may be an organized world religion like Christianity or Islam. It may be more Western and focus on a personal God and on living life to the fullest; or, it may be more Eastern and focus on relinquishing personal existence to become one with a nonpersonal greater power. More information on various religions can be found online at BeliefNet.com. Hospital chaplains may consult with both the client and the health care professional about how to work effectively within a client's religious framework. If outside spiritual leaders are requested by the client, either the client should contact them or the in-house chaplain should make the consultative call.[24]

Spiritual Practices

In a study in the late 1990s, a national sample of persons with AIDS reported using several spiritual practices frequently for their own health promotion. Activities ranking among the top 10 complementary therapies used by this group included prayer (56%), meditation (46%), support groups (42%), and other spiritual activities (33%).[25] When practiced, such activities are often described by the self-identified religious client as religious and by the self-identified nonreligious client as spiritual.

Prayer

Providers should be aware that prayer may take many silent or vocal forms, including meditation, thankfulness for things received, requesting needs be met, reading written prayers, conversing with God, and expressing anger or emotion. Appropriate prayers of meditation, adoration, invocation, and celebration from many faiths and cultures can be found at the World Prayers Project (www.worldprayers.org). Regardless of recent controversies about the role of prayer in physical healing, most individuals (72%) pray daily.[26] Many seriously ill persons use prayer to promote relaxation, hope, and comfort, and some health care providers use prayer to deal with their concerns about particular clients. Many health care professionals may wish to seek an appropriate spiritual leader to assist a client when that client desires prayer, but sometimes, clients may ask their health care professional personally to pray with or for them. The clinician may comply if comfortable with the request or make a referral if appropriate while assuring respect for the client's practices.

Spiritual Meditation

Silence, prayer, music, or other practices may facilitate meditation. Clinicians should be aware of activities that conflict with the religious beliefs of some, in addition to the meditative practices used or adapted by Hindus, Jews, and Christians to promote health.

Music

Music helps to express deep spiritual feelings, is present in all religions, and can be calming or enlivening. Some of music's positive effects include relaxation, lower blood pressure, improved mood, enhanced cognitive function, relief of boredom, and pain control. Evidence also exists that music timed to the individual's biological rhythms (like a heartbeat) can have a soothing effect. Recordings of religious music are readily available in bookstores and online and may include nature sounds, calming and meditative Buddhist or Taize chants, classical works, traditional Christian hymns, or rock and roll.

Devotional Supports

Health-promoting devotion, an act of prayer or private worship, may be facilitated by silence, music, prayer, devotional items, and readings. Examples of devotional items may include a small Buddhist altar, rosary beads, a prayer card, religious jewelry, or a bead to protect against "evil eye." If clients request such items, chaplains or other spiritual leaders can be of assistance. Devotional items can provide clues about spiritual practice to the observant health care professional, opening the door to a discussion of belief systems. Devotional readings may enhance hope, peace, and relaxation. According to a Gallup poll, more than 75% of Americans regard the Bible as inspired scripture.[26] Multiple translations of audio and print scripture online resources are available, including the Koran, Sikh scriptures, the Bible, and Christian devotional e-books.

PLAN Model

If a client seems to be having difficulty with a particular spiritual need, such as forgiveness, hope, or supportive relationships, the health care professional may find the PLAN model helpful when used along with specific resources. A modified version of PLAN includes giving *P*ermission for the individual to express concerns; providing *L*imited information or *A*ctivating past coping resources; and, if the issue is beyond the health care professional's time, comfort, or competence, referring the client to *N*on–health care disciplines, such as social work, psychology, or clergy. PLAN can be coupled with some of the following information.[27]

Forgiveness and Compassion

Forgiveness is "letting go of negative feelings"[28] toward others in a way that restores and repairs relationships. Clients may focus more on forgiving than on being forgiven because they realize their negative feelings toward another person can cause harm to themselves. Health care professionals can facilitate this health-promoting process by listening empathetically to the client through 4 forgiveness stages of anger: (1) inability to forgive, (2) wondering if he or she should forgive, (3) letting go of negative feelings, but (4) not forgetting.[28]

Compassion is the understanding or empathy for the suffering of others and helping them to come out from the suffering. This characteristic is considered in many religious traditions as among the greatest of virtues. The *Harvard Business Review* reported, "Studies show that people who practice 'self-compassion' are happier, more optimistic, and less anxious and depressed. A dose of self-compassion when things are at their most difficult can reduce your stress and improve your performance, by making it easier to learn from your mistakes. So remember that to err is human, and give yourself a break."[29] As His Holiness the Dalai Lama said: "If you want others to be happy, practice compassion. If you want to be happy, practice compassion."[30]

Hope

Hope may be best evidenced by the person's ability to imagine and participate in the enhancement of a positive future. Hope has been associated with lower anxiety, higher functional status, and better physical health. The health care professional can build an individual's hope by promoting client confidence that he or she is not alone; sharing a vision for the client of a mutually established, achievable, positive future; and committing energy to helping the person achieve wellness goals.

Cognitive Reserve and Lifestyle

A lifestyle characterized by social and intellectual engagement may be a buffer to the stresses in life and, ultimately, pathologies affecting the brain. Although social support can be a stress resource, the development of a *cognitive reserve*, formulated through years of life experience coupled with innate intellectual ability, may slow the cognitive decline in healthy older adults and may reduce the risk of dementia, including Alzheimer's disease. Risk factors for Alzheimer's disease include advanced age, lower intelligence, small head size, history of head trauma, and female sex.[31] Evidence from functional imaging studies indicates that individuals engaged in cognitively challenging activities can clinically tolerate more Alzheimer's disease pathology, suggesting that life experience can provide cognitive reserves that delay the onset of clinical manifestations of dementia.[31]

Complementary and Alternative Medicine

Nontraditional resources for health and wellness are being investigated by researchers funded by the National Institutes of Health and other public and private institutions interested in expanding options for health care. *Complementary and alternative medicine* (CAM) includes forms of treatment used in addition to, or instead of, standard or usual medical treatments. These practices cover a wide range of treatment approaches, such as special diets, vitamins, herbs, acupuncture, massage therapy, magnetic therapy, spiritual healing, and meditation. Their use increased from 34% in 1990 and 42% in 1997 to over 50% in 2007.[32] In one study looking at a group of 453 cancer patients, 83% reported using at least one CAM, including special diets, psychotherapy, spiritual practices, and vitamin supplements. When psychotherapy and spiritual practices were excluded, 64% of patients used at least one CAM in their cancer treatments.[32] Because many of the CAM therapies have not been subjected to the same strict scientific evaluation for safety and effectiveness as conventional therapies, they may pose some risk. The National Cancer Institute and the National Center for Complementary and Alternative Medicine are sponsoring or cosponsoring various scientific studies of complementary and alternative medicine to determine which CAM therapies interfere with standard treatment or may be harmful when used with conventional treatment.

Making Lifestyle Changes

Many recommendations for intervention, although proven effective in reducing the risk of disease, are often unheeded. The United States Preventive Services Task Force (USPSTF)[33] recommends the following steps for helping individuals change poor health habits:

- Identify an individual's beliefs about specific behaviors and adjust advice to the individual's lifestyle.
- Provide the rationale for each recommendation and develop a realistic time frame for achieving results. As the individual achieves small successes, propose larger but achievable goals.
- Add new behaviors. Adopting good habits is often easier than discarding bad ones.
- Link positive behaviors with the daily routine. Have the individual explain how the behavior will be integrated into daily activities.
- Subspecialists in many chronic diseases have trained teams that can educate patients far more effectively than individual health care providers. Another form of referral is sending novice patients to talk with successful patients.
- According to research findings, a call from a health professional to inquire about progress is effective in changing a behavior.

Ideally, unhealthy behaviors should be prevented before they develop into lifestyle habits. Unfortunately, unhealthy behaviors often develop in response to the inability to react to the many stresses individuals encounter across the lifespan. To best manage stress, it is important to understand what stress is and how it is most effectively managed.

Summary

There is an incredible range of resources for managing health and wellness to prevent disease or to reduce the effect of pathology on the quality of life. Although maintaining a balanced lifestyle is important, certain stressors in life can present barriers to good health and wellness. In 1960 the life expectancy was 69.77 (66.60 for males and 73.10 for females); the life expectancy in 2012 rose to 78.74 (76.40 for males and 81.20 for females).[30] Using resources wisely for health and wellness promises to prolong healthy living and, hopefully, enrich the quality of life throughout the life span.

References

1. Lazarus RS. *Psychological Stress and the Coping Process.* New York, NY: McGraw-Hill; 1966.
2. Lazarus RS, Cohen, JB. Environmental stress. In: Altman I, Wohlwill JF, eds. *Human Behavior and Environment.* Vol 2. New York, NY: Plenum; 1977:90-127.

3. "hypokinesia." Merriam-Webster.com. http://www.merriam-webster.com/medical/hypokinesia. Accessed May 30, 2013.
4. Chapman DP, Perry GS, Strine TW. The vital link between chronic disease and depressive disorders. *Prev Chronic Dis* [serial online]. http://www.cdc.gov/pcd/issues/2005/jan/pdf/04_0066.pdf. Accessed May 20, 2014.
5. The National Institute for Occupational Safety and Health (NIOSH). Centers for Disease Control and Prevention. http://www.cdc.gov/niosh/. Accessed May 30, 2013.
6. Stress in the workplace. American Psychological Association. http://www.apa.org/news/press/releases/phwa-survey-summary.pdf. Accessed May 20, 2014.
7. Holmes TH, Rahe RH. The social readjustment rating scale. *J Psychosom Res.* 1967;11(2):213-221.
8. Yeaworth RC, McNamee MJ, Pozehl B. The Adolescent Life Change Event Scale: its development and use. *Adolescence.* 1992;27(108):783-802.
9. Cohen S, Kamarck T, Mermelstein R. A global measure of perceived stress. *J Health Soc Behav.* 1983;24(4):385-396.
10. Hamilton M. The assessment of anxiety states by rating. *Br J Med Psychol.* 1959;32:50-55.
11. Maier W, Buller R, Philipp M, Heuser I. The Hamilton Anxiety Scale: reliability, validity and sensitivity to change in anxiety and depressive disorders. *J Affect Disord.* 1988;14(1):61-68.
12. Hergenhahn BR. Early diagnosis, explanation, and treatment of mental illness. In: *An Introduction to the History of Psychology.* 7th ed. Belmont, CA: Wadsworth; 2013:486-514.
13. Schafer W. *Stress Management for Wellness.* 3rd ed. Dumfries, NC: Holt, Rinehart and Winston; 1996.
14. Stress...at work. DHHS (NIOSH) Publication Number 99-101. Centers for Disease Control and Prevention. http://www.cdc.gov/niosh/docs/99-101/. Accessed May 23, 2013.
15. Rosch PJ. The quandary of job stress compensation. *Health and Stress.* 2001;3:1-4.
16. Glanz K, Rimer BK, Lewis FM. *Health Behavior and Health Education: Theory, Research and Practice.* San Francisco, CA: Wiley & Sons; 2002.
17. Antonovsky A. *Health, Stress, and Coping.* San Francisco, CA: Jossey-Bass; 1979.
18. Lin KC, Gau ML, Kuan CL, Chuang TH. Validation of the Braden Self-Help Model in women with systemic lupus erythematosus. *J Nurs Res.* 2010;18(3):206-214.
19. SWOT analysis: discover new opportunities. Manage and eliminate threats. MindTools. http://www.mindtools.com/pages/article/newTMC_05.htm. Accessed May 20, 2014.
20. Rahe RH, Taylor CB, Tolles RL, Newhall LM, Veach TL, Bryson S. A novel stress and coping workplace program reduces illness and healthcare utilization. *Psychosom Med.* 2002;64(2):278-286.
21. Backman CL. Occupational balance: exploring the relationships among daily occupations and their influence on well-being. *Can J Occup Ther.* 2004;71(4):202-209.
22. Questions and answers about Americans' religion. Gallup Poll. http://www.gallup.com/poll/159548/identify-christian.aspx. Accessed December 29, 2013.
23. Seven in 10 Americans are very or moderately religious. Gallup Poll. http://www.gallup.com/poll/159050/seven-americans-moderately-religious.aspx. Accessed December 29, 2013.
24. VandeCreek L. Collaboration between nurses and chaplains for spiritual caregiving. *Semin Oncol Nurs.* 1997;13(4):279-280.
25. MacIntyre RC, Holzemer WL. Complementary and alternative medicine and HIV/AIDS: part II: selected literature review. *J Assoc Nurses AIDS Care.* 1997;8(2):25-38.
26. Newport F. One-third of Americans believe the Bible is literally true. Gallup. http://www.gallup.com/poll/27682/onethird-americans-believe-bible-literally-true.aspx. Assessed May 20, 2014.
27. Highfield ME. *PLAN: A Spiritual Care Model for Every Nurse in Quality of Life: A Nursing Challenge.* Bala Cynwyd, PA: Meniscus Health Care Communications; 1996.
28. Mickley JR, Cowles K. Ameliorating the tension: use of forgiveness for healing. *Oncol Nurs Forum.* 2001;28(1):31-37.
29. Harvard Business Review. Management tip for the day: reduce stress with self-compassion. *Time.* http://business.time.com/2013/03/22/reduce-stress-with-self-compassion/. Accessed May 20, 2014.
30. Dalai Lama. Brainy Quote. http://www.brainyquote.com/quotes/quotes/d/dalailama105551.html. Accessed May 20, 2014.
31. Scarmeas N, Stern Y. Cognitive reserve: implications for diagnosis and prevention of Alzheimer's disease. *Curr Neurol Neurosci Rep.* 2004;4(5):374-380.
32. Cassileth B, Chapman C. Alternative and complementary cancer therapies. *Cancer.* 1996;77(6):1026-1033.
33. United States—life expectancy at birth. CountryEconomy.com. http://countryeconomy.com/demography/life-expectancy/usa. Accessed May 20, 2014.

11

Nutrition

Catherine Rush Thompson, PT, PhD, MS

"If we could give every individual the right amount of nourishment and exercise, not too little and not too much, we would have found the safest way to health."—Hippocrates, *Collected Works*

When working with individuals who are healthy, at risk for injury and disease, or experiencing pathological conditions, it is important to consider all the factors contributing to their health. Using the International Classification of Functioning, Disability and Health, health care professionals can identify personal and environmental factors that contribute significantly to a person's health status. Internal personal factors include sex, age, coping styles, social background, education, profession, past and current experience, overall behavior pattern, and character.[1]

Eating behavior and the resulting nourishment to the body are key personal factors that need to be screened during an interview with individuals seeking optimal health. Environmental factors, such as accessibility to healthy foods and adequate financial resources, may also contribute to an individual's nutritional status.

Nutrition

Nutrition is the intake of foods and beverages that provide energy to the entire body. *Good nutrition* involves receiving and using the optimal nutrients to manage variations in health and disease.[1] According to the World Health Organization, an adequate, well-balanced diet combined with regular physical activity is a cornerstone of good health. Poor nutrition can lead to reduced immunity, increased susceptibility to disease, impaired physical and mental development, and reduced productivity.[1,2] Health care professionals need to be aware of the basics of healthy nutrition and recognize the need for referral when a person engages in unhealthy eating and drinking behaviors.

The Centers for Disease Control and Prevention provides an educational website called Nutrition for Everyone listing the 5 basic food groups that can contribute to healthy nutrition.[3] These food groups include vegetables, fruits, grains, dairy, and protein foods, regardless of

Thompson CR.
Prevention Practice and Health Promotion: A Health Care Professional's Guide to Health, Fitness, and Wellness, Second Edition (pp 175-187).

whether they are fresh, canned, frozen, liquefied, or dried. This website lists a variety of healthy foods that can contribute to a healthy diet.

Healthy vegetables include broccoli, carrots, collard greens, split peas, green beans, black-eyed peas, kale, lima beans, potatoes, spinach, squash, sweet potatoes, tomatoes, and kidney beans. Any vegetable or 100% vegetable juice counts in this group. Healthy fruits include apples, apricots, bananas, dates, grapes, oranges, grapefruit, mangoes, melons, peaches, pineapples, raisins, strawberries, tangerines, and 100% fruit juice.

Whole grains are the preferred grains and include whole wheat, oatmeal, bulgur, and brown rice. Refined grains, such as white bread, white rice, pasta, flour tortillas, and most noodles, offer less nutritional value.

Dairy products include all milks and calcium-containing milk products, such as cheeses and yogurt, as well as lactose-free and lactose-reduced products and soy beverages.

Protein foods include meats and poultry, seafood, beans and peas, eggs, processed soy products, unsalted nuts, and seeds. Nutrients found in the various food groups contributing to a healthy diet include carbohydrates, proteins, dietary fats, vitamins and minerals, and water.[4]

CARBOHYDRATES

Carbohydrates provide a source of ready energy for muscle activity. The digestive system converts carbohydrates into blood glucose for immediate energy or into glycogen that is stored in the liver and muscles for later use. There are 2 types of carbohydrates: readily digestible *simple carbohydrates* with small molecular structures, and *complex carbohydrates* comprising long-chained molecules that take more time to digest.[5]

Simple carbohydrates include natural sugars and sugars added in food and beverage processing. Processed sugars can be readily identified on food labels and include brown sugar, corn sweetener, corn syrup, dextrose, fructose, fruit juice concentrates, glucose, high-fructose corn syrup, invert sugar, lactose, maltose, malt syrup, molasses, raw sugar, and sucrose.[5] These processed sugars can give a quick energy boost but are typically less healthy than natural carbohydrates found in fruits, vegetables, and milk. Sugar added to food now accounts for nearly 16% of the average American's daily intake, and sweetened soft drinks make up nearly 8%.[6]

Complex carbohydrates include starch and dietary fiber that must be converted to a glucose source over time. Starch is found in bread, cereals, and grains. Dietary fibers may be soluble (eg, oatmeal, nuts, seeds, dry beans, peas, and many fruits) or insoluble (eg, brown rice, couscous, bulgur, seeds, whole wheat, barley, and most fruits and vegetables).[4]

Carbohydrates converted to blood sugar or glucose travel in the bloodstream to reach all parts of the body. As blood sugar levels rise, the pancreas responds with *insulin*, a hormone signaling cells to absorb blood sugar, lowering glucose levels in the bloodstream. *Glucagon*, another hormone, is released from the pancreas when blood sugars are lowered, resulting in the release of stored glucose in the liver. This balance of insulin and glucagon helps to regulate the levels of glucose in the bloodstream. Some individuals have type 1 diabetes, a condition resulting in insufficient insulin for glucose absorption in cells. Others have type 2 diabetes, a condition causing insulin-resistant cells. Type 2 diabetes has been linked with high blood pressure, high levels of triglycerides, low high-density lipoprotein (HDL; good) cholesterol, and excess weight. Researchers estimate that 90% of type 2 diabetes cases could be prevented through a combination of a healthy diet and an active lifestyle.[7]

The glycemic index (GI) attempts to measure how quickly blood glucose levels rise after consuming various types of carbohydrates.[8] According to the American Diabetes Association:

> [F]oods with a high GI are rapidly digested and absorbed and result in marked fluctuations in blood sugar levels. Low-GI foods, by virtue of their slow digestion and absorption,

produce gradual rises in blood sugar and insulin levels, and have proven benefits for health. Low-GI diets have been shown to improve both glucose and lipid levels in people with diabetes (types 1 and 2). These diets have benefits for weight control because they help control appetite and delay hunger. Low-GI diets also reduce insulin levels and insulin resistance.[9]

Foods with a score of 70 or higher are defined as having a high GI, whereas those with a score of 55 or below have a low GI.[9] Factors that can affect the GI include processing (eg, refined grains have a higher GI than whole grains), type of starch (eg, potato starch is readily digested), fiber content (eg, sugars linked to fibers are less digestible and deliver less glucose), ripeness (eg, ripe fruits and vegetables have higher sugar), fat content and acid content (eg, foods with fat and acid require longer to digest), and physical form (eg, fine grains digest rapidly).[9] The University of Sydney in Australia maintains an updated, searchable international database at www.glycemicindex.com.

PROTEINS

Proteins, comprising amino acids, are considered the building blocks of the body because they contribute to the development of muscles, bone, tendons, skin, hair, and other tissues. In addition, amino acids provide nutrient transportation and contribute to enzyme production.[10] Although there are 20 different amino acids that compose proteins, certain amino acids, called *essential amino acids,* must be provided through diet.[11]

Protein sources are identified by how many essential amino acids they provide. For example, a *complete* protein or high-quality protein source contains all of the essential amino acids. Examples of these complete proteins include meat, poultry, fish, milk, eggs, and cheese.[4] An *incomplete* protein source is one that is low in one or more of the essential amino acids, and *complementary* proteins have 2 or more incomplete protein sources that combine to provide all the essential amino acids. Two incomplete proteins that combine as complementary proteins are rice and beans, popular staples in many diets.[4] The Recommended Dietary Allowances (RDA) for proteins range from 13 g daily for children 1 to 3 years of age to 56 g daily for men aged 19 to 70 years and 46 g daily for women of the same age.[4]

FATS

Dietary fat, along with carbohydrates and proteins, provides energy for the body. Fats contain 9 calories per gram compared with carbohydrates and protein, both with 4 calories per gram.[12,13] There are several types of dietary fat.

Healthy Fats

- *Unsaturated fats*: Polyunsaturated and monounsaturated fats are the 2 unsaturated fats that are found in oils from plants (eg, soybean, corn, safflower, canola, olive, and sunflower), nuts (eg, walnuts), seeds, and many fish (eg, salmon, trout, and herring).[14] These fats may help lower blood cholesterol level when used in lieu of saturated and trans fats.[14] There is growing evidence that polyunsaturated omega-3 (found in salmon, mackerel, and tuna) and omega-6 fatty acids (commonly found in corn oil, soybean oil, and sunflower oil, as well as in nuts and seeds) are essential fats (ie, they help maintain nerve and brain function, as well as lower the risk of heart disease and protect against type 2 diabetes, Alzheimer's disease, and age-related brain decline).[15]

Unhealthy Fats

- *Trans fatty acids and hydrogenated oils*: While producing certain foods, such as margarine and shortening, fats may undergo a chemical process called *hydrogenation*, creating trans fatty acids and hydrogenated oils.[14] According to the American Heart Association, trans fatty acids or hydrogenated fats tended to raise total blood cholesterol levels, raise low-density lipoprotein (LDL; bad) cholesterol, and lower HDL cholesterol.[14]
- *Saturated fats*: These fats are found in many meats and poultry (eg, beef, veal, lamb, pork, and chicken), dairy products (eg, butter, cream, milk, cheeses, and other dairy products made from whole and 2% milk), and other foods (eg, coconut, coconut oil, coconut butter, and palm oil). All of these foods also contain dietary cholesterol that can be harmful to the body.[14] Diets high in saturated fat have been linked to chronic heart disease.[14]

The *Dietary Guidelines for Americans* recommend that Americans consume less than 10% of calories from saturated fats, replace solid fats with oils when possible, limit trans fatty acid consumption, eat fewer than 300 mg of dietary cholesterol per day, and reduce intake of calories from solid or saturated fats. Total fat limits are 30% to 40% in children 2 to 3 years of age, 25% to 35% in children 4 to 18 years of age, and 20% to 35% in adults 19 years of age and older.[16]

Vitamins and Minerals

Vitamins and minerals contribute to many of the biochemical processes that enable the body to function and grow. For example, vitamin D helps the body absorb calcium, a mineral needed for bone strength and nerve conduction.[17] Vitamins are organic (made by plants and animals) and minerals are inorganic (absorbed by plants).[17] A healthy diet typically provides enough vitamins and minerals, although many individuals take supplemental vitamins and minerals to enhance their health. Dietary supplements may be taken as tablets, capsules, powders, or energy drinks and bars. During pregnancy, additional vitamins and minerals are commonly recommended. A pregnant woman taking a multivitamin with 400 µg of folic acid reduces the risk of having a child with spinal defects by up to 70%.[18] It is important to note whether an individual is taking dietary supplements, particularly if he or she is also taking prescribed medications or using the supplements in lieu of prescribed medications, because these supplements may have strong side effects that can affect his or her health. For example, a person using vitamin K may be unaware that this dietary supplement reduces certain blood thinners to prevent blood from clotting.

One preventable problem that is common in many Americans is using too much sodium. Although the majority of salt is added in processed foods (75%), a large percent is added while cooking and eating. On average, the more salt a person eats, the higher his or her blood pressure.[17] For more information about specific vitamins and minerals, the National Institutes of Health provides facts sheets at http://ods.od.nih.gov/factsheets/list-vitaminsminerals/.

Water

Water is essential for balancing the bodily fluids, facilitating energy production in cells, hydrating body tissues (eg, the skin), and aiding in bowel and bladder function. The body is composed of approximately 60% water, which contributes to multiple body functions, including digestion, absorption, circulation, creation of saliva, transportation of nutrients, and maintenance of body temperature.[19] Water is present in most foods, in liquids, and in its natural form, so individuals typically consume some water with every meal. The Institute of Medicine determined that an adequate intake for men is roughly 3 L (approximately 13 cups) of total beverages a day. The adequate intake for women is 2.2 L (approximately 9 cups) of total beverages a day.[20]

When exercising, additional water is needed to replace fluid lost in perspiration. The American College of Sports Medicine recommends that people drink approximately 17 ounces of fluid 2 hours before exercise. During exercise, they recommend that people start drinking fluids early and drink them at regular intervals to replace fluids lost by sweating.[19]

According to the Healthy Eating Plate created by nutrition experts at Harvard School of Public Health,[21] individuals should fill half of their plate with vegetables and fruits with a wide variety of color; fill one-fourth of their plate with whole grains, such as whole wheat, brown rice, and foods made with them, such as whole wheat pasta; and fill the remaining one-fourth of the plate with a healthy source of protein, including fish (containing heart-healthy omega-3 fatty acids), chicken, beans, or nuts. Red meats and processed meats, including bacon, cold cuts, and hot dogs, should be limited because they can raise the risk of heart disease, type 2 diabetes, and colon cancer. Also, a healthy diet should include plant oils (eg, olive, canola, soy, corn, sunflower, and peanut) and restrict butter and hydrogenated oils. Finally, a healthy meal should be accompanied by water, coffee, or tea.

Milk and dairy products should be limited to 1 to 2 servings per day because high intakes are associated with increased risk of prostate cancer and possibly ovarian cancer. The Healthy Eating Plate's placemat also recommends staying active and eating modest portions that meet caloric needs.[21]

Signs of Nutritional Status

Signs of good nutrition include a toned and well-developed body, ideal body weight for body composition, smooth skin, clear and bright eyes, glossy hair, and an alert facial expression.[22] Although other factors contribute to these healthy features, good nutrition is essential for optimal health. *Undernutrition* refers to a diet that lacks a full complement of healthy nutrients.[22] Individuals who are undernourished are limited in their physical work capacity, immune function, mental activity, and ability to recover from illness and injury. *Malnutrition* occurs when nutritional stores are depleted and the body lacks sufficient nutrients for the demands of daily living.[22] Although malnutrition is commonly reported in distressed and impoverished conditions, individuals with chronic disease may also lack sufficient stores of nutrients for their daily needs. *Overnutrition,* which literally refers to an overabundance of nutrients exceeding health guidelines, may mask malnutrition in severely obese individuals.[22] Certain lifestyle habits affect the body's ability to absorb and process nutrients appropriately. For example, those who drink alcohol heavily or smoke inhibit the body's ability to absorb vitamins B_6, B_{12}, A, D, thiamin, folic acid, and niacin.[22] Table 11-1 provides a list of the types of tests and measures used to assess nutritional status, and Table 11-2 includes typical signs and symptoms that suggest the need for referral.[22]

Need for Referral

Health care professionals should screen for possible nutritional deficits or conditions that pose nutritional risks for their clients and make proper referrals to the client's physician or a registered dietitian. Any dietary recommendations should be made by the individual's physician or a registered dietitian. It is important to consider not only a person's food, but also the cleanliness of its preparation and presentation. Foods and their containers may be contaminated by environmental toxins, food additives, or hormones. For instance, exposure to chemicals that mimic estrogen

Table 11-1. ABCD Assessment of Nutritional Status

	TEST AND MEASURES	FACTORS IDENTIFIED	INDICATORS OF NUTRITIONAL RISK
Anthropometrics	Anthropometrics	Weight Height Circumferential measurements Skinfold measurements Hip-to-waist ratio Body mass index	Values falling outside of normal ranges for age and sex
Biochemical, laboratory methods	Plasma protein From a blood sample	Hemoglobin Hematocrit Serum albumin Serum transferrin Total iron-binding capacity Ferritin	Decreased values indicate nutritional deficiencies
	Protein metabolism Based on a 24-hour urine test	Urinary creatinine Urea nitrogen	Increased levels indicate an increased breakdown of body tissue
	Immune system integrity	Lymphocyte count Skin testing	Elevated lymphocyte count Allergic response to nutrients
	Skeletal system integrity	Radiographs	Skeletal system integrity
	Gastrointestinal function	Radiographs	Malformation of structures
Clinical methods	Interview Clinical examination	Nutritional history Examination: note clinical signs of poor nutrition	
Dietary evaluation methods	Nutritional history Dietary diary 24-hour recall	Activity-associated food pattern of a typical day (food eaten for breakfast, lunch, evening meal, and additional meals, noting place and hour of meal)	Food preparation (eg, fried) and preferences that do not meet recommended guidelines

(continued)

Table 11-1 (continued). ABCD Assessment of Nutritional Status

	TEST AND MEASURES	FACTORS IDENTIFIED	INDICATORS OF NUTRITIONAL RISK
Dietary evaluation methods (continued)		Food preparation Food preferences Environmental factors (eg, access to food, socialization related to food)	

Adapted from Elamin A. Assessment of Nutritional Status. College of Medicine, Sultan Qaboos University, Oman. www.pitt.edu/~super7/19011-20001/19801.ppt. Accessed May 20, 2014.

(known as *xenoestrogens*) have been found in some plastic food containers and linked to early puberty in humans.[23]

A variety of issues surround healthy nutrition, including access to food, ability to consume food, eating behaviors, food allergies, and medical conditions affecting appetite. The following are examples of common issues encountered with individuals across the lifespan.

Infants

Newborns may experience a failure to thrive for a wide range of reasons related to eating difficulties, feeding patterns, breastfeeding issues, and/or other problems. These infants are generally identified in early screenings of anthropometrics with a growth pattern well below normal. Infants may also present with food allergies that may be difficult to recognize early in life.

Childhood

Early in life, children may develop eating patterns that lead to obesity and type 2 diabetes. Early parental education is essential for helping families develop healthy eating habits and for teaching children to prepare healthy snacks.

Prader-Willi syndrome is a rare genetic condition resulting in an insatiable appetite and obsessive overeating.[24] This condition requires medical attention and is managed by a comprehensive team approach. Autism commonly presents with food aversions.[25] Professionals working with children should be alert to their eating substances that are largely nonnutritive, such as clay, chalk, dirt, or sand. Although this is not uncommon in early childhood, it is considered *pica* if it is a persistent behavior because it may reflect a mineral deficiency.[26] If pica is suspected, the individual needs to have blood testing.

Adolescence

Two significant problems seen in adolescence relate to eating disorders: *anorexia nervosa* and *bulimia*. According to the American Academy of Child and Adolescent Psychology,[27] the symptoms and warning signs of anorexia nervosa and bulimia include the following:

- "A teenager with anorexia nervosa is typically a perfectionist and a high achiever in school. At the same time, she suffers from low self-esteem, irrationally believing she is fat regardless of how thin she becomes. Desperately needing a feeling of mastery over her life, the teenager with anorexia nervosa experiences a sense of control only when she says 'no' to the normal food demands of her body. In a relentless pursuit to be thin, the girl starves herself. This often

Table 11-2. Clinical Signs of Nutritional Status

BODY AREA	SIGNS OF GOOD NUTRITION	SIGNS OF POOR NUTRITION
General appearance	Alert, responsive	Listless, apathetic, cachectic (ie, appearing wasted and emaciated)
Weight	Normal for height, age, and body build	Overweight or underweight (special concerns if underweight)
Posture	Erect posture, arms and legs straight	Sagging shoulders, sunken chest, humped back
Muscles	Well developed, firm, good tone; some fat under skin	Flaccid, poor tone, underdeveloped, tender, wasted appearance, cannot walk properly
Nervous control	Good attention span, not irritable or restless, normal reflexes, psychological stability	Inattentive, irritable, confused, burning and tingling of hands and feet, loss of position and vibratory sense, weakness and tenderness of muscles, decrease or loss of ankle and knee reflexes
Gastrointestinal function	Good appetite and digestion, normal regular elimination, no palpable organs or masses	Anorexia, indigestion, constipation or diarrhea, liver or spleen enlargement
Cardiovascular function	Normal heart rate and rhythm, no murmurs, normal blood pressure for age	Tachycardia, enlarged heart, abnormal rhythm, elevated blood pressure
General vitality	Good endurance, energetic, sleeps well, vigorous	Easily fatigued, no energy, falls asleep easily, looks tired, apathetic
Hair	Shiny, lustrous, firm, not easily plucked, healthy scalp	Stringy, dull, brittle, thin and sparse, depigmented, can be easily plucked
Skin (general)	Smooth, slightly moist, good color	Rough, dry scaly, pale, pigmented, irritated, bruises, petechiae
Face and neck	Skin color uniform, smooth, pink, healthy appearance, not swollen	Greasy, discolored, scaly, swollen, skin dark over cheeks and under eyes, lumpiness or flakiness of skin around nose and mouth
Lips	Smooth, good color, moist, not chapped, not swollen	Dry, scaly, swollen, or angular lesions at corners of the mouth or fissures

(continued)

TABLE 11-2 (CONTINUED). CLINICAL SIGNS OF NUTRITIONAL STATUS

BODY AREA	SIGNS OF GOOD NUTRITION	SIGNS OF POOR NUTRITION
Mouth and oral membranes	Reddish pink mucous membranes in oral cavity	Swollen, boggy oral mucous membranes
Gums	Good pink color or deep reddish in appearance, not swelling or bleeding	Spongy, bleed easily, marginal redness, inflamed, gums receding
Tongue	Good pink color or deep reddish in appearance, not swollen or smooth, surface papillae present, no lesions	Swelling, scarlet and raw, magenta color, beefy, hyperemic and hypertrophic papillae, atrophic papillae
Teeth	No cavities, no pain, bright, straight, no crowding , well-shaped jaw, clean, no discoloration	Unfilled cavies, absent teeth, worn surfaces, mottled, malpositioned
Eyes	Bright, clear, shiny, no sores at corner of eyelids, membranes moist and healthy pink color, no prominent blood vessels or amount of tissue or sclera, no fatigue circles beneath	Eye membranes pale, redness of membrane, dryness, signs of infection, redness and fissuring of eyelid corners, dryness of eye membrane, dull appearance of cornea
Neck (glands)	No enlargement	Thyroid enlargement
Nails	Firm, pink	Spoon-shaped, brittle, ridged
Legs, feet	No tenderness, weakness, or swelling; good color	Edema, tender calf, tingling weakness
Skeleton	No malformations	Bowlegs, knock-knees, deformity of chest wall, abnormally shaped ribs, prominent scapula

Adapted from Overview of undernutrition. The Merck Manual. http://www.merckmanuals.com/professional/nutritional_disorders/undernutrition/overview_of_undernutrition.html#v882544. Accessed May 20, 2014.

reaches the point of serious damage to the body, and in a small number of cases may lead to death.

- "The symptoms of bulimia are usually different from those of anorexia nervosa. The patient binges on huge quantities of high-caloric food and purges her body of dreaded calories by self-induced vomiting or by using laxatives. These binges may alternate with severe diets, resulting in dramatic weight fluctuations. Teenagers may try to hide the signs of throwing up by running water while spending long periods of time in the bathroom. The purging of bulimia presents serious threats to the patient's physical health, including dehydration, hormonal imbalance, the depletion of important minerals, and damage to vital organs."[27]

In addition to anorexia nervosa and bulimia, adolescents are at an increased risk for obesity associated with unhealthy nutrition, commonly associated with the consumption of sodas. From 1989 to 2008, calories from sugary beverages increased by 60% in children aged 6 to 11 years, from 130 to 209 calories per day, and the percentage of children consuming them rose from 79% to 91%.[28]

Adulthood

According to the Centers for Disease Control and Prevention,[29] obesity has reached epidemic proportions, affecting 37% of adults, depending on the region of the country. Adult obesity is associated with a number of serious health conditions, including heart disease, diabetes, and some cancers.[30] Promoting regular physical activity and healthy eating while creating an environment that supports these behaviors is essential to reducing this epidemic. A common condition associated with obesity is type 2 diabetes. This condition may develop over time and is often preceded by *prediabetes*, a condition with elevated blood glucose but below levels of diabetes. Prediabetes can put people at increased risk of developing type 2 diabetes, heart disease, and stroke. Individuals with prediabetes can prevent or delay the onset of type 2 diabetes by losing 5% to 7% of their body weight and getting at least 150 minutes per week of moderate physical activity.[31]

Older Adults

Healthy nutrition and lifestyle habits need to be maintained across the lifespan to ensure optimal health. Problems that develop with aging, including osteopenia, osteoporosis, and sarcopenia, can be reduced with proper nutrition and exercise. According to the National Institutes of Health, "extra weight is a concern for older adults because it can increase the risk for diseases such as type 2 diabetes and heart disease and can increase joint problems."[32] Another concern for older adults is vitamin deficiencies resulting from a poor diet. This problem is common among the frail and institutionalized elderly.[33] Mild vitamin deficiencies can contribute to anemia, cognitive impairment, increased risk for infections, and problems with wound healing; severe deficiencies can lead to irreversible organ damage.[33] Common vitamin deficiencies in older adults include vitamin B_{12}, folic acid, vitamin C, and vitamin D.[33] A nutritional screening tool for older adults can be found in Chapter 9.

Popular Diets

Many individuals select specific diets to manage their daily nutrition for various reasons, including weight management, food allergies, and philosophical beliefs. Lifestyle behaviors, such as weight loss of 5% to 10% body weight and modest physical activity (30 minutes daily), significantly affect the development of diabetes in patients with prediabetes.[34]

Some of the more common diets are listed below:

- *Vegetarian diets*, although limited in animal sources for protein and relying primarily on plant sources of protein, vary according to underlying philosophies or dietary needs of the individual. Vegetarian eating patterns usually fall into the following groups: The *vegan diet* excludes all meat and animal products; the *lacto-ovo vegetarian diet* excludes red meats but allows dairy products, eggs, and, in some cases, fish and poultry; and the *lacto-vegetarian diet* includes dairy products and plant sources of proteins but does not allow meat, fish, or poultry.[35] Vegetarians need to ensure adequate amino acid balance through well-planned diets. It is important to ask clients if they are getting adequate vitamin B_{12} and zinc in their diet because these 2 deficiencies are often noted.[35]
- *Gluten-free diets* are necessary for individuals with celiac disease who cannot tolerate the protein gluten found in grains such as wheat, rye, and barley. This diet is also becoming popular with individuals with gluten sensitivity. There is reportedly no clear evidence indicating that this diet is beneficial for individuals with no gluten sensitivity. In a *Scientific American* article discussing gluten-free diets, the author states, "For most other people, a gluten-free diet won't provide a benefit."[36]

- *Lactose intolerance* suggests that the individual has intolerance to milk and some dairy products and that these foods should be avoided to reduce the risk of abdominal pain, diarrhea, and flatulence (gas). For these individuals, it is important to encourage adequate calcium and vitamin D through other supplementation.[37]
- *Vitamin-enriched diets* include fortified cereal and other prepared foods. These individuals should be cautioned about taking more than 100% RDA for each nutrient—especially niacin, pyridoxine, and vitamins A, D, and E.
- *Low-carbohydrate diets* have proven effective for short-term weight reduction but are controversial for long-term use. Recent studies involving over 80,000 women examined the relationship between low-carbohydrate diets and heart disease and risk of diabetes. Overall, women eating low-carbohydrate diets high in vegetable sources of fat or protein had a 30% lower risk of heart disease and a modestly lower risk of type 2 diabetes compared with those eating high-carbohydrate, low-fat diets. Women eating low-carbohydrate diets high in animal fats or proteins did not have a reduced risk of heart disease or diabetes.[38]

Importance of Physical Activity and Good Nutrition

Athletes need a healthy diet to maintain their strength and endurance and repair injured tissue. According to the Dietitians of Canada, the American Dietetic Association, the American College of Sports Medicine, and the *Canadian Journal of Dietetic Practice and Research*[10]:

> Athletes need protein primarily to repair and rebuild muscle that is broken down during exercise and to help optimize carbohydrate storage in the form of glycogen. Protein is not an ideal source of fuel for exercise, but can be used when the diet lacks adequate carbohydrate. This is detrimental, though, because if used for fuel, there isn't enough available to repair and rebuild body tissues, including muscle.

Athletes in strength training require more carbohydrates and glycogen stores for their workouts, yet no additional protein, as popularly believed. Carbohydrates fuel high-energy workouts, such as power lifting, by meeting the immediate energy demands through rapid oxidization and by restoring glycogen storage for future muscle contraction demands. Neither fat nor protein can be oxidized rapidly enough to meet the demands of high-intensity exercise. Adequate dietary carbohydrate must be consumed daily to restore glycogen levels.[10]

Recommended protein intake for the average adult is 0.8 g per kg (2.2 lb) of body weight per day; 1.4 to 1.8 g per kg (2.2 lb) of body weight per day for athletes engaged in strength training, and 1.2 to 1.4 g per kg (2.2 lb) of body weight per day for athletes engaged in endurance training.[10]

Dental Health

Another key factor that relates to healthy nutrition is dental health. The need for dental care is ongoing to ensure proper function for eating and other oromotor skills. Although public health policies encourage the fluoridation of water to prevent cavities, daily brushing and flossing, as well as periodic cleaning (ideally every 3 months), should be encouraged to prevent cavities and gum disease.

In addition, health care professionals need to remind individuals to wear protective mouth gear when engaging in sports. Teeth protection may also be needed for individuals who tend to exhibit *bruxism* (grinding of the teeth). A dentist can determine the need for special guards to protect the teeth from excessive stress that can wear down dental surfaces. All individuals should have their teeth examined annually for potential dental problems resulting from injury, disease, poor hygiene, or teeth grinding.

Another common problem seen by doctors, dentists, and physical therapists is *temporomandibular joint* (TMJ) *dysfunction*. TMJ is involved in any movements involving the jaw, including eating, drinking, and yawning. Generally, individuals complain of pain that travels along the jawline down the neck or through the face on the involved side, as well as limitations in movement, painful clicking in the joint, stiff muscles surrounding the joint, or jaw malalignment.[39] If the pain persists, a referral should be made to a specialist who deals with TMJ dysfunction.

Summary

Overall, managing one's physical health through a well-rounded, nutritious diet and maintaining dentition for healthy eating habits contribute to general health across the lifespan. In addition, regular physical activity works in conjunction with a healthy diet to ensure physical fitness. Health care professionals should be observant of clinical signs of poor nutrition and dental decay and inquire about each individual's daily diet and dental care habits. A simple screen of nutrition and dental health adds a safety net to overall health care. A variety of websites offer helpful resources that can guide individuals and their families in the areas of nutrition and dental care. If problems are suspected, referrals should be made for specialized medical care, assessment by a registered dietician, or examination by a dental specialist to curtail ongoing problems, prevent further oromotor damage, and promote healthier lifestyle habits.

References

1. WHO guidelines on nutrition. World Health Organization. http://www.who.int/publications/guidelines/nutrition/en/. Accessed May 22, 2013.
2. Katz D. *Nutrition in Clinical Practice: A Comprehensive, Evidence-Based Manual for the Practitioner.* Baltimore, MD: Lippincott Williams & Wilkins; 2008.
3. Nutrition for everyone. Centers for Disease Control and Prevention. http://www.cdc.gov/nutrition/everyone/basics/foodgroups.html. Accessed May 22, 2013.
4. National Research Council. *Dietary Reference Intakes for Energy, Carbohydrate, Fiber, Fat, Fatty Acids, Cholesterol, Protein, and Amino Acids (Macronutrients).* Washington, DC: The National Academies Press; 2005.
5. Carbohydrates. Harvard School of Public Health Nutrition Source. http://www.hsph.harvard.edu/nutritionsource/carbohydrates/. Accessed May 22, 2013.
6. Vartanian LR, Schwartz MB, Brownell KD. Effects of soft drink consumption on nutrition and health: a systematic review and meta-analysis. *Am J Public Health.* 2007; 97:667-675.
7. The nutrition source. Harvard School of Public Health. http://www.thenutritionsource.org. Accessed May 22, 2013.
8. Glycemic index defined. Glycemic Research Institute. http://www.glycemic.com/GlycemicIndex-LoadDefined.htm. Accessed May 22, 2013.
9. The glycemic index of foods. American Diabetes Association. http://www.diabetes.org/food-and-fitness/food/planning-meals/the-glycemic-index-of-foods.html. Accessed May 22, 2013.
10. The Position Statement from the Dietitians of Canada, the American Dietetic Association, and the American College of Sports Medicine. *Can J Diet Pract Res.* 2000;61(4):176-192.
11. Protein in diet. MedlinePlus. http://www.nlm.nih.gov/medlineplus/ency/article/002467.htm. Accessed May 22, 2013.
12. Diseases and conditions. Cleveland Clinic. http://my.clevelandclinic.org/disorders/obesity/hic_fat_and_calories.aspx. Accessed May 22, 2013.
13. ChooseMyPlate.gov. US Department of Agriculture. http://www.choosemyplate.gov. Accessed May 22, 2013.
14. Know your fats. American Heart Association. http://www.heart.org/HEARTORG/Conditions/Cholesterol/PreventionTreatmentofHighCholesterol/Know-Your-Fats_UCM_305628_Article.jsp. Accessed May 22, 2013.
15. Understanding the omega fatty acids. WebMD. http://www.webmd.com/diet/healthy-kitchen-11/omega-fatty-acids. Accessed May 22, 2013.

16. Dietary guidelines for Americans, 2010. US Department of Health and Human Services. http://www.health.gov/dietaryguidelines/2010.asp. Accessed May 22, 2013.
17. Vitamins and minerals. Centers for Disease Control and Prevention. http://www.cdc.gov/nutrition/everyone/basics/vitamins/. Accessed May 22, 2013.
18. Spina bifida. American Pregnancy Association. http://americanpregnancy.org/birthdefects/spinabifida.html. Accessed May 22, 2013.
19. 6 reasons to drink water. WebMD. http://www.webmd.com/diet/features/6-reasons-to-drink-water?page=2. Accessed May 22, 2013.
20. Water: how much should you drink every day? Mayo Clinic. http://www.mayoclinic.com/health/water/NU00283. Accessed May 22, 2013.
21. Healthy eating plate. Harvard Medical School. http://www.health.harvard.edu/plate/healthy-eating-plate. Accessed May 22, 2013.
22. Nutritional disorders. The Merck Manual. http://www.merckmanuals.com/professional/nutritional_disorders.html. Accessed May 22, 2013.
23. Talsness CE, Andrade AJ, Kuriyama SN, Taylor JA, vom Saal FS. Components of plastic: experimental studies in animals and relevance for human health. *Philos Trans R Soc Lond B Biol Sci.* 2009;364:2079-2096.
24. Prader-Willi syndrome. Prader-Willi Syndrome Association. http://www.pwsausa.org/. Accessed May 22, 2013.
25. Schreck K, Williams K, Smith A. A comparison of eating behaviors between children with and without autism. *J Autism Dev Disord.* 2004;34(4):433-438.
26. Rose EA, Porcerelli JH, Neale AV. Pica: common but commonly missed. *J Am Board Fam Pract.* 2000;13(5):353-358.
27. Teenagers with eating disorders. American Academy of Child and Adolescent Psychiatry. http://aacap.org/page.ww?name=Teenagers+with+Eating+Disorders&section=Facts+for+Families. Accessed May 25, 2013.
28. Lasater G, Piernas C, Popkin BM. Beverage patterns and trends among school-aged children in the US, 1989-2008. *Nutr J.* 2011;10:103.
29. Overweight and obesity. Centers for Disease Control and Prevention. http://www.cdc.gov/obesity/data/adult.html. Accessed May 22, 2013.
30. National Institutes of Health. *Clinical Guidelines on the Identification, Evaluation, and Treatment of Overweight and Obesity in Adults: The Evidence Report.* Bethesda, MD: National Institutes of Health; 1998.
31. Knowler WC, Barrett-Connor E, Fowler SE, et al. Reduction in the incidence of type 2 diabetes with lifestyle intervention or metformin. *N Engl J Med.* 2002;346(6):393-403.
32. Eating as you get older. National Institutes of Health. http://nihseniorhealth.gov/eatingwellasyougetolder/benefitsofeatingwell/01.html. Accessed May 22, 2013.
33. Beers MH, Berkow R, eds. *The Merck Manual of Geriatrics.* 3rd ed. Whitehouse Station, NJ: Merck Research Laboratories; 2000.
34. American Diabetes Association. Position statement: Prevention or delay of type 2 diabetes. *Diabetes Care.* 2004;27(Suppl 1):S47-S54.
35. Vegetarian diet. National Institutes of Health. http://www.nlm.nih.gov/medlineplus/vegetariandiet.html. Accessed May 22, 2013.
36. Rettner R. Most people shouldn't eat gluten-free. *Scientific American.* http://www.scientificamerican.com/article.cfm?id=most-people-shouldnt-eat-gluten-free. Accessed May 22, 2013.
37. Lactose intolerance. MedicineNet.com. http://www.medicinenet.com/script/main/art.asp?articlekey=7809&questionid=507. Accessed May 25, 2013.
38. Hu F, Manson J, Stampfer M, et al. Diet, lifestyle, and the risk of type 2 diabetes mellitus in women. *N Engl J Med.* 2001;345(11):790-797.
39. Temporomandibular joint dysfunction. National Institutes of Health. http://www.nlm.nih.gov/medlineplus/temporomandibularjointdysfunction.html. Accessed May 25, 2013.

12

Health Protection

Catherine Rush Thompson, PT, PhD, MS

"The scars of others should teach us caution."—Saint Jerome

One of the major goals of Healthy People 2020 is to reduce the incidence of injury and infection across the lifespan through health protection strategies. As part of the health care team, all professionals provide an important safety net for injury prevention and infection control through screenings and health education. Health care professionals have an opportunity to provide primary prevention in a variety of community settings through (1) comprehensive health screenings to identify injury or infection risk factors, (2) education to address risk factors, and (3) collaboration with others to provide health protection resources designed to reduce injuries and infection.

Infection Control

Healthy People 2020 aims to "increase immunization rates and reduce preventable infectious diseases."[1] *Infectious diseases* are considered those diseases caused by microbes that can be passed to or among humans by several methods, including contact with infectious agents that gain entry to the body through a variety of portals, including the skin, mouth, nose, and body parts engaged in sexual contact. Many infections may be transmitted from person to person, but some cases involve infection transmission through shared objects (eg, drinking glasses) or infected animals (eg, rodents). Infectious diseases, many of which are preventable, are the leading cause of death in the world.[1] Epidemics, such as severe acute respiratory syndrome (SARS), which spread among 29 countries in 2003,[2] remind the public of the possible fatal outcomes of uncontrolled infections. The Healthy People 2020 website provides specific information and resources about infectious diseases.

The best prevention from infection is adopting a risk-free or low-risk lifestyle that includes protective devices, immunizations, and sanitary health habits. Health care professionals should remind their clients to use protection when engaged in activities that pose any risk of infection (eg, condoms when engaged in sexual activity). In addition, clients should be advised to maintain their immunizations for prevention. Up-to-date vaccination information for professionals is located at the Centers for Disease Control and Prevention (CDC) website.

Thompson CR.
Prevention Practice and Health Promotion: A Health Care Professional's Guide to Health, Fitness, and Wellness, Second Edition (pp 189-207).

Table 12-1. 10 Leading Causes of Death and Injury by Age Group, Highlighting Unintentional Injury Deaths Per Year, United States

Rank	*<1 y*	*1 to 4 y*	*5 to 9 y*	*10 to 14 y*	*15 to 24 y*
1	Unint suffocation 905	Unint drowning 436	Unint MV traffic 354	Unint MV traffic 452	Unint MV traffic 7024
2	Homicide unspecified 154	Unint MV traffic 343	Unint drowning 134	Suicide suffocation 168	Homicide firearm 3889
3	Homicide other spec, classifiable 82	Homicide unspecified 163	Unint fire/burn 89	Unint drowning 117	Unint poisoning 3183
4	Unint MV traffic 76	Unint fire/burn 151	Homicide firearm 58	Homicide firearm 107	Suicide firearm 2046
5	Undet suffocation 39	Unint suffocation 134	Unint suffocation 31	Suicide firearm 80	Suicide suffocation 1824
6	Unint drowning 39	Unint pedestrian, other 103	Unint other land transport 26	Unint suffocation 48	Unint drowning 656
7	Undet unspecified 35	Homicide other spec, classifiable 84	Unint pedestrian, other 20	Unint fire/burn 46	Homicide cut/pierce 420
8	Adverse effects 22	Unint natural/environment 52	Adverse effects 14	Unint other land transport 42	Suicide poisoning 371
9	Unint fire/burn 22	Homicide firearm 43	Unint natural/environment 14	Unint poisoning 40	Undet poisoning 282
10	Unint natural/environment 22	Unint struck by or against 37	Unint poisoning 14	Unint firearm 26	Unint other land transport 221

(continued)

Health care professionals should promote sanitary habits whenever working with clients. One example of increasing awareness of healthy sanitary habits is providing signage that encourages frequent hand washing and cleaning of areas likely to spread infections through hand or mouth contact. Clients should be reminded that skin that is broken by abrasions, burns, or wounds is particularly vulnerable to infection and needs to be kept free of infection through cleanliness and appropriate medical precautions.

Injury Prevention Through Education

The Healthy People 2020 initiative provides health care professionals with a framework to collaboratively work toward injury prevention goals. These goals range from reducing injuries and deaths from

Table 12-1 (continued). 10 Leading Causes of Death and Injury by Age Group, Highlighting Unintentional Injury Deaths Per Year, United States

Rank	*25 to 34 y*	*35 to 44 y*	*45 to 54 y*	*55 to 64 y*	*65+ y*	*Total*
1	Unint poisoning 6767	Unint poisoning 7476	Unint poisoning 9662	Unint poisoning 4451	Unint fall 21,649	Unint MV traffic 33,687
2	Unint MV traffic 5558	Unint MV traffic 4552	Unint MV traffic 5154	Unint MV traffic 4134	Unint MV traffic 6037	Unint poisoning 33,041
3	Homicide firearm 3331	Suicide firearm 2914	Suicide firearm 4092	Suicide firearm 3387	Unint unspecified 4596	Unint fall 26,009
4	Suicide firearm 2594	Suicide suffocation 1839	Suicide poisoning 2061	Unint fall 2011	Suicide firearm 4276	Suicide firearm 19,392
5	Suicide suffocation 1910	Homicide firearm 1673	Suicide suffocation 1965	Suicide poisoning 1382	Unint suffocation 3400	Homicide firearm 11,078
6	Suicide poisoning 787	Suicide poisoning 1279	Unint fall 1283	Suicide suffocation 1130	Adverse effects 1544	Suicide suffocation 9493
7	Undet poisoning 580	Undet poisoning 712	Homicide firearm 1097	Unint suffocation 613	Unint poisoning 1402	Suicide poisoning 6599
8	Unint drowning 476	Unint fall 493	Undet poisoning 955	Homicide firearm 533	Unint fire/burn 1088	Unint suffocation 6165
9	Homicide cut/pierce 43	Unint drowning 409	Unint drowning 578	Undet poisoning 480	Suicide poisoning 709	Unint unspecified 5688
10	Unint fall 299	Homicide cut/pierce 349	Unint suffocation 464	Unint fire/burn 479	Suicide suffocation 648	Unint drowning 3782

Abbreviations: MV, motor vehicle; undet, undetermined; unint, unintentional.
Source: Ten leading causes of death and Injury. Centers for Disease Control and Prevention. http://www.cdc.gov/injury/wisqars/LeadingCauses.html. Accessed May 20, 2014.

head injuries, poisonings, and firearms to increasing the number of states that collect data on causes of injury.[1] Health care providers need to increase public education about health risks in a variety settings, including schools and universities, occupational settings, and the home. The CDC recommends increasing health education in the areas of unintentional injury, violence, and suicide for youth and adults.

The National Center for Injury Prevention and Control provides information for understanding and preventing violence at its website http://www.cdc.gov/violenceprevention/pdf/dvp-research-summary-a.pdf. Violence and injuries "kill more people ages 1 to 44 in the United States than any other cause" and "cost more than $406 billion in medical care and lost productivity each year."[3] The CDC collects data on the most common types of injuries based on sex, race, and age group.[3] Table 12-1 lists the leading causes of death by age group, highlighting unintentional injury deaths.

Health care professionals can screen for potential risks for injury and educate the public about injury risks using the data provided in Table 12-1.

Injury Prevention for Children and Adolescents

Unintentional or Undetermined Suffocation

The top cause of infant death is unintentional suffocation, which may occur from a variety of causes but is attributed to sudden infant death syndrome (SIDS) in some cases. The Back to Sleep campaign[4] has reduced deaths from SIDS in part attributed to sleeping prone. Many educational resources for families are available from http://www.healthychildcare.org/sids.html, which recommends the following:

- Promoting the Back to Sleep message in child care programs
- Raising awareness and change practices in child care settings
- Disseminating information on national child care recommendations/standards related to SIDS risk reduction
- Supporting states to enhance existing and establish new child care regulations

It is essential to offset time supine during sleep with time spent prone during waking hours. Changing positions enables the infant to develop both physically and motorically through activities in various positions. Due to the pliability of an infant's skull, a small child can develop deformities of the skull if he or she remains in one position over long periods of time.[5] Various campaigns include the Prone to Play and Tummy to Play program endorsed by the American Academy of Pediatrics.[6] All health care professionals working with families of young infants need to educate their clients about these essential developmental programs.

Unintentional Poisonings

Children under the age of 4 are particularly vulnerable to poisoning. Parents should be advised to remove or lock up any hazardous agents and to store drugs (securing the safety cap) carefully in the home at all times.

Unintentional Drownings

Three children die every day as a result of drowning.[7] Safety tips to pass on to parents include the following:

- Teaching all family members life-saving skills as soon as possible, including the basics of swimming (floating, moving through the water) and cardiopulmonary resuscitation (CPR)
- Fencing off swimming pools
- Using life jackets around natural bodies of water
- Taking extra precautions around bodies of water, ensuring that all are on the lookout for those at risk and not distracted by activities such as talking on the phone or reading a book[7]

Unintentional Motor Vehicle Accidents

"Every hour, nearly 150 children between ages 0 and 19 are treated in emergency departments for injuries sustained in motor vehicle crashes."[8] Prevention tips based on the age of the child are as follows:

- "Birth through age 2—Rear-facing child safety seat. For the best possible protection, infants and children should be kept in a rear-facing child safety seat, in the back seat buckled with the seat's harness, until they reach the upper weight or height limits of their particular seat. The weight and height limits on rear-facing child safety seats can accommodate most children through age 2. Check the owner's manual for details.
- "Between ages 2 to 4 or until 40 pounds—Forward-facing child safety seat. When children outgrow their rear-facing seats (the weight and height limits on rear-facing car seats can accommodate most children through age 2), they should ride in forward-facing child safety seats, in the back seat buckled with the seat's harness, until they reach the upper weight or height limit of their particular seat (usually around age 4 and 40 pounds). Many newer seats have higher weight limits. Check the owner's manual for details).
- "Between ages 4 to 8 or until 4'9" tall—Booster seat. Once children outgrow their forward-facing seats (by reaching the upper height and weight limits of their seat), they should ride in belt positioning booster seats. Remember to keep children in the back seat for the best possible protection.
- "After age 8 and/or over 4'9" tall—Seat belt. Children should use booster seats until adult seat belts fit them properly. Seat belts fit properly when the lap belt lays across the upper thighs (not the stomach) and the shoulder belt fits across the chest (not the neck). When adult seat belts fit children properly, they can use the adult seat belts without booster seats. For the best possible protection, keep children in the back seat and use lap and shoulder belts."[8]

In all cases, the back seat is the safest because airbags can pose a risk to a small child.

Unintentional Burns

Every day, 2 children die from burns, and over 300 children and adolescents are treated in emergency departments for burns.[9] Prevention tips to share with families include ensuring that homes are equipped with smoke alarms, creating and practicing escape plans, cooking with care (restricting children's use of stoves, ovens, or microwaves), and lowering the water heater temperature to below 120°F.[9]

Unintentional Homicides

Unfortunately, firearm death is a leading cause of mortality in children.[10] The Community Preventive Services Task Force has a community guide that has useful evidence-based recommendations for laws that can mediate firearm violence.[11] The community guide can be found at http://www.thecommunityguide.org/violence/firearms/firearmlaws.html.

Environment

The CDC has a wide array of resources for its trademark purpose: "Saving Lives. Protecting People." Health care professionals should review this site for additional causes of morbidity and mortality for infants and children (eg, playground injuries and bicycle accidents) and share prevention tips offered for each problem noted.

Health care professionals working in early intervention should educate families about how to make the home environment as risk free as possible for accidents. Several ways to childproof the home include blocking dangerous entrances (eg, place a fence in front of staircases) and keeping children away from electrical outlets, cords, heaters, fans, and other electrical devices. BabyCenter recommends additional measures to childproof the environment and provides a helpful checklist at its website http://www.babycenter.com/0_childproofing-checklist-before-your-baby-crawls_9446.bc.[12]

Sports-Related Injuries

Health care professionals are often involved in providing services to young athletes. The unique knowledge, skill, and expertise of the health care professional complements the knowledge of others who may be involved in managing a team, including the athletic trainer, coach, and team physician. The American Physical Therapy Association and the Sports Physical Therapy Section provide valuable resources to guide health care professionals in providing current information for children and adults engaged in sports. Before engaging in any sport, it is important for each child or youth to have a thorough preparticipation physical examination. The form typically includes demographic information (name, date of birth, sex), personal information (address, school, sports, emergency contacts), medical history, height, weight, percent body fat, vision (specifying correction, as needed), papillary status, and clinical observations of the eyes, ears, nose, throat, lymph nodes, heart, pulses, lungs, genitals (males only), skin, neck, back, shoulder/arm, elbow/forearm, wrist/hand, hip/thigh, knee, leg/ankle, and foot.[13] The musculoskeletal examination focuses on joints that may be stressed by the particular physical activity or sport. For example, the physician might examine the shoulder joint of a pitcher more thoroughly than his ankle joint.

The American Heart Association (AHA) recommends that preparticipation cardiovascular screenings for high school and collegiate athletes are "justifiable and compelling, based on ethical, legal, and medical grounds."[13,14] According to recent studies, "preparticipation screening by history and physical examination alone (without noninvasive testing) is not sufficient to guarantee detection of many critical cardiovascular abnormalities in large populations of young trained athletes." The prevalence of athletic field deaths nationally range from 1:100,000 to 1:300,000 high school–age athletes and is disproportionately higher in males, with the majority of deaths associated with undetected congenital heart defects.[13,14] To reduce this risk of athletic field deaths, one study recommends a comprehensive cardiovascular history addressing the following[14]:

> (1) prior occurrence of exertional chest pain/discomfort or syncope/near-syncope as well as excessive, unexpected, and unexplained shortness of breath or fatigue associated with exercise; (2) past detection of a heart murmur or increased systemic blood pressure; and (3) family history of premature death (sudden or otherwise) or significant disability from cardiovascular disease in close relative(s) younger than 50 years old or specific knowledge of the occurrence of certain conditions (eg, hypertrophic cardiomyopathy, dilated cardiomyopathy, long QT syndrome, Marfan syndrome, or clinically important arrhythmias). These recommendations are offered with the awareness that the accuracy of some responses elicited from young athletes may depend on their level of compliance and historical knowledge. Indeed, parents should be responsible for completing the history forms for high school athletes. The cardiovascular physical examination should emphasize (but not necessarily be limited to): (1) precordial auscultation in both the supine and standing positions to identify, in particular, heart murmurs consistent with dynamic left ventricular outflow obstruction; (2) assessment of the femoral artery pulses to exclude coarctation of the aorta; (3) recognition of the physical stigmata of Marfan syndrome; and (4) brachial blood pressure measurement in the sitting position.

In addition to screening for health status, the health care professional should monitor the use of protective gear appropriate for the client's sport of choice. For example, individuals engaged in soccer need shin guards and properly fitted soccer shoes. Nearly each sport has recommended protective gear that should be required of participants to prevent or reduce injury. Those with proper training can use appropriate athletic taping and strapping to provide support and prevent sports injuries. Warm-up and cool-down exercises, such as stretching and light jogging, also may reduce the risk of tissue injury. Head protection is especially important in contact sports because head injury is potentially a lethal injury. All personnel working with children in sports should be aware of signs of concussion and their immediate management. The Children's Hospital of Philadelphia has a helpful website (http://www.chop.edu/service/concussion-care-for-kids/home.html) that "promotes the prompt recognition of a concussion and immediate treatment with cognitive and physical rest to promote recovery." This site offers a wide range of resources about the recognition and management of concussion designed for health care professionals, coaches, school staff, and families with children. Additional information about concussion is presented in Chapter 15.

Any physical activity, particularly summer sports, can lead to heat-related illnesses. Adequate fluids should be made available at all times to prevent *dehydration*, or deficient body fluids. Children are especially vulnerable to heat-related illness because their thermoregulatory system is not fully developed. Preventable heat-related illnesses include dehydration, *heat exhaustion* (characterized by nausea, dizziness, weakness, headache, pale and moist skin, heavy perspiration, normal or low body temperature, weak pulse, dilated pupils, disorientation, fainting spells), and *heat stroke* (characterized by a fever of 104°F or higher, severe headache, dizziness and feeling lightheaded, a flushed or red appearance to the skin, lack of sweating, muscle weakness or cramps, nausea, vomiting, tachycardia or fast heart rate, tachypnea or fast breathing, feeling confused, anxious or disoriented, and possibly seizures).[13] Health care professionals should caution young athletes and children in sports to maintain adequate hydration and cease activity if they show signs or experience symptoms of heat-related illness. Additionally, athletes need to be aware that certain medications increase the risk of heat-related illness, including beta-blockers and vasoconstrictors, amphetamines, laxatives, antidepressants and antipsychotics, anticonvulsants, and diuretics.[15]

An excellent reference for prevention of sports-related injuries developed by the National Institute of Arthritis and Musculoskeletal and Skin Diseases is located at http://www.niams.nih.gov/hi/topics/childsports/child_sports.htm.[16]

Certain sports pose specific risks to players. Note the concerns that should be addressed for each of the following sports[16]:

- *Football:* Football tends to cause a large number of injuries, especially among males. The most common injuries in football include soft tissue injuries (sprains and strains), as well as damaged bones and internal organs. Knee and ankle injuries are the most common injury sites.[17] To reduce the incidence of injuries, football players should be encouraged to use the proper equipment (helmet, mouth guard, shoulder pads, athletic supporter for males, chest pads, arm pads, thigh pads, shin guards, and the proper shoes for the play surface).
- *Basketball:* The most common injuries in basketball are sprains, strains, bruises, fractures, dislocations, abrasions, and dental injuries. Females have a higher incidence of knee injuries secondary to their lower extremity alignment. Other vulnerable joints include the ankles and shoulders (eg, a *rotator cuff injury*, which is a tear or inflammation of the rotator cuff tendons in the shoulder).[18,19] Basketball players should wear protective gear, including eye protection, mouth guard, elbow and knee pads, basketball shoes, and athletic supporters (for males).[18,19]
- *Soccer:* Soccer injuries include primarily abrasions, lacerations, and bruises. Proper attire includes soccer cleats, shin guards, and athletic supporters (for males). Recent studies have indicated that heading (using the head to strike the ball) may cause head injury or concussion. Players with the highest lifetime estimates of heading had poorer scores on scales measuring attention, concentration, cognitive flexibility, and general intellectual functioning.[18] One suggestion for reducing the risk of head injuries from heading the ball is ensuring the proper proportion of the ball to the player.
- *Baseball and softball:* Baseball and softball share common injuries that relate to sliding into a base or being hit by a ball, resulting in soft tissue injuries and possible fracture.[19] Recommended attire for baseball and softball includes batting helmet, mouth guard, elbow guards, shin guards, and athletic supporters (for males).
- *Track and field:* The most common injuries from running, jumping, and throwing events include sprains, strains, and abrasions from falls.[19] As with most sports, the proper shoes are needed, along with athletic supporters for males.

Injury Prevention for Adults

Sports and Recreation

Sports and recreation can provide much-needed physical activity but can also pose a risk to those who exercise without the proper precautions and protective gear. The CDC estimates that approximately 3.7 million emergency department visits occur each year for injuries related to participation in sports and recreation.[20] The most common sports- and recreation-related injuries include bicycling, basketball, baseball/softball, exercise/running, skiing, weightlifting, football, golf, inline skating, soccer, swimming, volleyball, tennis, horseback riding, and snowboarding, as well as injuries from recreational fires, avalanches, and bites from insects, snakes, and other animals.[20] Wearing protective gear, such as helmets and teeth guards, and using proper techniques can help reduce these injuries in adults.

An excellent resource for injury prevention and care for injured athletes is *Sports Medicine for the Primary Care Physician* by Richard Birrer and Francis O'Connor. This book offers preparticipation examination details, details of common injuries and their management, as well as resources for injury surveillance and prevention.

Fire and Burn Safety

Health care professionals often work with burn patients in acute care, but few offer prevention education to protect against burn injuries. Smoking is the leading cause of fire-related deaths, and cooking is the primary cause of residential fires.[21] Health care professionals can share these facts with their clients and suggest that fire detectors be placed in the home of their clients and teach the "Stop, Drop, and Roll" technique to extinguish fires in case someone encounters flames. Educational media is readily available at local fire stations, as well as the National Fire Protection Association, located at http://www.nfpa.org/, a website that offers various educational media for fire protection education.[22]

Unintentional Poisonings

The CDC states that 87 people die daily as a result of unintentional poisoning, and nearly 2500 require treatment in emergency departments.[23] Medications should be checked each time they are taken, noting the correct name, dosage, and precautions on the label and avoiding alcohol use while using selected medications. Additional helpful tips for preventing medication poisoning are listed at www.poisonprevention.org.[23] Websites with updated drug information include the Food and Drug Administration (FDA) Center for Drug Evaluation and Research (www.fda.gov/cder/index.html) and the National Center for Complementary and Alternative Medicine (NCCAM) (http://nccam.nih.gov/health/decisions).[24] NCCAM offers information about dietary supplements and other alternative treatments that may affect the effectiveness or toxicity of medications.[25]

The CDC estimates that each year roughly 1 in 6 Americans (or 48 million people) get sick, 128,000 are hospitalized, and 3,000 die of foodborne diseases.[26] One helpful resource, *Diagnosis and Management of Food-borne Illnesses: A Primer for Physicians and Other Health care Professionals*, contains charts, scenarios, and a continuing medical education section, and is free to health care professionals (http://www.cdc.gov/mmwr/preview/mmwrhtml/rr5304a1.htm).[27] The primer was created through a partnership of the American Medical Association (AMA) and the American Nurses Association (ANA)–American Nurses Foundation (ANF), in conjunction with the CDC Food Safety Office, the FDA Center for Food Safety and Applied Nutrition, and the US Department of Agriculture (USDA) Food Safety and Inspection Service.

Botulism is a muscle-paralyzing disease caused by a toxin made by a bacterium called *Clostridium botulinum*. Botulism can become foodborne when a person ingests preformed toxin that leads to illness. With foodborne botulism, symptoms begin within 6 hours to 2 weeks (most commonly between 12 and 36 hours) after eating toxin-containing food.[28] Symptoms of botulism include double vision, blurred vision, drooping eyelids, slurred speech, difficulty swallowing, dry mouth, and muscle weakness that always descends through the body (shoulders are affected first, then upper arms, lower arms, thighs, and calves).[28] Paralysis of breathing muscles can cause a person to stop breathing unless mechanical ventilation is provided. If a client presents with these signs and symptoms, botulism should be suspected and the individual should seek immediate medical attention.

Tobacco Use

Cigarette smoking is the leading preventable cause of death in the United States, but the health consequences extend beyond smokers to nonsmokers who are involuntarily exposed to environmental tobacco smoke or secondhand smoke. The statistics for smoking are alarming[29]:

- Smoking causes cancer, heart disease, stroke, and lung diseases (including emphysema, bronchitis, and chronic airway obstruction).
- For every person who dies from a smoking-related disease, 20 more people suffer with at least one serious illness from smoking.
- Cigarette smoking is responsible for approximately 1 in 5 deaths annually (ie, more than 440,000 deaths per year), and an estimated 49,000 of these smoking-related deaths are the result of secondhand smoke exposure.
- On average, smokers die 10 years earlier than nonsmokers.

A helpful website with evidence-based programs to facilitate smoking cessation, jointly offered by the National Cancer Institute, the CDC, the National Institutes of Health, and the US Department of Health and Human Services, is located at www.smokefree.gov.[30]

Pesticides

Pesticides are substances used to kill pests: *herbicides* are pesticides used to kill weeds, *insecticides* are pesticides used to kill insects, and *fungicides* are pesticides used for controlling disease on crops and seed. Farmers are relatively heavy users of pesticides, and they appear to experience an excess of certain types of cancer. Cancers more commonly seen in farmers include non-Hodgkin's lymphoma, soft tissue sarcoma, and cancers of the lip, stomach, brain, and prostate.[31] Non-Hodgkin's lymphoma and sarcomas are also increasing in the general population of the United States, suggesting that a common set of exposures may be involved.[31]

> Results from the Agricultural Health Study, an ongoing study of pesticide exposures in farm families, show that farmers who used agricultural insecticides experienced an increase in headaches, fatigue, insomnia, dizziness, hand tremors, and other neurological symptoms. Evidence suggests that children are particularly susceptible to adverse effects from exposure to pesticides, including neurodevelopmental effects. People may also be exposed to pesticides used in a variety of settings including homes, schools, hospitals, and workplaces.[31]

If exposed to pesticides, individuals should exercise caution and try to avoid direct contact between pesticides and the sites of body entry (the skin and eyes). A wide variety of toxins surround Americans daily, and health care professionals need to be acutely aware of the risks of these toxins, whether they are natural organisms or man-made agents designed to kill microorganisms or other pests, and educate the public about their risks. Using sanitary health habits can reduce the risk of toxicity when exposed to both natural and synthetic toxins.

Firearms: Homicide and Suicide

Many Americans have access to guns, increasing the risk of injury and death from firearms. For those using guns for recreation and sport, it is essential that firearm safety be taught. The risk of homicide and suicide are related to mental health issues that must be addressed through multifaceted approaches, including primary prevention of violence and recognition of those at risk for suicide or homicide.

One effective preventive strategy for suicide is promoting social connection. "Increasing connectedness among persons, families, and communities—including service, funding, and advocacy communities—is likely to have a universal as well as a targeted effect on suicidal behavior."[32] Health care professionals who note social isolation should also be aware of risk factors for suicide, including a family history of suicide or child maltreatment, previous suicide attempt(s), a history of mental disorders (particularly clinical depression), a history of alcohol and substance abuse, feelings of hopelessness, impulsive or aggressive tendencies, cultural and religious beliefs (eg, belief that suicide is a noble resolution of a personal dilemma), local epidemics of suicide, isolation, barriers to accessing mental health treatment, loss (relational, social, work, or financial), physical illness, easy access to lethal methods, and an unwillingness to seek help because of the stigma attached to mental health and substance abuse disorders or to suicidal thoughts.[32] Warning signs of suicide are sufficient evidence to make a referral to a doctor, psychologist, or psychiatrist. It is important to explore suicidal thoughts with depressed individuals in a nonjudgmental manner, and take thoughts of or plans for suicide seriously. If necessary, the health care professional may choose to contact 911 if the client has a serious plan for committing suicide.

Drowning

An average of 10 people die of drowning per day, and more than 80% of drownings occur among males.[33] Health care professionals should advise their clients to swim under the supervision of a qualified lifeguard and avoid swimming under risky conditions, such as while using alcohol.

Swimming

Health care professionals, particularly those who practice aquatic therapy, should keep these tips in mind when developing client regulations for their programs: (1) do not enter the water if you have diarrhea; (2) do not swallow the water; (3) wash hands and bottom thoroughly with soap and water after a bowel movement; and (4) notify the lifeguard if fecal matter is seen in the water or if someone changes diapers on nearby tables and chairs. These precautions can reduce preventable health hazards for community pools.

Sun and Heat

Reduced sun exposure can reduce the risk of skin cancer. Individuals are at the greatest risk when the sun's ultraviolent rays are strongest, generally between 10 AM and 4 PM.[34] Individuals should be encouraged to wear long sleeves and pants and apply sunscreen and protective lip balm with a comprehensive SPF of 30 or higher whenever exposed to sunlight. Sunscreen and lip balm should be reapplied frequently when swimming.

Safety and Occupational Health

The mission of the Occupational Safety and Health Administration is to ensure the safety and health of America's workers by setting and enforcing standards; providing training, outreach, and education; establishing partnerships; and encouraging continual improvement in workplace safety and health.[35] According to 2011 statistics, workers in transportation, construction, agriculture, fishing, forestry, and hunting have the highest number of fatal occupational injuries.[35] The most common injuries are sprains, strains, and tears, and the areas of the body most commonly injured are the back, upper extremities, lower extremities, and trunk.[35] Health care professionals can play a key role in preventing injuries by educating the public about proper posture and body position. Work ergonomics is a burgeoning area of physical therapy practice that can contribute significantly to injury prevention. See Chapter 13 for additional information about safety and occupational health.

Product Safety

Certain products must be recalled because of manufacturing flaws or designs flaws that put the public at risk. The US Consumer Product Safety Commission (CPSC) is charged with protecting the public from unreasonable risks of serious injury or death from consumer products under the agency's jurisdiction.[36] Health care professionals can help reduce the incidence of product injuries by keeping informed of product risks and discouraging their use. Updated information about specific products can be found at the CPSC website at http://www.cpsc.gov/.[36]

Motor Vehicle Accidents

In any given year, approximately 10 million Americans are involved in motor vehicle accidents (MVAs).[37] Simply encouraging individuals to buckle up when they leave the physical therapy setting is a brief, helpful reminder that could reduce fatal MVAs. Factors contributing to MVAs include alcohol, drugs, fatigue, and distractions such as texting, using a cellphone, eating and drinking, talking to passengers, grooming, reading (eg, looking at maps), using a navigation system, watching a video, adjusting a radio or music player, smoking, and eating. In 2011, 3331 people were killed in crashes involving a distracted driver.[38]

Those who survive MVAs may have multiple impairments affecting their ability to function and participate in daily life, such as posttraumatic stress, depression, and anxiety. Health care professionals treating patients post-MVA need to be aware of the need for psychological counseling if their clients show signs of posttraumatic stress disorder, including depression, substance abuse, problems with memory and cognition, and other problems of physical and mental health. The disorder is also associated with impairment of the person's ability to function in social or family life, including occupational instability, marital problems and divorces, family discord, and difficulties in parenting. It is helpful to encourage survivors of MVAs to maintain as much of their preaccident lifestyle as possible, with as much support from family and friends as available. Such coping strategies appear to be linked with positive mental health outcomes.

Spinal Cord Injuries

Spinal cord injuries (SCIs) can be caused by any number of injuries resulting from MVAs, falls, sports injuries (particularly diving into shallow water), industrial accidents, gunshot wounds, and assault. Individuals with rheumatoid arthritis or osteoporosis are vulnerable to even minor injuries due to their compromised skeletal system. Complications of SCI include respiratory complications, urinary tract infections, spasticity, and scoliosis. Prevention includes health education about physical activities that increase the risk the SCI, including participating in risky physical activities, not wearing protective gear during work or play, or diving into shallow water. Additional information about SCIs is provided in Chapter 15.

Traumatic Brain Injuries

Nearly 1.5 million people experience traumatic brain injury (TBI) annually in the United States, and approximately 50,000 people die, costing nearly $50 billion annually.[39] Precautions to reduce injuries caused by motor vehicles and bicycles can help reduce the incidence of TBI, including automobile airbags, seatbelts, and infant or child safety seats. Health care professionals should remind their clients that the risk of TBI and SCI warrant special attention to use of their vehicles. Chapter 15 provides additional information about prevention practice for individuals with TBI.

Dog Bite Injuries

Although seemingly minor, dog bites account for a large number of preventable injuries. Health care professionals may encounter clients with guide dogs or dogs trained to assist with mobility. It is important to recognize the risks posed by dogs and to encourage appropriate and respectful interaction with dogs to reduce injuries.

Violence Across the Lifespan

Violence is defined as "the intentional use of physical force or power, threatened or actual, against oneself, another person, or against a group or community, either resulting in or having a high likelihood of resulting in injury, death, psychological harm, maldevelopment, or deprivation."[40] Violence may be directed at an intimate partner, child, older adult, or community, such as a school or workplace. Additionally, some violence is motivated by hate and intolerance, such as racial bigotry and intolerance to sexual orientation. The health care professional should be aware of factors that put individuals at risk for violence. Although abuse is discussed in Chapters 5, 6, and 9, this section will provide additional information related to violence typically seen across the lifespan.

Intimate Partner Violence

Intimate partner violence affects women more than men and includes domestic abuse, spouse abuse, battering, domestic violence, courtship violence, marital rape, and date rape. Certain factors put women at an increased risk for intimate partner violence. These individual vulnerability factors include (1) a history of physical abuse, (2) prior injury from the same partner, (3) having a verbally abusive partner, (4) economic stress, (5) partner history of alcohol or drug abuse, (6) childhood abuse, and (7) being under the age of 24. In addition, research has identified several relational vulnerability factors related to intimate partner violence, including marital conflict, marital instability, male dominance in the family, and poor family functioning.[40] If these factors are suspected, the health care professional should make an attempt to interview the woman separately from her partner to inquire about her personal concerns and fears of domestic violence.

Sexual Violence

Sexual violence may be perpetrated by someone the individual does not know, such as rape by a stranger. Of rape victims who reported the offense to law enforcement, a large percentage are under the age of 18.[40] Alcohol is reported as a contributing factor in half of all reported rapes. Health care professionals need to be aware of such violence and ask open-ended questions that allow their clients to share their intimate lives. Children may be vulnerable to sexual violence and *sexual abuse* (fondling a child's genitals, intercourse, incest, rape, sodomy, exhibitionism, and commercial exploitation through prostitution or the production of pornographic material). In addition to sexual abuse and violence, children may endure *physical abuse* (infliction of physical injury as a result of punching, beating, kicking, biting, burning, shaking, or otherwise harming the child) or *neglect* (failure to provide for the child's basic psychological, medical, emotional, or physical needs).[40] Children at an increased risk for neglect include those with mothers who are angry, have low self-esteem, lack confidence, are impulsive, and have unrealistic expectations.[40] Mothers and children in disadvantaged communities may be at higher risk for child neglect. If any type of violence against a child is suspected, the health care professional must report the suspected abuse to the Child Protective Services agency in the state in which the abuse occurred. The Childhelp USA National Child Abuse Hotline (1-800-4-A-CHILD) can help locate the appropriate agency for reporting suspected abuse or negligence and provide counseling.[41]

Individuals of all ages are vulnerable to rape. Behaviors exhibited post-rape may include, but are not limited to, chronic headaches, fatigue, sleep disturbances, recurrent nausea, decreased appetite, eating disorders, menstrual pain, sexual dysfunction, and suicidal behavior.[41] Individuals who present with unusual behaviors or factors that put them at risk for violence should be examined thoroughly by an appropriate health care professional, such as a physician, social worker, or psychologist.

Elder Abuse

Elder abuse is a term referring to any knowing, intentional, or negligent act by a caregiver or any other person that causes harm or a serious risk of harm to a vulnerable adult.[42] According to National Center on Elder Abuse, the laws for elder abuse vary from state to state but generally include the following: (1) *physical abuse* (inflicting, or threatening to inflict, physical pain or injury on a vulnerable elder or depriving them of a basic need), (2) *emotional abuse* (inflicting mental pain, anguish, or distress on an elder person through verbal or nonverbal acts), (3) *sexual abuse* (nonconsensual sexual contact of any kind), (4) *exploitation* (illegal taking, misuse, or concealment of funds, property, or assets of a vulnerable elder), (5) *neglect* (refusal or failure by those responsible to provide food, shelter, health care, or protection for a vulnerable elder), and (6) *abandonment* (the desertion of a vulnerable elder by anyone who has assumed the responsibility for care or custody of that person).[42] The health care professional should be alert to signs of elder abuse, including the following[42]:

- Physical signs of abuse, neglect, or maltreatment, such as bruises, pressure marks, broken bones, abrasions, and burns. Bruises around the breasts or genital area can occur from sexual abuse.
- Unexplained withdrawal from normal activities, a sudden change in alertness, and unusual depression may be indicators of emotional abuse.
- Sudden change in financial situation may be the result of exploitation.
- Bedsores, unattended medical needs, poor hygiene, and unusual weight loss are indicators of possible neglect.
- Behaviors such as belittling, threats, and other uses of power and control by spouses are indicators of verbal or emotional abuse; frequent arguments between the caregiver and elderly person are a common sign.

In addition, individuals who are incapable of self-care may exhibit self-neglect or behaviors that indicate the need for intervention. These behaviors include, but are not limited to, hoarding; poor hygiene; confusion; wearing inappropriate clothing; leaving stoves, irons, or other devices unattended; poor housekeeping; and dehydration. Often, self-neglect is coupled with declining health, isolation, Alzheimer's disease or dementia, or drug and alcohol dependency.[42] The health care professional is responsible for reporting suspected abuse or neglect for adults at increased risk for elder abuse. Reports can be made by calling 911 for individuals who are at immediate risk.

Ideally, health care professionals should work together to prevent violence to all populations at risk.

Falls

Every hour, an older adult dies or is injured as the result of a fall. Chapter 9 discusses how health care professionals can help screen older adults who are at increased risk for falling and address problems contributing to falls. The CDC has published an online resource, the *Compendium of Effective Fall Interventions: What Works for Community-Dwelling Older Adults*, that describes evidence-based interventions along with relevant details about these interventions for organizations that want to implement fall prevention programs.[43] This compendium includes interventions ranging from exercise and home modifications to multifaceted programs.

A comparable resource is offered for children at risk for falls. Unintentional falls are the leading cause of nonfatal injury in children younger than 19 years of age in the United States.[44] Interestingly, many infants fall while supervised by their caregiver. The age of the child dictates the most likely cause of falling: infants tend to fall from furniture, stairs, or walkers; toddlers more often fall from windows and balconies; and older children fall from bicycles, skateboards, scooters, and playground equipment.[44] Boys are more than twice as likely as girls to die from fall-related injuries. Each year, 2.9 million children are treated in emergency rooms for fall-related injuries, with children younger than 5 years representing the largest proportion of visits.[44] Falls are also the most frequent cause of any injury during infancy due to immature motor skills and novel movements. Falls by children occur mainly in the warmer months and in the home for younger children; as children grow, more falls occur at school or on playground equipment. The location and mechanism of injuries caused by falls vary depending on the age of the child. Health care professionals should remind parents to be especially vigilant when children learn how to climb furniture and explore their new freedoms at increased heights.

Alcoholism

Alcohol has been touted as a healthy drink in a limited amount but is deleterious if overconsumed. According to the Harvard Medical School of Public Health:

> Moderate drinking seems to be good for the heart and circulatory system and probably protects against type 2 diabetes and gallstones. Heavy drinking is a major cause of preventable deaths and is implicated in about half of fatal traffic accidents. Heavy drinking can damage the liver and heart, harm an unborn child [blocks folate], increase the chances of developing breast and some other cancers, contribute to depression and violence, and interfere with relationships. Excessive drinking includes heavy drinking, binge drinking, and any drinking by pregnant women or underage youth.[45]

Heavy drinking refers to consuming more than an average of 1 drink per day for women and more than 2 drinks for men. One drink is comparable to 12 ounces of regular beer or wine cooler, 8 ounces of malt liquor, 5 ounces of wine, or 1.5 ounces of 80-proof distilled spirits or liquor (eg, gin, rum, vodka, or whiskey).[46] *Binge drinking*, by definition, is 4 or more drinks during a single occasion for women and 5 or more drinks during a single session for men.[46]

Research has implicated a gene (D2 dopamine receptor gene) that, when inherited in a specific form, might increase a person's chance of developing alcoholism.[47] Usually, a variety of factors contribute to the development of a problem with alcohol. Social factors, such as the influence of family, peers, and society and the availability of alcohol; and psychological factors, such as elevated levels of stress, inadequate coping mechanisms, and reinforcement of alcohol use from other drinkers, can contribute to alcoholism. Once the disease develops, the factors that contributed to initial alcohol use may vary from those maintaining it.[47]

Ideally, individuals who are prone to alcoholism would avoid drinking alcohol; however, alcohol consumption and drug abuse are prevalent in society, and it is difficult to eradicate the source of the problem. Prevention activities may require a multifaceted approach among health

Table 12-2. Screening for Adult Hearing Loss
"Yes" answers to 3 or more questions indicate the need for a medical referral.
1. Do I have a problem hearing on the telephone?
2. Do I have trouble hearing when there is noise in the background?
3. Is it hard for me to follow a conversation when 2 or more people talk at once?
4. Do I have to strain to understand a conversation?
5. Do many people I talk to seem to mumble (or not speak clearly)?
6. Do I misunderstand what others are saying and respond inappropriately?
7. Do I often ask people to repeat themselves?
8. Do I have trouble understanding the speech of women and children?
9. Do people complain that I turn the TV volume up too high?
10. Do I hear a ringing, roaring, or hissing sound a lot?
11. Do some sounds seem too loud?
Source: Hearing, ear infections, and deafness. National Institute on Deafness and Other Communication Disorders. National Institutes of Health. http://www.nidcd.nih.gov/health/hearing. Accessed February 2, 2006.

care providers. If alcoholism is suspected, an immediate referral to the physician or psychologist is necessary.

Hearing Loss

Major causes of deafness and hearing impairment result from congenital or early-onset childhood hearing loss, chronic otitis media (ie, chronic middle ear infection from viruses or bacteria), injury, tumors, and ototoxic drugs that damage the inner ear.[48]

Some individuals lose their hearing slowly as a result of *presbycusis* (a progressive, age-related hearing loss that may be caused by changes in the blood supply to the ear because of heart disease, high blood pressure, vascular conditions caused by diabetes, or other circulatory problems).[49] Approximately 25% to 30% of people aged 65 to 74 years and 40% to 50% over age 75 are estimated to have impaired hearing associated with genetics, environmental noise, drugs, diet and metabolism, and stress, among other factors.[49] With presbycusis, sounds often seem less clear and lower in volume and higher-pitched sounds are difficult to distinguish.

Another common cause is noise exposure. Avoiding loud noises or protecting the ears with foam earplugs can help protect against hearing loss, especially for individuals who use loud machinery (eg, lawn mowers or power tools) or firearms. Screenings for hearing loss can alert individuals of their hearing ability so that proper treatment can be sought. Table 12-2 provides a list of questions that can help an individual recognize the onset of hearing loss. If hearing loss is suspected, a medical referral should be made to an audiologist, otolaryngologist, or primary physician for further examination. Often, hearing aids can be used to augment hearing in the case of hearing loss.

Because communication is so important in daily living, it is important to prevent the psychosocial isolation that can accompany hearing loss. The following suggestions are offered by the National Institute on Deafness and Other Communication Disorders[50]:

- Face the person who has a hearing loss so your face can be seen when you speak.

- Be sure that lighting is in front of you when you speak. This allows a person with a hearing impairment to observe facial expressions, gestures, and lip and body movements that provide communication clues.
- During conversations, turn off the radio or television.
- Avoid speaking while chewing food or covering your mouth with your hands.
- Speak slightly louder than normal, but don't shout. Shouting may distort your speech.
- Speak at your normal rate, and do not exaggerate sounds.
- Clue in the person with hearing loss about the topic of the conversation whenever possible.
- Rephrase your statement into shorter, simpler sentences if it appears you are not being understood.
- In restaurants and social gatherings, choose seats away from crowded or noisy areas.

General Safety

Health care providers must be prepared to act decisively when evacuating an area during an emergency. Easter Seals provides the following S.A.F.E.T.Y. tips to guide those aiding in evacuation during emergency situations[51]:

- *S*tart preparing an evacuation plan now. If you have a disability, identify yourself to building managers and help devise an effective emergency procedure. People of all abilities must be equally prepared for an emergency evacuation. It is critical that everyone works together.
- *A*sk family, friends, and coworkers with disabilities—including those with vision, hearing and mobility issues—about their personal evacuation concerns and needs. Keep in mind that the needs of pregnant women, older adults, and people with injuries or illnesses are often similar to specific needs of people with disabilities.
- *F*ind "buddies." These can be coworkers or friends with whom you plan and practice. Buddies find you in an emergency and can provide planned assistance in the event of an emergency or evacuation.
- *E*valuate the area. Predetermine and practice your evacuation route with your buddies, who also know how to operate any special equipment needed to evacuate someone safely.
- *T*est smoke detectors, public announcement systems, fire extinguishers, and flashlights to assure proper function when needed. Make sure alternate alert systems are available for individuals with special needs, especially for people with vision and hearing disabilities.
- *Y*ou can help Easter Seals by making this important issue top-of-mind in your community—talking to business leaders, building management, government officials, and police and fire departments.

The following considerations should be taken into account when talking to individuals with disabilities about their plans for evacuation[51]:

- Do you need help with personal care or use adaptive equipment to meet your personal care needs?
  - What assistance would you need in an emergency?
  - What would you do if water or electricity were cut off?
- Do you need accessible transportation?
- Do you need assistance to leave your home or office?
- How will you need to be alerted to an emergency?

- If elevators are not working, do you have a backup plan?
- Who will be available and know how to help you exit?
- Will you need mobility aids to exit?
    - Will you need backup mobility aids when you reach a safe place?
- Do you need medical supplies available in a safe place?
- Will you need assistance in training and caring for a service animal?
- Who needs to know where you will be after an emergency evaluation?

Share answers and the plan for evacuation with families, caretakers, and others working with individuals with disabilities.

SUMMARY

The success of Healthy People 2020 relies on the expertise of health care professionals to identify individual and community risk factors that potentially lead to preventable accidents and diseases. As part of a team, health care professionals can contribute to the identification of risk factors and developing health problems resulting from inadequate protection from infections and injury. They can also avert catastrophes for those with disabilities by planning ahead. Health care professionals play an essential role in providing health education and screenings to their clients, who are often at increased risk for hazards that further jeopardize health and wellness. As advocates, health care professionals can work to improve communities by developing accurate health protection information, detecting risks, recognizing at-risk populations, and locating resources for transforming communities into healthy, safe living environments.

REFERENCES

1. Immunizations and infectious diseases. Healthy People 2020. http://www.healthypeople.gov/2020/topicsobjectives2020/overview.aspx?topicid=23. Accessed May 5, 2013.
2. Lam WK, Zhong NS, Tan WC. Overview on SARS in Asia and the world. *Respirology.* 2003;8(Suppl):S2-S5.
3. Injury and violence prevention. Centers for Disease Control and Prevention. http://www.cdc.gov/injury/. Accessed May 5, 2013.
4. HCCA safe sleep campaign. American Academy of Pediatricians. http://www.healthychildcare.org/sids.html. Accessed May 5, 2013.
5. Jones MW. Supine and prone infant positioning: a winning combination. *J Perinat Educ.* 2004;13(1):10-20.
6. Back to sleep, tummy to play. Healthy Child Care America. http://www.healthychildcare.org/pdf/SIDStummytime.pdf. Accessed May 5, 2013.
7. Drowning: the reality. Centers for Disease Control and Prevention. http://www.cdc.gov/SafeChild/Drowning/. Accessed May 5, 2013.
8. Road traffic injuries: the reality. Centers for Disease Control and Prevention. http://www.cdc.gov/safechild/Road_Traffic_Injuries/index.html. Accessed May 5, 2013.
9. Burn safety: the reality. Centers for Disease Control and Prevention. http://www.cdc.gov/Safechild/Burns/. Accessed May 5, 2013.
10. Violence prevention: firearms laws. Community Preventive Services Task Force. http://www.thecommunityguide.org/violence/firearms/firearmlaws.html. Accessed May 5, 2013.
11. Hahn RA, Bilukha O, Crosby A, et al. Firearms laws and the reduction of violence: a systematic review. *Am J Prev Med.* 2005;28(2S1):40-71.
12. Childproofing checklist: before your baby crawls. BabyCenter. http://www.babycenter.com/0_childproofing-checklist-before-your-baby-crawls_9446.bc. Accessed May 5, 2013.
13. Maron B, Thompson P, Puffer J, et al. Cardiovascular pre-participation screening of competitive athletes. *Circulation.* 1996;94:850-856.
14. Damlo S. AHA releases recommendations on pre-participation screening in student athletes. *Am Fam Physician.* 2007;76(10):1568-1569.

15. Heat exhaustion and heatstroke. FamilyDoctor.org. http://familydoctor.org/familydoctor/en/prevention-wellness/staying-healthy/first-aid/heat-exhaustion-an-heatstroke.html. Accessed May 5, 2013.
16. Childhood sports injuries and their prevention: a guide for parents with ideas for kids. National Institute of Arthritis and Musculoskeletal and Skin Diseases. http://www.niams.nih.gov/hi/topics/childsports/child_sports.htm. Accessed May 8, 2013.
17. Requa R. The scope of the problem: the impact of sports-related injuries. In: Proceedings of Sports Injuries in Youth: Surveillance Strategies. Bethesda, MD: National Institues of Health; 1992:19.
18. Messina DF, Farney WC, DeLee JC. The incidence of injury in Texas high school basketball. *Am J Sports Med.* 1999;27(3):294-299.
19. Powell JW, Barber-Foss KD. Injury patterns in selected high school sports: a review of the 1995-1997 seasons. *J Athl Train.* 1999;34(3):277-284.
20. Preventing injuries in sports, recreation, and exercise. Centers for Disease Control and Prevention. http://www.cdc.gov/ncipc/pub-res/research_agenda/05_sports.htm. Accessed May 8, 2013.
21. Ahrens M. *Home Structure Fires.* Quincy, MA: National Fire Protection Association; 2011.
22. Safety information. National Fire Protection Association. http://www.nfpa.org/. Accessed May 8, 2013.
23. Prevent unintentional poisonings. Centers for Disease Control and Prevention. http://www.cdc.gov/features/poisonprevention/. Accessed May 8, 2013.
24. Safety information. Food and Drug Administration's Center for Drug Evaluation and Research. http://www.fda.gov/cder/index.html. Accessed May 8, 2013.
25. Health supplements. National Center for Complementary and Alternative Medicine. http://nccam.nih.gov/health/supplements. Accessed May 8, 2013.
26. Estimates of foodborne illness in the United States. Centers for Disease Control and Prevention. http://www.cdc.gov/foodborneburden/. Accessed May 8, 2013.
27. Diagnosis and management of foodborne illnesses: a primer for physicians and other health care professionals. American Medical Association. http://www.ama-assn.org//ama/pub/physician-resources/medical-science/foodborne-illnesses/diagnosis-management-foodborne.page. Accessed May 8, 2013.
28. Hatheway CL. Botulism: the present status of the disease. *Curr Top Microbiol Immunol.* 1999;195:55-75.
29. Smoking and tobacco use. Centers for Disease Control and Prevention. http://www.cdc.gov/tobacco/data_statistics/fact_sheets/fast_facts/index.htm. Accessed May 8, 2013.
30. Resources for health professionals. Smokefree.gov. http://www.smokefree.gov/hp.aspx. Accessed May 8, 2013.
31. Pesticides. National Institute of Environmental Health Science. http://www.niehs.nih.gov/health/topics/agents/pesticides/. Accessed May 8, 2013.
32. Strategic direction for the prevention of suicidal behavior: Promoting individual, family, and community connectedness to prevent suicidal behavior. National Center for Injury Prevention and Control. http://www.cdc.gov/ViolencePrevention/pdf/Suicide_Strategic_Direction_Full_Version-a.pdf. Accessed May 8, 2013.
33. Unintentional drowning: get the facts. Centers for Disease Control and Prevention. http://www.cdc.gov/homeandrecreationalsafety/water-safety/waterinjuries-factsheet.html. Accessed May 8, 2013.
34. Skin cancer facts. American Cancer Society. http://www.cancer.org/cancer/cancercauses/sunanduvexposure/skin-cancer-facts. Accessed May 8, 2013.
35. Occupational health and safety. US Department of Labor. http://www.osha.gov/about.html. Accessed May 8, 2013.
36. CPSC overview. US Consumer Product Safety Commission. http://www.cpsc.gov. Accessed May 8, 2013.
37. Transportation: motor vehicle accidents and fatalities. US Census Bureau. http://www.census.gov/compendia/statab/cats/transportation/motor_vehicle_accidents_and_fatalities.html. Accessed May 8, 2013.
38. What is distracted driving? Distraction.gov. http://www.distraction.gov/content/get-the-facts/facts-and-statistics.html. Accessed May 8, 2013.
39. Traumatic brain injury. Health Communities.com. http://www.healthcommunities.com/traumatic-brain-injury/overview-of-tbi.shtml. Accessed May 8, 2013.
40. Injury, violence & safety. Centers for Disease Control and Prevention. http://www.cdc.gov/features/injuryviolencesafety.html. AccessedMay 8, 2013.
41. ChildHelp National Abuse Hotline. http://www.childhelp-usa.com/. Accessed May 8, 2013.
42. Types of abuse: self-neglect. Department of Health and Human Services National Center on Elder Abuse. http://www.ncea.aoa.gov/FAQ/Type_Abuse/index.aspx#self. Accessed May 20, 2014.
43. CDC compendium of effective fall interventions: what works for community-dwelling older adults. Centers for Disease Control and Prevention. http://www.cdc.gov/HomeandRecreationalSafety/Falls/compendium.html. Accessed May 8, 2013.
44. Falls: the reality. Centers for Disease Control and Prevention. http://www.cdc.gov/safechild/falls/. Accessed May 8, 2013.
45. Alcohol: balancing risks and benefits. Harvard School of Public Health. http://www.hsph.harvard.edu/nutritionsource/alcohol-full-story/. Accessed May 8, 2013.
46. Alcohol and public health. Centers for Disease Control and Prevention. http://www.cdc.gov/alcohol/fact-sheets/alcohol-use.htm. Accessed May 8, 2013.

47. Alcoholism. University of Maryland Medical Center. http://www.umm.edu/patiented/articles/what_causes_alcoholism_000056_2.htm. Accessed May 8, 2013.
48. Strategies for prevention of deafness and hearing impairment. World Health Organization. http://www.who.int/pbd/deafness/activities/strategies/en/index.html. Accessed May 8, 2013.
49. Presbycusis. Medscape. http://reference.medscape.com/article/855989-overview. Accessed May 8, 2013.
50. Hearing loss and older adults. National Institute on Deafness and Other Communication Disorders. http://www.nidcd.nih.gov/health/hearing/pages/older.aspx. Accessed May 8, 2013.
51. Emergency preparedness. Easter Seals. http://www.easterseals.com/. Accessed May 5, 2013.

13

Prevention Practice for Musculoskeletal Conditions

Amy Foley, DPT, PT; Gail Regan, PhD, MS, PT; and Catherine Rush Thompson, PT, PhD, MS

"Pain is the only way the musculoskeletal system can protect itself."—Vladimir Janda, MD, *Assessment and Treatment of Muscle Imbalance: The Janda Approach*

Musculoskeletal conditions involve pathologies of connective tissue and bone that impair joint mobility and range of motion, limit motor function, and affect motor performance. Common pathologies covered in this chapter include musculotendinous injuries due to cumulative, repetitive stress syndromes; chronic low back pain; and osteoarthritis. Familiarity with the normal development of body systems, in particular the musculoskeletal system, helps health care professionals make keen observations during screenings across the lifespan.

Risks to the Musculoskeletal System During Development

For children younger than age 1, it is important to note the development of body systems that enable motor function. During the first 6 months of life, the infant's skeleton is exposed to dynamic muscle activity and gravitational forces that provide the forces needed to grow long bones and develop proper alignment of skeletal structures.[1] The skull grows with forces exerted by the developing brain, and teeth emerge from the mandible as early as 6 months. As the child develops head control, the primary curve in the cervical region develops; with developing sitting posture, the secondary curve is evident in the lumbar spine. Rapid growth and development of the skeleton continues from 7 to 12 months, sufficient to support the infant's weight on all fours and in standing.[1] Table 13-1 summarizes the musculoskeletal changes during the first year of life.[1]

Thompson CR.
Prevention Practice and Health Promotion: A Health Care Professional's Guide to Health, Fitness, and Wellness, Second Edition (pp 209-224).

Table 13-1. Musculoskeletal Changes in the First Year of Life

	1 TO 6 MONTHS	7 TO 12 MONTHS
Skeletal muscles	Muscle fibrils grow by multiplication Muscle length is stimulated by skeletal growth Muscle is growing in size by accumulating cytoplasm rather than growing in numbers (after 4 to 5 months)	
Cardiac muscle	Cells of the visceral muscle increase in number and in size with growth Cardiac muscle also increases by enlarging existing muscle fibers	
Facial muscles	Muscles of the face and respiration are well developed at birth	
Postural patterns and functional movement associated with muscle development	Second month characterized by decreased flexion and increased extension and asymmetry Third month characterized by the beginning of symmetry and the beginning of bilateral control of neck muscles By 6 months, baby can extend the neck against gravity	By 7 months, baby can pivot around in prone using symmetrical upper extremity movement By 8 months, baby can creep as the primary means of locomotion By 12 months, baby is capable of rising to stand by sole use of legs By 12 months, finger opposition is present

Adapted from Kaywood K, Hetchell N. *Life Span Motor Development*. Champaign, IL: Human Kinetics; 2001; and Linn JP, Brown JK, Walsh EG. Physiological maturation of muscles in childhood. *Lancet*. 1994;343:1386-1389.

Muscular Changes During the First Year

Skeletal muscle fibers grow by multiplication as the infant uses the body to explore the environment. The stress of skeletal growth elongates the muscles, and cellular changes after 4 to 5 months cause an increase in fiber size.[1] Likewise, cardiac muscle tissue grows in size, and the myocardium (heart muscle) increases in size as existing muscle fibers grow, with increasingly stronger heartbeats to match demands by physical activity. The normal resting heart rate for an infant is 100 to 160 beats per minute.[1] The muscles of the face and respiration are both well developed at birth, enabling the infant to eat and cry for attention.

Muscular Changes in Years 1 to 6

In the first 3 years of life, the child increases muscle strength to support bipedal locomotion. The cardiac muscle subsequently increases in size, especially the left ventricle, to accommodate the increasing workload associated with the motor activity of an infant and toddler. Children from 1 to 10 years of age have resting heart rates of 70 to 120 beats per minute, slightly slower than that of newborn babies.[1] As the child develops sphincter control, the child may begin toilet training

Table 13-2. Muscular Changes in Years 1 to 6

	1 TO 3 YEARS	4 TO 6 YEARS
Skeletal muscles	Early in this stage, muscular strength of the trunk and lower extremities increases to support bipedal locomotion	Creatinine in urine increases as muscle mass increases Muscle fibers increase in diameter as strength increases Muscle strength increases as activity increases
Cardiac muscle	Muscles of the left ventricle of the heart grow more than the right to accommodate the increase in workload	
Sphincter muscles	Sphincter muscles develop to allow toilet training	
Postural patterns associated with muscle development	With continued weight bearing, growth of intrinsic feet muscles causes the once fat, thick, and archless foot to become arched with the development of the longitudinal arch At 2 years, toddler displays a mature grasp pattern that enables prehension and the manual exchange of objects	Muscle strength depends on body proportions (adult normative values are not accurate for children) Children may experience growth pains as muscle growth accompanies bone growth By age 5, children have adequate manipulation skills to begin handwriting

Adapted from Kaywood K, Hetchell N. *Life Span Motor Development.* Champaign, IL: Human Kinetics; 2001.

and eliminate the need for diapers. With continued motor activity, particularly weight-bearing activities like walking and running, the child increasingly develops the strength of foot intrinsic muscles that support the longitudinal arches of both feet. More sophisticated reach and grasp patterns enable prehension and manipulation of objects for play.

Strength from ages 4 to 6 is dependent on the child's body proportions but can generally be determined by the child's ability to perform functional activities that are normal for a specific age. Growth can be variable and rapid, sometimes contributing to growth pains that emanate from muscles being stretched on growing bones.[1] By age 5, the child has sufficient postural control and fine motor strength to begin handwriting activities. Table 13-2 provides a summary of muscular changes from ages 1 to 6.[1]

Skeletal Changes in Years 1 to 6

Dramatic changes take place in the skeletal system as the body assumes an upright posture (Table 13-3). The leg growth accelerates with the increased weight bearing performed by the ambulating toddler, and height increases as much as 5 inches in the second year of life and 2 inches during the third year.[1] The structural changes of long bones are the greatest when the child is 2.5 years old. The skull is completely ossified at age 2, and dentition continues to emerge.[1] With growth and gravitational forces affecting postural alignment, the toddler commonly stands with slightly bowed legs (*genu varus*) that become knock-kneed (*genu valgum*) with the remodeling of the pelvis. Increased walking realigns the lower extremities, causing the feet to become more

TABLE 13-3. SKELETAL CHANGES IN YEARS 1 TO 6		
	1 TO 3 YEARS	4 TO 6 YEARS
Spine and extremities	Leg growth accelerates in toddler years Height increases 5 inches in the second year and 2 inches during the third year Structural changes of long bone are greatest at 2.5 years of age	Primary ossification centers appear in the patella and the carpal bones by age 3 to 3.5 years Height increases from 5 to 6 cm/year
Skull	All bones of the skull are ossified by age 2	
Dentition	At approximately 6 months of age, the mandibular incisors are the first primary teeth to erupt	By age 6, child has developed primary dentition and has had some teeth replaced by the secondary dentition (permanent teeth)
Skeletal alignment/curvature	Toddler stands bowlegged (genu varus) at age 18 months and knock-kneed (genu valgus) at 3 years because of remodeling of the pelvis With increased walking, the lower limbs realign, the feet evert, and the angle made by the neck of the femur with the shaft gradually decreases from approximately 160 degrees to the adult value of 125 degrees	At age 3, nearly 75% of children develop genu valgum, which is resolved by 6 to 7 years of age
Adapted from Kaywood K, Hetchell N. *Life Span Motor Development.* Champaign, IL: Human Kinetics; 2001.		

everted and the femoral neck to decrease its angle with the shaft from 160 to 125 degrees.[1] Between the ages of 4 and 6, the primary ossification centers appear in the patella and are evident in the carpal bones of the wrists. Height continues to increase at a rate of approximately 2 to 3 inches per year. By age 6, the child has developed all the primary dentition and has some teeth replaced by secondary dentition (permanent teeth). Of all children with genus valgum at age 3, 75% have no evidence of it by age 7.

Skeletal Changes During Preadolescence and Adolescence

At age 6, the child's posture is characterized by a protruding abdomen and lumbar lordosis that eventually evolves into normal postural alignment as growing muscles support the skeleton.[1] The abdominal muscles increase in strength, supporting the lower trunk and reversing the lordotic curve. The child's growth in height during preadolescence results from the ossification of cartilage at the end of long bones, which is vulnerable to injury in sports activities.

As the child becomes an adolescent, posture resembles that of an adult. Rather than increasing in height, skeletal changes become more lateral and sex specific. Males tend to increase their shoulder width through growth of the clavicle, and females increase their pelvic width, which

Table 13-4. Musculoskeletal Changes During Preadolescence and Adolescence

	PREADOLESCENCE	ADOLESCENCE
Overall posture	6-year-old's silhouette characterized by a protruding abdomen and lordosis By age 10, the spine is better aligned, the abdomen is flatter, and the body is generally more slender and long-legged	Posture resembles adult posture
Cartilage	Skeletal growth is primarily linear, increasing the child's height Cartilage is being replaced by bone at the epiphyses (at ends of long bones and wrists)	Skeletal growth is more lateral Males increase their shoulder width through growth of the clavicle (one of the last bones to stop growing) and females increase width of the pelvis, which differentially becomes wider, shallower, and roomier (presumably for childbearing) Facial features become more prominent as the profile becomes more mature with the nose more projecting
Skeletal maximum growth	Skeletal growth occurs earlier in females than in males Skeletal growth occurs more rapidly in Blacks than Whites Maximal skeletal growth occurs between ages 10 to 14 in females and 12 to 14 in males	Linear growth is complete Lateral growth during the adolescent spurt is most evident

Adapted from Kaywood K, Hetchell N. *Life Span Motor Development*. Champaign, IL; Human Kinetics; 2001; and Linn JP, Brown JK, Walsh EG. Physiological maturation of muscles in childhood. *Lancet*. 1994;343:1386-1389; and Hay M, Levin M, Sondheimer J, Deterding R. *Current Pediatric Diagnosis and Treatment*. 17th ed. New York, NY: Lange Medical Books/McGraw Hill; 2005:4-5.

differentially becomes wider, shallower, and roomier for subsequent childbearing.[1] The facial features appear more adult, with the mature nose projecting to its adult length. Overall, the maximum skeletal growth occurs between the ages of 10 to 14 in females and between the ages of 12 to 14 in males.[1] Also, skeletal growth occurs differently in Blacks and Whites, with skeletal growth occurring more rapidly in Blacks (Table 13-4).[1]

Health care providers play a key role in identifying skeletal problems through musculoskeletal screenings. By adolescence, the upper spine normally has a gentle rounded posterior curve *(normal kyphosis)* and the lower spine has the reverse curve *(normal lordosis)*. Certain amounts of *cervical* (neck) *lordosis, thoracic* (upper back) *kyphosis*, and *lumbar* (lower back) *lordosis* are normally present and are needed to maintain appropriate trunk balance over the pelvis.

Deviations from this normal alignment may reflect abnormal kyphosis, lordosis, or, more commonly, scoliosis in this population. *Scoliosis* refers to a lateral curvature of the spine, or a side-to-side deviation from the normal frontal axis of the body. According to the Scoliosis Research Society, in over 80% of cases, the cause of scoliosis is unknown and is referred to as *idiopathic scoliosis*.[2] A comprehensive screening for scoliosis is critical and involves a thorough medical history, developmental history, and family history. The physical screening centers on assessing the spinal alignment and symmetry both when standing erect and when bending forward with both knees extended, noting muscular vs skeletal asymmetries. The spinal asymmetry may be accompanied by uneven shoulder height when standing erect, unequal leg length, or the presence of asymmetry of sacral dimples, sinuses, hairy patches, and skin pigmentation changes, typically in the lumbosacral area. Suspected scoliosis should be reported to the family physician for further diagnostic testing.

Typical Changes Associated With Aging in the Musculoskeletal System

Muscle Strength

Muscle strength and postural alignment are critical to efficient and effective function in adults. Loss of isometric and dynamic strength has been documented in individuals as young as 50 to 59 years old.[3] Decline in strength is closely associated with age, loss of type II fast twitch muscle fibers, and loss of muscle mass. Normal aging is characterized by loss of muscle mass *(sarcopenia)* and integrity of the skeletal system.[4] Changes in the aging musculoskeletal system can be compounded by physical inactivity. Generally, within 2 weeks of discontinuance of resistance training, more than 50% of the benefits gained are greatly diminished.[5]

Not only can physical inactivity accelerate the physiologic decline that can be associated with aging, it can also hamper an individual's ability to cope with acute physiologic stressors.[6] If older persons are forced by illness or injury to spend days or weeks exclusively on bedrest, muscle strength as well as aerobic capacity swiftly decline.[6] Following disuse due to injury or inactivity, muscle strength is lost at approximately twice the rate it takes to regain it.[7] Older women who do not exercise risk losing one-quarter pound of skeletal muscle per year from age 40 on.[7]

Less muscle mass can lead to increased rates of disability. The dramatic decline in physical activity over the lifespan does not completely explain the age-related loss of bone mass, and additional research is needed to determine whether the relationship of muscle mass with bone density is a direct one or is due to additional factors such as circulating hormone levels.[8]

The concept of threshold values for strength necessary for independent function is an interesting one. For example, there is a threshold value for quadriceps strength necessary to rise from a chair or toilet seat.[9] At worst, when deterioration of function prevents an older adult from carrying out essential daily activities independently, professional assistance either in the home or a care center is warranted. On the other hand, a small strength gain may translate to a considerable functional improvement. For example, an increase in muscle strength that allows one to transfer independently can make a substantial difference in quality of life, not to mention residential setting. When strength increases are achieved by previously deconditioned older adults, there is a corresponding improvement in physical function.[10]

Numerous studies have suggested that loss of muscle strength may be slowed or reversed with progressive resistive exercise programs. For example, healthy older adults trained for 12 weeks using a universal gym experienced a 109% increase in their 1-repetition max.[11] Frail elders living in long-term care participated in a 3-times-per-week strengthening program, resulting in a 174% increase in strength and a 9% increase in muscle mass. Even less strenuous exercise programs have resulted in modest gains in strength in a variety of older adult populations.[12] Although loss of muscle strength appears typical in the older adult, regular strength training has been shown to minimize and, in some instances, reverse this common change associated with aging. Physical therapists are well equipped to screen for muscle strength in the older adult and make recommendations related to specific exercise programs to address weakness in all muscle groups.

Skeletal System

Age-related bone density differs from site to site. More peripheral sites, such as the radius, experience relative stability in density until menopause, whereas more central skeletal structures, such as the spine and the neck of the femur, show bone loss 5 to 10 years earlier.[13] Recent research has demonstrated that bone loss may be reversed in men and women aged 65 years and older. Researchers gave 500 mg of calcium and 700 IU of vitamin D to both women and men older than 65 years.[14] These individuals were also receiving calcium in their diets. At the end of 3 years, participants had a 3% increase in hip bone mineral density. More importantly, fractures were prevented.

Weight-bearing exercise has also been found to minimize bone loss and, in some instances, halt the decrease in bone density commonly seen with advancing age.[15] Although decreases in bone density appear to be common in the older adult population, some research suggests that this trend can be reversed with appropriate nutritional/dietary changes and exercise. Loss of joint fluid commonly associated with aging also adds to the wear and tear on the joint. Joint changes seem almost inevitable with advanced age; in fact, osteoarthritis is one of the conditions nearly all 100-year-old people develop.[16] Over time, wear and tear on the joints will result in some changes. Numerous studies suggest the positive effects of glucosamine and chondroitin for reducing joint pain when taken for short periods of time. Exercise and activity that promote optimal postural alignment and strength assist in delaying the occurrence of these changes until very late in life.

Postural Changes

Changes associated with the spine are the primary reason behind the postural changes typically noted in the older adult. With aging, the intervertebral disks essentially lose water and undergo other deleterious changes on a cellular level. As the intervertebral disks are flattening, the bones of the spine become more porous. This accounts for loss of disk height and compression of the spinal column, hence the inevitable height loss for all older adults. Spinal compression, combined with decrease in strength of intrascapular muscles and gradual wedging of the thoracic vertebrae, are contributing factors in increased thoracic spine *kyphosis* (rounding of the shoulders with a forward lean), commonly seen in the elderly.

Ergonomics: Prevention Practice in Adulthood

Ergonomics is the field of study devoted to how work gets done, especially in terms of body position, motion, and equipment used in the workplace. Ergonomics encompasses changes in job processes and equipment to allow for pain-free work.

A certain amount of fatigue is normal at the end of a physically demanding workday. Usually, normal fatigue dissipates with adequate rest. Fatigue or pain that is always present is a warning sign that an injury is likely to occur or has already occurred. These types of warning signs are typical of injuries contributed to by less-than-sound ergonomic practices. Physical therapists have long been treating repetitive use injuries and addressing job-related injuries. However, the term *ergonomics* has not always been applied to this type of work. As is the case for other venues of physical therapy education/clinical work, ergonomics is not solely addressed by physical therapists. Exercise physiologists, occupational therapists, occupational safety specialists, and specially trained businesspersons are among the professionals who may see clients or employees with work-related injury and/or pain problems. The main certification presently available, Certified Professional Ergonomist, is obtained from the Board Certification in Professional Ergonomics, a nonprofit organization established in 1990.[17]

In the United States, the Occupational Health and Safety Administration (OSHA), is responsible for regulations of the workplace, ensuring the welfare of workers. OSHA's responsibilities include enforcing the laws governing employee safety and providing information to employers about how to interpret workplace legislation. Educational Resource Centers that are operated by the National Institute for Occupational Safety and Health (NIOSH) furnish training and outreach services. Regional offices of OSHA also provide free consultation services on ergonomic problems.

Especially in light of the ever-increasing use of computers and automated processes in the workplace and the home, it behooves physical therapists to apply principles of ideal posture and body mechanics to educate people about injury prevention and to determine whether work spaces are configured properly to avoid strain or stress. The goal of an ergonomics program or an individual ergonomic assessment is to reduce *musculoskeletal disorders* (MDS), or what now may be termed *cumulative trauma injuries* (CTI). CTIs are caused by too-frequent, uninterrupted repetitions of an activity or motion, unnatural or awkward motions such as twisting the arm or wrist, overexertion, incorrect and sustained postures, or muscle fatigue. CTIs occur most commonly in the hands, wrists, elbows, and shoulders but are also present in the neck, back, hips, knees, feet, legs, and ankles.[18] These disorders are characterized by pain, tingling, numbness (due in part to the end-range strains applied to the tissue), visible swelling or redness of the affected area, and the eventual loss of flexibility and strength. Over time, CTIs can cause temporary or permanent damage to the soft tissues in the body (such as the muscles, nerves, tendons, and ligaments) and compression of nerves or tissue. In addition, CTIs affect individuals who perform mechanical loading of tissues in a repetitive, imbalanced fashion. These clients typically perform such work-related tasks as assembly line work, meatpacking, sewing, playing musical instruments, and computer work. The disorders may also affect individuals who engage in recreational activities, such as gardening and tennis.[18] Cumulative trauma injuries may be precipitated by problems in 3 major areas: (1) posture, (2) repetitive motion, and (3) force or pressure (including vibration). Posture also may induce pain/stiffness when a position is either awkward or is maintained for a long time. Some posture problems may be created by repeated twisting, bending, kneeling, reaching, or moving the arms overhead. Repetitive motions occur in a number of ways, including continual typing at a computer, working steadily on an assembly line, or doing a monotonous stocking job.

Muscles and tendons are especially stressed with repetitive motion, with severity of potential risk dependent on the frequency of the motion and its speed and requisite force. Force or pressure exerted to complete a certain activity can involve sustained muscle contractions, repeated application of pressure over long durations, or holding onto and maneuvering vibrating equipment. Force is a factor in tasks such as heavy lifting and controlling equipment or tools that are not necessarily heavy but require a precision grip. Even the way in which a person sleeps and moves during exercise may play a role in CTI. As is true for most physical and mental health issues, there is a wide variation in both the capacity to perform work and the ability to respond to external work factors. This variation is a composite result of factors such as sex, age, lifestyle, physique, and individual strength and flexibility.

One of the most common repetitive use injuries affecting the upper extremity is *carpal tunnel syndrome*. This is a condition involving compression of the median nerve caused by swelling tendons in the carpal tunnel. The tunnel is bounded by the transverse carpal ligament on the palmar surface and the carpal bones on the dorsal surface. As a result of poor wrist position and/or repetitive motion, the tendons or the tendon sheath running through this tunnel may become inflamed. A common mechanism of injury is sustained flexion or extension while typing for many hours per day. A preferable position is keeping the wrist in neutral as much as possible. Signs may include *anesthesia* (numbness), *paresthesia* (tingling), pain, and increased temperature sensitivity. Too much pressure on the median nerve can limit movement and sensation in the thumb and fingers. Symptoms reported may include dropping things due to decreased strength or control, pain at night, and stiffness similar to osteoarthritis.

A *herniated spinal disk* is a condition in which part or all of the soft, gelatinous central portion of an intervertebral disk (the *nucleus pulposus*) is forced through a weakened part of the disk, resulting in back and leg pain caused by nerve root irritation. A herniated spinal disk may also be referred to as a *ruptured disk, lumbar radiculopathy* (pain in the low back region), *cervical radiculopathy* (pain in the neck region), a *prolapsed intervertebral disk*, or a *slipped disk*. *Tension neck syndrome*, also known as *costoscapular syndrome*, is characterized by muscle tightness, palpable hardening, and tender spots with pain on resisted neck lateral flexion and rotation.[19] *Sciatica* is a term used to describe pain along the sciatic nerve, which runs along the back of the leg. When this nerve is irritated, it can result in decreased ability to flex the knee, decreased ability to move the foot and toes in certain directions, numbness, burning or tingling in the leg, or pain in the lower back that may travel to the back of the thigh and calf.

Epicondylitis is a painful inflammatory condition of the muscles and soft tissues around an epicondyle or bony prominence. *Tennis elbow* refers to lateral epicondylitis of the humerus and is characterized by elbow pain that gradually worsens, pain radiating from the outside of the elbow to the forearm and back of the hand when grasping or twisting, and a weakened grasp. This condition can result from any type of overuse of the upper extremity.

Hand-arm vibration syndrome has also been referred to as *vibration-induced white finger, traumatic vasospastic disease, dead fingers,* and *spastic anemia*. It is a chronic and progressive disorder that affects the vascular, sensory, and musculoskeletal structures of the hand. It can result in permanent, painful numbness and tingling in the fingers and hands, damage to bones in hands and arms, painful joints, and muscle weakness. Prevalence increases with increasing exposure time and vibration intensity.[19]

CTI can be costly to treat and debilitating for the worker. Worksite evaluation with the goal of injury prevention is an efficient intervention approach and will be discussed later in the chapter. Potential costs avoided are not simply those of medical treatment and possible hospitalization, but also workers' compensation benefits, the indefinite cost of disability, and the replacement cost of that worker. Those on the business side of the workforce are concerned with implementation of an ergonomics program or worksite improvement and medical management of injuries that occur.

Prevention Practice for Back Pain and Back Injuries

Close to 35% of the US population has musculoskeletal symptoms and impairments, with back pain being the most common area of complaint.[20] The prevalence of low back pain tends to increase with age, reaching 50% in people over age 60.[20] A strong etiological factor in the occurrence of low back pain and extremity pain is repetitive motion. Back pain and back injuries are the most common CTIs. As the term implies, most back injuries are not caused by a single event, but rather the cumulative effect of poor body mechanics or external factors imposing repetitive posture problems. Keeping the back in anatomical position (natural curves) is best for spine health. Natural curves can be viewed as a concave "C" for the cervical and lumbar regions, and a convex "C" for the thoracic region. Lifting heavy objects while twisting is probably the most dangerous motion as far as causing injuries. In general, lifting rather than pulling or pushing objects may be a potential problem. Weight that has to be moved with arms overhead is also dangerous, particularly with respect to spinal compression. Standing for the day or for an entire shift, particularly on concrete or tile, can cause lower back pain. That pain may be induced not only by the hard surface of the floor but by poor job design with infrequent changes in position. For less physically demanding jobs, posture while sitting or standing is equally important to prevent upper back and neck pain. When typing or viewing a computer screen for much of the day, it is important for the screen to be at a height where the neck is in a neutral position and the keyboard is placed so the

TABLE 13-5. SIGNS AND SYMPTOMS OF UPPER LIMB DYSFUNCTION
• Change in color of skin or nails
• Pain
• Swelling
• Discomfort
• Limited active and passive joint movement
• Tenderness
• Sensory: numbness, tingling, pins and needles, burning sensation, feeling of warmth
• Muscle: cramp, stiffness, weakness, reduced grip, muscle spasms, muscle fasciculations

wrist is in neutral position or slightly flexed, rather than extended. The work station should not be too high or too low.

PREVENTION PRACTICE USING SCREENING TOOLS

To address the staggering number of clients with musculoskeletal symptomology due to repetitive motion or cumulative trauma, physical therapists must screen for impaired posture and improper arthrokinetics at adjacent joints, examine job analysis and redesign, assess ergonomic principles at home and work, and identify the psychosocial factors that complicate the care of the client with CTI and potentially lead to chronic pain. Table 13-5 provides potential signs and symptoms of common work-related problems of the upper extremities.

OSHA provides screening tools that address the major risk factors previously discussed: repetition, force, awkward or unnatural postures, and vibration. General questions for the employee include areas and level of pain, level of fatigue, and whether the fatigue is greater in one area of the body than another. If management permits, one approach for evaluating stresses and risk factors of a job involves replicating the physical job demands. This option may include photographing or videotaping people performing their typical tasks for movement analysis and examination of the ergonomics. Other tools for assessment include a scale to weigh items lifted or moved and a dynamometer to measure grip strength.

Posture screening is a useful feedback mechanism for clients and, more importantly, a recognized tool to prevent the prolonged positioning in poor posture, leading to pain and dysfunction. Postural impairments can be performed by the *Matthias Posture Test* (also known as the *Alexander Technique*), which is based on the principle that the mind and body form one continuous unit.[21] The theory contends that habits of poor posture result in many of the everyday aches and pains commonly experienced and can be caused by imbalances created by the incorrect positioning of the head in relation to the neck and torso. Poor postural alignment results in inefficient or misplaced muscular effort and unnecessary muscle tension, diminishing both the physical health and the mental attitude of an individual.[21] To perform this quick screen, the therapist positions the client standing with feet and back placed against a wall. The client flexes his or her shoulders to 90 degrees, then holds the pose for 30 seconds. If the client has poor muscle control and inefficient postural responses, he or she will begin to exhibit those patterns of poor posture during the 30-second standing trial.

A more conventional postural screening technique, developed by Kendall et al,[22] involves looking at each segment of the body responsible for posture and teasing out the most common faults of each area. Any position contributing to the increase in joint stress is termed *faulty posture* and is thought to cause excessive wearing of the articular surface of the joint. Excessive wearing of the joint results in (1) the production of *osteophytes* (projections of bone occurring at sites of cartilage degeneration near joints), (2) *traction spurs* (abnormal bone growths), (3) soft tissue stretch, and (4) weakening.[21]

Prevention Practice Using Job Analysis and Design

NIOSH is the agency established to help assure safe and healthy working conditions by providing research, information, education, and training in the field of occupational safety and health. NIOSH recommends several ways to prevent cumulative trauma disorders and the sequelae from these repetitive motion disorders and outlines the primary mechanisms for secondary prevention of cumulative trauma disorders, including (1) redesigning tools, workstations, and job duties; (2) educating the employee regarding care of joints, proper lifting techniques, and posture; and (3) recommending that employees take frequent and scheduled breaks from static positioning.[23] NOISH also recommends 7 elements of an effective program for evaluating and addressing musculoskeletal concerns in an individual workplace, including the following[24]:

1. Looking for signs of a potential musculoskeletal problem in the workplace, such as frequent worker reports of aches and pains or job tasks that require repetitive, forceful exertions
2. Showing management commitment in addressing possible problems and encouraging worker involvement in problem-solving activities
3. Offering training to expand management and worker ability to evaluate potential musculoskeletal problems
4. Gathering data to identify problematic conditions using injury and illness logs, medical records, and job analyses
5. Identifying effective controls for tasks that pose a risk of musculoskeletal injury and evaluating various approaches to determine their effectiveness in injury prevention
6. Establishing health care management to emphasize the importance of early detection and treatment of musculoskeletal disorders
7. Minimizing risk factors for musculoskeletal disorders when planning new work processes and operations because it is less costly to build than to redesign or retrofit later

Health care professionals may find it helpful to use a quick questionnaire to determine the likelihood for potential musculoskeletal problems in the workplace (Table 13-6).

After evaluating the worksite and its potential for musculoskeletal problems, the redesign phase should begin. This can be accomplished by recommending the client's company have a qualified ergonomist or a qualified physical or occupational therapist perform a careful analysis of the risk factors in each job. Both worker input and input by the local union's health and safety committee should be incorporated into this analysis. In addition, worker and union input is critical in developing the best redesign solutions. There are several ergonomic guidelines on lifting and materials-handling tasks to help physical therapists provide ranges of activity alterations at work. These guidelines are based on various biomechanical assumptions and theoretical equations to build a margin of safety for individuals who have to lift at work or perform repeated movements over prolonged periods of time.[25] When recommending activity modifications for clients who work, the clinician should obtain a written description of the physical demands of required job tasks. The nature and duration of limitations will depend on the clinical status of the patient and the physical requirements of the job. Activity modifications must be time limited, clear to both patient and employer, and reviewed by the clinician on a regular basis. It is also helpful to establish activity goals in consultation with the client and the employer, when applicable. Such goals are particularly

Table 13-6. Screening for Repeated Motion Disorders

DOES YOUR JOB REQUIRE YOU TO:	HOW OFTEN DOES YOUR JOB REQUIRE YOU TO PERFORM THIS TASK?
1. Repeatedly bend and twist your wrists?	
2. Repeatedly twist your arm?	
3. Repeatedly hold your elbows away from your body?	
4. Repeatedly use a pinch grip?	
5. Repeatedly reach behind your body?	
6. Repeatedly reach or lift things above your body?	
7. Repeatedly reach or lift items above shoulder level?	
8. Repeatedly use a tool that vibrates?	
9. Repeatedly use your hand as a hammer?	
10. Repeatedly twist or flex your body?	
11. Repeatedly lift objects from below knee level?	
12. Repeatedly work with your neck bent?	
13. How much time is spent in a static position?	
14. How many hours are spent in front of a visual display terminal or computer?	

important for the small percentage of clients who are still not able to overcome activity intolerance after 1 to 2 months of symptoms.

The literature is rich with suggestions and discussion regarding physical ergonomics of the work area and workstation and potential modifications for both. Only recently have data supported the importance of frequent breaks during the workday for employees and especially for those employees susceptible to cumulative trauma or repetitive motion disorders.

The most significant factor associated with symptoms of CTI was the length of time workers spent in a static position with unchanging postures (eg, keyboarding or prolonged standing activities).[26] An optimal work-rest schedule of a 45-minute shift/15-minute break is ideal when considering the viscoelastic deformation of the spine and the prevention of secondary changes from faulty posture changes.[26] Rest breaks decrease musculoskeletal soreness and discomfort, decrease levels of eyestrain and visual blurring, and slightly increase the work rate after rest breaks.[26,27] Scheduled breaks were found to be generally more effective than allowing workers to take breaks on their own.[27] Rest breaks should be short and frequent to avoid fatigue (eg, 5 to 10 seconds taken every 5 to 10 minutes of continuous use).[28]

Activity modifications, including rest breaks and job redesign (based on principles of ergonomics), are important options for the clinician who is treating clients with repetitive motion disorders to reduce the impairment, functional limitations, and potential sequelae.

Prevention Practice by Screening for Psychosocial Factors Leading to Chronic Pain

All health care professionals need to be mindful of the psychological consequences of chronic pain. Many health care professionals are adept at examining clients for mechanical injury, faulty posture, and clinical manifestation of pathology but may not be as prepared to recognize the psychosocial factors contributing to these disorders. For example, when a physical therapist performs the examination portion of an evaluation of someone with repetitive motion disorders, back pain from repetitive mechanical stress, or degenerative joint conditions, attention must be paid to psychological and socioeconomic problems in that individual's life. These nonphysical factors can complicate both assessment and treatment.[29]

Emotional distress, low work satisfaction, and depression can affect an individual's symptoms and response to treatment. Clinicians should question their clients regarding sociodemographic indices, stressors, moderators in work and nonwork settings, psychological symptoms, attitudes about health care, and symptom reporting because these are potential extenders of the client's initial complaints. Objective indices of *work characteristics* (lighting, job essentials, hours in static position, worksite description) as well as *subjective work stressors* (psychological demands, decision latitude, work and social support, and job satisfaction) should be included in the initial history of a client with repetitive motion symptoms or chronic low back pain. These nonwork stressors, in addition to financial problems and social support, have a huge effect on patient functioning and outcomes and need to be screened.[29]

The Job Demand-Control-Support (D-C-S) model has served as a research tool for several years to assess the interaction of 2 main dimensions in the work environment: *psychological demands* and *job control*.[30] Job control, also called decision latitude, includes 2 components: decision authority and skill discretion. These terms are further defined as *decision authority* (the worker's ability to make decisions on the job) and *skill discretion* (the breadth of skills used by the worker).

Most health care professionals have a high/high rating when looking at decision authority and skill discretion compared with meat packers or persons on assembly lines. According to the D-C-S model, the highest strain, most work-related injuries, and lowest job satisfaction arises in a work environment when demands are high, control is low, and social support is low.[30] The combination of job demand and job control determined stress ratings, whereas decision latitude predicted energy ratings on the job. In addition, social support was related to both stress and energy ratings. Stress ratings were significantly related to symptoms of shoulder, neck, and back pain. These findings indicate that perceived job stress, an employee's ability to control his or her environment by making decisions, and the latitude of those decisions have a direct effect on work-related injuries. These data raise the issue of the effect of job characteristics on a worker's health in a specific work environment. The better understanding of the interactions between workers and their work conditions will be significant for reconstruction of the work environment, helping to improve productivity in industry and quality of life for workers.

Depression is by far the most common emotion associated with pain syndromes, particularly back pain. Major depression is thought to be 4 times greater in people with chronic back pain than in the general population.[31] In research studies on depression in chronic low back pain clients seeking treatment at pain clinics, prevalence rates are even higher, with 32% to 82% of clients showing some type of depression or depressive problem (average, 62%).[31] The rate of major depression increases in a linear fashion with greater pain severity.[32] Also, the combination of chronic pain and depression is associated with greater disability than either depression or chronic pain alone.[32] Given these staggering findings, it is imperative that health care professionals screen for depression in their populations with any pain syndrome. In a study examining the accuracy of therapists' screening for depressive symptoms in clients with low back pain, the therapists did not accurately identify symptoms of depression—even symptoms of severe depression. The examiners recommend that clinicians managing clients with low back pain use the 2-item depression screening test featured in the PRIME-MD patient health questionnaire (Table 13-7). Administration of this screening test would improve health care professionals' ability to screen for symptoms of depression, enable referral for appropriate management, and potentially lessen the secondary effects from musculoskeletal conditions.

Using the World Health Organization's International Classification of Functioning, Disability and Health model,[33] health care professionals can develop programs to address musculoskeletal problems that affect body function and body structure impairments. For example, muscle strengthening exercises can improve weakened muscles, and injured muscles can be protected from overuse injuries by adapting the environment and the tasks that are causing the injuries. Environmental factors can be addressed using splints or supports to improve alignment and limit use of injured muscles. Better seating for low back pain and improved ergonomics at the workplace can reduce risks contributing to chronic musculoskeletal problems. Daily living activities and work tasks can be modified to reduce overuse of affected structure and to alter factors contributing to musculoskeletal disorders. Finally, encouraging individuals to eat nutritious meals, sleep soundly, and manage stress can contribute to healthy lifestyle behaviors that promote healing and reduce the risk of further injury.

Summary

Health care professionals need to be aware of the changes in muscular and skeletal systems across the lifespan. This baseline knowledge serves as a foundation for providing optimal preventive care for children, adults, and older adults as they engage in work and leisure activities. Application of ergonomic principles, combined with a background in biomechanics, kinesiology, and preventive care, gives health care professionals the opportunity to reduce the high incidence of cumulative trauma injuries and back pain in the workplace. Chapter 20 provides additional information about how to manage a prevention practice business that focuses on corporate wellness.

References

1. Sinclair D, Dangerfield P. *Human Growth After Birth*. 6th ed. Oxford, UK: Oxford Publishers; 1998.
2. Scoliosis Research Society Terminology Committee. A glossary of scoliosis terms. *Spine*. 1976;1:57-58.
3. Brown M, Kern F, Barr J. How do we look? Functional Aging within the physical therapy community. *J Geriatr Phys Ther*. 2003;26(2):17-21.
4. Carlson JE, Ostir GV, Black SA, Markides KS, Rudkin L, Goodwin JS. Disability in older adults 2: physical activity as prevention. *Behav Med*. 1999;24(4):157-168.
5. Turner CH, Robling AG. Designing exercise regimens to increase bone strength. *Exercise Sports Sci Rev*. 2003;31:45-50.

Table 13-7. PRIME-MD Screening Tool

Evaluation questions:

- Depressed mood: Have you felt sad, low, down, depressed, or hopeless? On a scale of 0 to 10 (0=most depressed, 10=least depressed), how have you been feeling lately?
- Loss of interest: Have you lost interest or pleasure in the things you usually like to do? Have you been as social as usual? Have you been less interested in interacting with others (family, coworkers)?

If you answered yes to one or both of the above symptoms, continue.

Symptom questions:

- Sleep disturbance: Have you been sleeping much more than usual or had difficulty falling asleep or staying asleep?
- Appetite disturbance: Have you lost your appetite or had an unusual increase in appetite? Any cravings for junk food?
- Loss of energy: Have you been feeling tired or having little energy?
- Difficulty concentrating: Does your thinking seem slower or more confused than usual? Are you making more mistakes?
- Feelings of worthlessness: Have you felt that you are a failure or that you let yourself or your family down? What are you looking forward to? Have you felt guilty about things that happened in your life?
- Psychomotor retardation: Have you been moving or talking more slowly than usual? Have you felt agitated or on edge? Do you feel like you have to keep talking or moving all the time? (Also can be observed.)
- Suicidal thoughts (bored with life): Have you thought that you or your family would be better off if you were dead? Have you thought of killing yourself? Have you tried to hurt/kill yourself before? When? How many times? What did you do? Are you thinking of killing yourself? Do you have a plan? How will you do it? What stops you from acting on your thoughts?

Scoring:

- Score one point for each positive category.
- Cutoff value is 5/9, but patients who answer positively to suicide questions are at high risk and need urgent attention. Observed and reported behavior should be incorporated into the evaluation.
- If the individual has experienced 5 or more symptoms for at least 2 weeks, diagnosis is major depressive disorder. If fewer than 5 symptoms are present, consider other depressive disorders.

Adapted from Spitzer RL, Kroenke K, Williams JB. Validation and utility of a self-report version of PRIME-MD: the PHQ primary care study. Primary Care Evaluation of Mental Disorders. Patient Health Questionnaire. *JAMA*. 1999;282(18):1737-1744.

6. Colcombe S, Kramer AF. Fitness effects on the cognitive function of older adults: a meta-analytic study. *Psychol Sci*. 2003;14(2):125-130.
7. Mazzeo RS, Cavanagh P, Evans WJ, et al. Exercise and physical activity for older adults: American College of Sports Medicine Position Stand. *Med Sci Sports Exerc*. 1998;30(6):992-1008.

8. Kohrt WM, Snead DB, Slatopolsku E, Birge SJ Jr. Additive effects of weight-bearing exercise and estrogen on bone mineral density in older women. *J Bone Miner Res.* 1995;10:1303-1311.
9. Jones CJ, Rikli RE, Beam WC. A 30-second chair-stand test as a measure of lower body strength in community-residing older adults. *Research Q Exerc Sport.* 1999;70(2):113-119.
10. Spirduso WW. *Physical Dimensions of Aging.* Champaign, IL: Human Kinetics; 1995.
11. Stevenson JS, Topp R. Effects of moderate and low intensity long-term exercise by older adults. *Res Nurs Health.* 1990;13(4):209-218.
12. Brown M, Sincacore DR, Host HH. The relationship of strength to function in the older adult. *J Gerontol.* 1995;50:A55-A59.
13. Iwamoto J, Takeda T, Ichimura S. Effect of exercise training and detraining on bone mineral density in post-menopausal women with osteoporosis. *J Orthop Sci.* 2001;6(2):128-132.
14. Nutrition and osteoporosis. International Osteoporosis Foundation. http://www.iofbonehealth.org/sites/default/files/PDFs/nutrition_fact_sheet.pdf. Accessed May 20, 2014.
15. Turner CH, Robling AG. Designing exercise regimens to increase bone strength. *Exercise Sports Sci Rev.* 2003;31:45-50.
16. Ettinger WH Jr, Burns R, Messier SP, et al. A randomized trial comparing aerobic exercise and resistance exercise with a health education program in older adults with knee osteoarthritis. *JAMA.* 1997;277(1):25-31.
17. How to certify. Board of Certification in Professional Ergonomics (BCPE). http://www.bcpe.org/how-to-certify/. Accessed June 10, 2014.
18. Vibration syndrome. DHHS (NIOSH) Publication No. 83-110. Centers for Disease Control and Prevention. http://www.cdc.gov/niosh/docs/83-110/. Accessed March 13, 2014.
19. Kumar S. *Biomechanics in Ergonomics.* London, UK: Taylor & Francis; 1999.
20. Cunningham LS, Kelsey JL. Epidemiology of musculoskeletal impairments and associated disability. *Am J Public Health.* 1984;74(6):574-579.
21. Kodish B. *Back Pain Solutions.* Pasadena, CA: Extensional Publishing; 2001.
22. Kendall F, McCreary E, Provance P, Rodgers M, Roman W. *Muscles: Testing and Function With Posture and Pain.* Baltimore, MD: Lippincott Williams & Wilkins; 2005.
23. Battachrya A, McGlothlin JD. *Occupational Ergonomics: Theory and Applications.* New York, NY: Marcel Dekker, Inc; 2012.
24. Elements of ergonomic programs: a primer based on workplace evaluations of musculoskeletal disorders. US Department of Health and Human Services, National Institute for Occupational Safety and Health. http://www.cdc.gov/niosh/docs/97-117/pdfs/97-117.pdf. Accessed June 10, 2014.
25. Green N. The benefits of breaks and micropauses: a survey of the literature [white paper]. Christchurch, NZ: Wellnomics; 2000.
26. Luczak H, Cakir A, Cakir G. Musculoskeletal disorder, visual fatigue and psychological stress of working with display units: current issues and research needs. Proceedings of the Third International Scientific Conference on Work With Display Units. Berlin, Germany; Technische Universitat Berlin:1992:288-289.
27. Mclean L, Tingley M, Scott RN, Rickards J. Computer terminal work and the benefit of micro-breaks. *Appl Ergon.* 2001;32(3):225-237.
28. Ergonomics: work breaks, exercises and stretches. Stanford University Environmental Health & Safety. http://www.stanford.edu/dept/EHS/prod/general/ergo/microbreaks.html. Accessed June 10, 2014.
29. Skov T, Borg V, Orhede E. Psychosocial and physical risk factors for musculoskeletal disorders of the neck, shoulders, and lower back in salespeople. *Occup Environ Med.* 1996;53(5):351-356.
30. Srunin L, Bodin LI. Family consequences of chronic back pain. *Soc Sci Med.* 2004;58:1385-1893.
31. Sullivan MJ, Reesor K, Mikail S, Fisher R. The treatment of depression in chronic low back pain: review and recommendations. *Pain.* 1992;50(1):5-13.
32. Haggman S, Maher CG, Refshauge KM. Screening for symptoms of depression by physical therapists managing low back pain. *Phys Ther.* 2004;84(12):1157-1166.
33. International Classification of Function, Disability and Health. World Health Organization. http://www.who.int/classifications/icf/en. Accessed June 10, 2014.

14

Prevention Practice for Cardiopulmonary Conditions

Amy Foley, DPT, PT; Gail Regan, PhD, MS, PT; and Catherine Rush Thompson, PT, PhD, MS

"If you can't breathe, you can't function."—Mary Massery, PT, DPT, Canadian Physiotherapy Association Manitoba Branch Newsletter, June 2005

Our vitality is dependent on the cardiopulmonary system because each breath oxygenates tissue, generates energy, and cleanses our bodies. Not only does breathing sustain life, but it brings the sense of smell to our consciousness, capturing the scents of home-baked cookies and delicate roses. Each heartbeat carries oxygenated blood through every limb, organ, and tissue, nourishing and sustaining life. But the heart also activates our unconscious reactions to threats, feelings of excitement, and signals of attraction. Cardiopulmonary function is central to the quality of a person's life.

Cardiopulmonary conditions, many preventable, are literally a matter of life or death—sometimes immediate, other times slow and suffocating. Health care professionals should help individuals understand the importance of these vital systems and encourage self-responsibility for preventive practice (ie, practicing lifestyle habits that can help prevent these conditions). Cardiopulmonary pathologies include the broad spectrum of cardiovascular diseases (CVDs) and pulmonary conditions that affect millions of Americans.

Recent statistics for the United States show that coronary heart disease is the single leading cause of death in America. Coronary artery disease causes *angina* (pains associated with poor heart circulation) and, ultimately, *myocardial infarctions* (heart attacks). "From 1999 to 2009, CVD deaths declined by 33%. However, CVD still takes the lives of more than 2150 Americans each day, an average of 1 death every 40 seconds. Women often experience a more 'silent' form of heart disease—one lacking significant angina or discomfort prior to myocardial infarction."[1]

Pulmonary pathology is nearly as prevalent in America. Overall, 6.3% of American adults (an estimated 15 million) are diagnosed with chronic obstructive pulmonary disease (COPD), one of the most common conditions.[2]

Thompson CR.
Prevention Practice and Health Promotion: A Health Care Professional's Guide to Health, Fitness, and Wellness, Second Edition (pp 225-239).

Cardiopulmonary conditions may be primary impairments or secondary complications resulting from pathologies affecting other body systems. These conditions include heart disease, hypertension, hyperlipidemia, arteriosclerosis, coronary artery disease, congestive heart failure, peripheral vascular disease, bronchitis, asthma, and emphysema. Impairments include limited aerobic capacity and endurance, impaired ventilation, ventilator pump dysfunction, and impaired respiration and gas exchange, all contributing to activity limitations and difficulties participating in social roles.[3] This chapter describes the health care professional's role in the prevention of some of these disease states and their sequelae because many cardiopulmonary diseases are preventable or managed with medical care combined with healthy lifestyle habits. Using the World Health Organization's International Classification of Functioning, Disability and Health model[4] can help the clinician consider the multiple factors contributing to cardiopulmonary health conditions as they relate to prevention and the management of patients.

Changes in the Cardiopulmonary System Across the Lifespan

The cardiopulmonary system begins functioning in utero and continues throughout the lifespan. During fetal development, the heart differentiates and enlarges, then begins beating at approximately 4 months' *gestational age* (in utero).[5] Congenital heart defects, such as *atrial* or *ventricular septal defects* (leaks in the inner heart), may reduce heart efficiency yet remain asymptomatic until vigorous activity later in life.

Typically, respiratory and pulse rates decline as a child matures into adulthood, while blood pressure concomitantly rises to meet the demands of increased physical activity. The more forceful *myocardium* (heart muscle) progressively uses more efficient contractions to deliver blood to the body. The resting heart rate of children older than 10 is comparable with an adult's rate of 60 to 100 beats per minute. Beginning at approximately age 25, aerobic capacity generally begins to decline as one ages, but the rate of decline can be diminished through physical activity.[5] *Maximum ventilatory uptake* (the maximum amount of oxygen the body inhales) usually drops between 5% and 10% per decade between the ages of 20 and 80.[5] Aerobic capacity, as measured by maximal rate of oxygen consumption (VO_2 *max*), declines with aging; however, the rate may be modulated by exercise training.

Decline in VO_2 max can be attributed to a decrease in maximum heart rate with aging and to decreased muscle mass and decreased muscle demands, which require less oxygen.[6] The metabolizing tissue that contributes to VO_2 max measurement is almost exclusively muscle tissue, and, unless exercising to preserve muscle mass and strength, older adults experience a gradual loss of both.[6]

Improving the lung's *vital capacity* (the volume of air that can be exhaled from the lungs after the deepest possible breath has been taken) and the *functional residual capacity* (functional reserve, or the volume of air present in the lungs at the end of passive expiration) are the keys to slowing the rate of decline of VO_2 max. Consistent physical activity over the course of one's life has been found to maintain ventilatory oxygen uptake at a higher level than being inactive. In the absence of regular physical activity, there is an increased risk of cardiopulmonary pathology and generalized deconditioning over the lifespan. Additional factors contribute to pathologies of the cardiopulmonary system and should be identified to reduce the risk of disease.

Screening for Cardiopulmonary Conditions

The cardiopulmonary system should be screened through client observation and testing of vital signs. Chapter 5 discusses simple tools for screening an individual for potential pathology and the need for referral. Table 14-1 provides an overview of screening information for common cardiovascular and pulmonary pathologies and positive findings warranting special attention. For example, if an individual has general health problems and is not being seen regularly by a physician, a referral is warranted. If another individual has a chronic medical condition that is stable and under medical care, consultation for a prevention program is appropriate. If an individual is in general good health and has no health complaints, a prevention program should begin immediately through health education and advisement on appropriate physical activity.

Common Cardiovascular Pathologies

Heart Disease

Heart disease includes a wide variety of cardiac and vascular conditions affecting the entire body. Congenital heart disease is caused by abnormal heart development before birth and is responsible for more deaths in the first year of life than any other birth defects.[5] Although there may be genetic factors contributing to congenital heart disease, prevention focuses on maternal health education to reduce risks associated with drug use, alcohol consumption, and prescribed medicines.

Common heart diseases of adulthood include coronary artery disease, congestive heart failure, ischemic heart disease, rheumatic heart disease, and myocardial infarction. Heart disease is the leading cause of death for both men and women. More than half of the deaths due to heart disease in 2009 were in men.[1] According to an estimate from the American Heart Association (AHA), the prevalence of heart disease in the United States may double by 2050.[1]

Because heart disease is one of the primary preventable causes of death, a thorough screening of the cardiovascular system is essential. Chest pain near the heart before, during, or after exercise warrants special attention. Although diseases such as *pleurisy* (inflamed membranes around the lungs) and *indigestion* (difficulty digesting food, often causing heartburn) may present with chest pain, this symptom is usually a cardinal sign of heart pathology. Another common symptom of cardiac pathology is dizziness when standing up, potentially due to inadequate venous return to the heart. *Orthostatic hypotension* (a condition associated with dizziness when changing position from lying to upright) may be caused by low blood pressure from other types of pathology as well.

Although rheumatic heart disease is best prevented through infection control to reduce the incidence of rheumatic fever, other types of heart disease are more amenable to preventive practice. Nonmodifiable factors contributing to this high prevalence rate, such as advanced age and a family history of early heart disease, should be noted, along with modifiable risk factors that can be affected by preventive care (Table 14-2).

Individuals with a personal or family history of heart problems are particularly vulnerable to heart pathology. Heredity plays a major role in determining blood lipid profile and heart rate variability (2 major risk factors for coronary artery disease). Across Whites and Blacks, lipid levels (high-density lipoprotein [HDL] cholesterol, low-density lipoprotein [LDL] cholesterol, and triglycerides) are 60% to 80% determined by genetics.[1] Prevention of cardiopulmonary disease involves recognizing and addressing the greatest risk factors.

According to a study at McMaster University with over 29,000 participants from 52 countries, cigarette smoking and an abnormal blood lipid profile are the 2 most important risk factors for myocardial infarction.[7] Other risk factors that contribute to heart disease include high blood

Table 14-1. Screening for Cardiopulmonary Conditions		
SCREENING INFORMATION	**RESOURCES NEEDED**	**POSITIVE FINDINGS**
Family history Hypertension Hypotension Heart disease Pulmonary conditions Lifestyle behaviors of family, such as smoking	Screening form	History of congenital, genetic, or family heart or pulmonary conditions Consider the possibility of secondhand smoke exposure
Prior history of individual Pulmonary illness Cardiac illness	Screening form	Note any history of congenital, genetic, or prior pulmonary conditions (eg, asthma)
Lifestyle habits of individual	Screening form	Note smoking, exercise, and diet information; detail FITTE (frequency, intensity, type[s], time, and enjoyment of exercise)
Anthropometrics of individual Body weight Body height Location of body fat		Check body mass index for body composition Note distribution of body fat, including presence of central obesity
General health of individual Blood pressure Pulse Respiratory rate	Screening form Stethoscope Sphygmomanometer	Note evidence of fatigue, weakness, malaise, fever, or illness Measures of blood pressure, pulse, and/or respiration rates outside of age- and sex-matched norms
Medication/drugs	Screening form	Note use of any prescribed or over-the-counter medications or supplements
Nose and sinuses	Screening form Otoscope	Note nasal or sinus discharge, sinus pain, unusual and frequent colds, changes in smell
Mouth and throat	Screening form Otoscope	Note any reports of pain, lesions or sores on the mouth or throat, altered taste
Neck	Screening form Palpation	Note pain, limitations in movement, lumps, swelling, tenderness, or discomfort
Respiratory system	Screening form Auscultation	Note chest pain, shortness of breath, or cough wheezing

(continued)

Table 14-1 (continued). Screening for Cardiopulmonary Conditions

SCREENING INFORMATION	RESOURCES NEEDED	POSITIVE FINDINGS
Cardiovascular system	Screening form Auscultation	Note pain with or without exertion, dizziness when standing, problems breathing while sleeping
Peripheral vascular system	Screening form Observation Auscultation	Note any coldness, numbness, tingling, swelling of legs or hands, pain in the legs, discolored hands or feet, varicose veins

Table 14-2. Modifiable Contributors to Heart Disease

- High blood pressure
- High blood cholesterol
- High low-density lipoprotein (LDL) cholesterol
- Low high-density lipoprotein (HDL) cholesterol
- Diabetes (adults with diabetes have heart disease death rates approximately 2 to 4 times as high as those of adults without diabetes)
- Obesity
- Overweight
- Smoking
- Physical inactivity (doubles the risk of heart disease)
- Apple-shaped body (worse than a pear-shaped body)
- High blood homocysteine
- Atherosclerosis
- High-fat diet
- High levels of stress
- Depression

pressure, diabetes, abdominal obesity, stress, lack of consumption of fruit and vegetables, and lack of regular exercise. On the other hand, protective factors include regular consumption of small amounts of alcohol. According to this study, more than 90% of heart attacks are predictable based on these risk factors. Additional symptoms that may suggest heart disease include problems with breathing when sleeping, fatigue, a racing heart rate, or feeling winded after exercise. Individuals complaining of these symptoms should have a more thorough medical examination before initiating a regular exercise program.

Suggested secondary prevention interventions include the following[7]:

- Controlling weight
- Eating a healthy diet low in saturated fat

- Quitting smoking
- Controlling diabetes
- Controlling blood pressure
- Controlling cholesterol
- Controlling homocysteine
- Taking antioxidants
- Considering the benefits and risks of hormone replacement therapy (HRT)
- Taking low-dose aspirin if you are a woman. In a study of more than 87,000 women, those taking low-dose aspirin were less likely to suffer a first heart attack than those without aspirin.[8] Women older than 50 appeared to benefit most. However, aspirin can increase the risk of ulcers, kidney disease, liver disease, and hemorrhagic stroke, so this intervention should be supervised by the client's physician.
- Engaging in physical activity. Physical activity can indirectly decrease LDL cholesterol levels, known to play a key role in the development of fatty depositions.[1] According to the Centers for Disease Control and Prevention, over 50% of Americans do not engage in regular physical activity,[1] so health care professionals can advocate for increased physical activity levels across all populations to help decrease the incidence of cardiovascular disease. When the heart condition is stabilized, the training should continue outside the hospital. Suitable activities are daily walks, jogging, cycling, swimming, aerobics, and dance, depending on the individual's interest and physical condition. Even patients with chronic heart failure benefit from controlled physical training, leading to increased cardiovascular function, load tolerance, and muscular strength.[1]
- Using healthy interventions to manage stress. One study demonstrated that patients with stable ischemic heart disease who engaged in aerobic exercise and stress management training reduced emotional distress and cardiovascular risk more than typical medical care alone. One effective intervention included aerobic exercise training for 35 minutes 3 times per week for 16 weeks, plus 1.5-hour stress management training for 16 weeks.[9]
- Reducing hostility. Younger patients with heart disease have a higher prevalence of hostility symptoms that adversely affect their condition.[9] Health care professionals should encourage younger patients who present with these symptoms to seek psychological counseling to reduce these symptoms and other psychological stressors contributing to their unhealthy condition.

Hypertension

Normal blood pressure, a vital sign easily assessed at home, should be below 120/80 (120 mm Hg systolic and 80 mm Hg diastolic), although 115/75 is recommended. *Prehypertension* values are 120 to 139 mm Hg systolic pressure and diastolic pressures ranging from 80 to 89 mm Hg; these tend to worsen with time. *Hypertension* is categorized in stages: (1) prehypertension with a systolic pressure ranging from 120 to 139 mm Hg or a diastolic pressure ranging from 80 to 89 mm Hg; (2) stage 1 with a systolic pressure ranging from 140 to 159 mm Hg or a diastolic pressure ranging from 90 to 99 mm Hg; and (3) stage 2, a more severe hypertension with a systolic pressure of 160 mm Hg or higher or a diastolic pressure of 100 mm Hg or higher.[10] Those taking antihypertensive medications also are included in clients with hypertension. Hypertension is prevalent in 50 million (ie, 1 in 5) Americans, with an additional 15 million Americans who are undiagnosed. Increased prevalence rates are seen in adults who are overweight.[11]

Compounding factors of obesity and metabolic disorders can put patients with hypertension at increased risk for more serious pathologies, such as coronary artery disease or enlargement of the heart's left ventricle. Various conditions and medications can lead to secondary hypertension, including kidney problems, adrenal gland tumors, congenital defects, certain medications (eg, birth control pills, cold remedies, decongestants, over-the-counter pain relievers, and some prescription drugs), and illegal drugs (eg, cocaine and amphetamines). Risk factors include age, family history, excess weight, tobacco use, excessive dietary sodium and potassium, vitamin D deficiency, alcoholism, stress, chronic illness, and physical inactivity.

Desired exercise includes regular aerobic physical activity, preferably at least 2 to 3 times per week for approximately 1 hour while carefully keeping a regular heart rate of 70% to 85% of the theoretic age-related maximum rate.[1] According to the AHA, "Physical inactivity is a major risk factor for developing coronary artery disease. It also increases the risk of stroke and such other major risk factors as obesity, high blood pressure, low HDL ('good') cholesterol, and diabetes."[1] The AHA recommends a daily combination of moderate and vigorous physical activity for both children and adults. "Specifically, we recommend a total of 30 minutes of moderate-intensity activities on most days of the week, and a minimum of 30 minutes of vigorous physical activity at least 3 to 4 days each week, to achieve cardiovascular fitness."[1] In addition, clients should discontinue, or at least sharply reduce, cigarette smoking, possibly replacing it with pipe smoking. All of these measures combined are effective in reducing tensive values in most patients.

Nonpharmacological measures to control hypertension, especially in those who are borderline or mildly hypertensive, include a combination of diet and lifestyle changes. Other measures, such as reduced coffee consumption to a maximum 2 cups per day; increased intake of potassium, calcium- or magnesium-rich substances (ie, some types of fruits and legumes and hard mineral water); increased intake of polyunsaturated fats (mainly contained in white meat and sea fish); and reduced saturated fat intake (mainly due to all animal-derived products), may also prove beneficial.

Obese patients can benefit from weight loss, and those consuming alcohol can reduce their intake to the recommended 20 to 30 g per day. A diet that is low sodium (a maximum 5 g of sodium chloride per day), low calorie, and high fiber (at least 30 g per day including 50% of soluble and 50% of insoluble fibers) is also recommended. Controlling associated diabetes by means of dietary and therapeutic measures and discontinuing any estroprogestinic contraceptive treatments are also required for both male and female hypertensive patients. Angiotensin-converting enzyme (ACE) inhibitors and calcium-antagonists are the drugs of choice because they may positively affect the development of vascular plaques and reduce the left ventricular mass, which may influence the outcome for hypertensive patients.[12]

Health care professionals should work closely with dietitians and psychologists to ensure that optimal prevention includes dietary, behavioral, and medical considerations. Whenever mild pressure increases are not monitored, arterial pressure values are likely to shift from moderate to considerably high in the relatively short term.

Hyperlipidemia

Hyperlipidemia is an increase in the blood levels of triglycerides and cholesterol that can lead to cardiovascular disease and other chronic pathologies. An estimated 101 million Americans have cholesterol levels greater than or equal to 200 mg/dL, which means 1 in 3 Americans have hyperlipidemia.[13] It has been shown that patients aged 65 to 75 years can benefit from intervention at least as much as younger patients.[14] Despite the clear demonstration that lowering LDL cholesterol improves cardiovascular risk, most adults who are eligible for cholesterol-lowering therapy do not receive it, including over half of those who qualify for drug therapy.[13] Lipid-lowering therapy can prevent cardiovascular mortality and morbidity for patients with known coronary artery disease and type 2 diabetes.[13] Risk factors for hyperlipidemia include fatty diets, diabetes, hypothyroidism, Cushing's syndrome, kidney failure, certain medications (including birth control pills, estrogen, corticosteroids, certain diuretics, and beta-blockers), and lifestyle factors (including habitual, excessive alcohol use and lack of exercise, leading to obesity). Clinicians working with individuals diagnosed with hyperlipidemia should encourage their clients to seek pharmacological management of this condition to complement nonpharmacological interventions, including screening for risk factors and providing education on disease and diet.

Although eating a healthy diet and following the AHA exercise guidelines for healthy populations can affect hyperlipidemia, one study demonstrated that intense lifestyle interventions are more effective for improving not only blood lipids but also other risk factors and the individual's quality of life. In one study, more intense supervised aerobic exercise (as opposed to unsupervised exercise) increased the participants' exercise capacity (1.6 to 1.9 metabolic equivalents), reduced body weight by 10%, and reduced LDL cholesterol by 7.6%.[15] Health care professionals can play a key role in secondary prevention by ensuring that sufficiently aggressive exercise training is coupled with a diet recommended by a registered dietitian and appropriate medical intervention. Clients taking statins to control cholesterol should be warned to avoid drinking grapefruit juice and other citrus fruits, which potentially have serious side effects. Not only can clients with hyperlipidemia reduce their cholesterol, but they can also increase their exercise capacity, lower their blood pressure, and lose weight, further reducing risk for pathology.

Arteriosclerosis

Arteriosclerosis describes several diseases characterized by the loss of elasticity and thickening of the arterial wall. The arteriosclerotic damage of the arterial endothelium is initiated by risk factors like dyslipidemia, hypertension, diabetes mellitus, and smoking, which account for the majority of vascular morbidity and mortality.[16] Because arteries supply the body with needed nourishment, vascular diseases caused by arteriosclerosis can affect all vital organs and ultimately lead to death. Coronary artery disease is an example of pathology resulting from arteriosclerotic processes affecting the myocardium. In the same manner, all body systems are vulnerable to arteriosclerosis, including the brain and peripheral vascular system. *Atherosclerosis*, a form of arteriosclerosis, is the most common vascular disease. Atherosclerosis is characterized by the deposition of plaques containing cholesterol and lipids on the innermost layer of the walls of large and medium-sized arteries. The deposition of plaques narrows the vessels, potentially leading to hypertension and impaired blood flow. The same lifestyle changes needed to prevent heart disease and hypertension can be used to reduce the risk of arteriosclerosis.

Peripheral Vascular Disease

People aged 50 years or older who have diabetes, smoke, have high blood pressure, or have high cholesterol levels are at risk for *peripheral vascular disease* (PVD), which is damage to their peripheral vascular system that impairs normal blood circulation.[17] PVD is a highly treatable disease in its early stages and can often be detected by the appearance of the extremities. The hands or feet may appear swollen or discolored. The individual may complain of coldness, numbness, tingling, or pain. Often, individuals will report a family history of vascular problems or will have evidence of varicose veins (spider veins) on their legs. Bruises and other skin discolorations may also be attributed to peripheral vascular pathology. PVD can be an early warning sign of a potential heart attack, stroke, or aneurysm, so individuals presenting with these clinical manifestations should be examined and followed by a physician.

Most people with PAD can be treated with lifestyle changes, medications, or both. Lifestyle changes are the same as the modifiable risk factors for heart disease. These lifestyle changes can be augmented by medications to improve vascular flow, antiplatelet drugs to slow blood clotting, and cholesterol-lowering agents (statins) (Table 14-3).[17]

Table 14-3. Examples of Common Cardiovascular Pathologies and Risk Factors

LIFESPAN	PATHOLOGY	MODIFIABLE RISK FACTORS	PREVENTION
Childhood	Congenital heart disease	Maternal health	Health education
Adulthood and older adulthood	Heart disease (including coronary artery disease, congestive heart failure, ischemic heart disease, rheumatic heart disease, and myocardial infarction)	Sedentary lifestyle, smoking, poor diet	Exercise, smoking cessation, diet modification, stress management
	Heart disease (rheumatic heart disease)	Prevent rheumatic fever	Education for infection control
	Hypertension	Sedentary lifestyle, smoking, poor diet	Exercise, smoking cessation, diet modification, stress management
	Hyperlipidemia	Sedentary lifestyle, smoking, poor diet, excessive and habitual alcohol use, certain medications	Exercise, reduce alcohol consumption, diet modification, medical management
	Arteriosclerosis	Hyperlipidemia, hypertension, diabetes, smoking	Exercise, smoking cessation, diet modification, stress management
	Peripheral vascular disease	Hyperlipidemia, hypertension, diabetes, smoking	Exercise, smoking cessation, diet modification, stress management
	Heart disease (myocardial infarction, congestive heart failure)	Sedentary lifestyle, smoking, poor diet	Exercise, smoking cessation, diet modification, stress management

Common Pulmonary Pathologies

Sudden Infant Death Syndrome

Sudden infant death syndrome (SIDS) is the sudden, inexplicable death of an infant younger than 1.[14] Although the Back to Sleep campaign urging parents to put their infants to sleep on their backs has reduced the incidence of this syndrome, thousands of babies in the United States die from this condition. Risk factors for this condition include the following[14]:

- Babies who sleep on their stomachs
- Babies who have soft bedding in the crib

- Multiple-birth babies
- Premature babies
- Babies with a sibling who had SIDS
- Mothers who smoke or use illegal drugs
- Teen mothers
- Short intervals between pregnancies
- Late or no prenatal care
- Poverty

The American Academy of Pediatrics (AAP) provides the following recommendations for preventing SIDS[18]:

- Always put a baby to sleep on its back. Allowing the baby to roll around on its tummy while awake can prevent a flat spot (due to sleeping in one position) from forming on the back of the head.
- Only put babies to sleep in a crib. NEVER allow the baby to sleep in bed with other children or adults, and do NOT put them to sleep on surfaces other than cribs, like a sofa.
- Let babies sleep in the same room (NOT the same bed) as parents. If possible, babies' cribs should be placed in the parents' bedroom to allow for nighttime feeding.
- Avoid soft bedding materials. Babies should be placed on a firm, tight-fitting crib mattress with no comforter. Use a light sheet to cover the baby. Do not use pillows, comforters, or quilts.
- Make sure the room temperature is not too hot. The room temperature should be comfortable for a lightly clothed adult. A baby should not be hot to the touch.
- Let the baby sleep with a pacifier. Pacifiers at naptime and bedtime can reduce the risk of SIDS. Doctors think that a pacifier might allow the airway to open more or prevent the baby from falling into a deep sleep. A baby that wakes up more easily may automatically move out of a dangerous position. However, do not force the infant to use a pacifier. Although pacifier use has been associated with dental problems and breastfeeding difficulties, researchers say the potential benefit (decreased SIDS risk) outweighs the risks. The AAP says that one SIDS death could be prevented for every 2733 babies who suck on a pacifier during sleep.
- Do not use breathing monitors or products marketed as ways to reduce SIDS. In the past, home apnea (breathing) monitors were recommended for families with a history of the condition, but research found that they had no effect, and the use of home monitors has largely stopped.

Asthma

Asthma is a chronic inflammatory pulmonary disorder characterized by reversible obstruction of the airways seen in nearly 7% of the population of the United States, including 12 million adults and 8 million children.[19] Annually, approximately 5,000 deaths are related to asthmatic attacks.[19] Almost all asthma patients can become free of symptoms with proper treatment. Removal of asthma triggers, as described in Chapter 6, can help reduce the incidence of asthma. For adults, workplace irritants need to be identified, along with home-based triggers of asthmatic reactions. A variety of products are available to help reduce the allergens in the individual's environment, including specialized bedding, water filtration, air filtration, and mold control products. The use of bronchodilators and exercise are also recommended.

Although breathing exercises may not result in significant reduction of bronchospasms, they contribute to improved quality of life. According to a study in the *Cochrane Database Systematic*

Review, "two studies demonstrated significant reductions in rescue bronchodilator use, three studies showed reductions in acute exacerbations, and two single studies showed significant improvements in quality of life measures. Overall, benefits of breathing exercises were found in isolated outcome measures in single studies."[20] Swimming is one type of exercise that is beneficial and has been shown to be less asthmogenic than other forms of exercise.[21] Exercise programs featuring whole-body exercise training and local resistance training have resulted in significant changes in perceived dyspnea and fatigue, use of health care resources, exercise performance, and health-related quality of life.[21]

For children who have asthma, the family should be advised to reduce or eliminate the triggers of asthma symptoms. Educating parents about recognized methods to address asthma triggers may help families use more effective measures. These triggers include airborne allergens; upper respiratory tract infections; smoke and other lung irritants; cold, dry air; intense emotional expressions; endocrine factors (menstrual cycle and thyroid disease); and various types of medications (aspirin and other nonsteroidal anti-inflammatory drugs and beta-blockers).[21]

Interdisciplinary teams can optimize secondary prevention strategies, enabling individuals with pulmonary pathology to exercise and improve their quality of life. Contact with the physician, pharmacologist, psychologist, social worker, and respiratory therapist may be appropriate when developing optimal secondary prevention for those with COPD and emphysema.

A simple and informative way to assess the pulmonary system is to check the respiratory rate. Simply watching the rate of chest expansions or shoulder elevations while an individual is resting provides baseline values. Irregularities in respiratory rates not caused by imposed exercise or activity suggest a problem that may need medical attention. For example, infections such as pneumonia commonly present with elevated respiratory rates. In addition, the respiratory system should be screened for common pathologies such as asthma. Individuals who present with chest pain, shortness of breath, a cough, or wheezing should receive a more comprehensive examination. Chronic smokers have an increased risk of developing lung, throat, and mouth cancers and should be examined more extensively for early detection. Other types of breathing problems may suggest either a respiratory or a cardiovascular problem.

Sleep Apnea

Sleep apnea is a common breathing problem that occurs while lying down. Sleep apnea is defined as the cessation of breathing for 10 or more seconds during sleep.[22] Consequences of sleep apnea range from simple annoyance to life threatening. A thorough medical examination is warranted if sleep apnea is suspected.

Early recognition and treatment of sleep apnea is important because it may be associated with irregular heartbeat, high blood pressure, heart attack, and stroke. According to the National Sleep Foundation, there are nearly 18 million Americans who have sleep apnea, 4% being middle-aged men and 2% being middle-aged women.[23] These individuals may complain of excessive daytime sleepiness, problems with their weight, high blood pressure, loud snoring, or possible obstructions in their airways. They may have additional symptoms, including depression, irritability, sexual dysfunction, learning problems, and memory difficulties, as well as falling asleep while at work, on the phone, or driving because of their excessive sleepiness. Obese patients with sleep apnea are at increased risk of death, so patients with possible sleep apnea, especially those with obesity, should be referred for a more extensive examination of their sleep problems.

Prevention of sleep apnea includes reducing risk factors that commonly cause the problem, including use of alcohol, excess body weight, smoking, and congestion. Recommended prevention measures for sleep apnea also include the following[22]:

- Avoiding the use of sedatives, which can relax throat muscles and slow breathing, and antihistamines that cause drowsiness. Decongestants can decrease drainage from colds or allergies without increasing sleep apnea.

- Changing sleeping posture to sidelying with pillows between the knees.
- Raising the head of the bed by 6 inches to reduce respiratory efforts.

In general, cardiovascular pathologies could be reduced significantly if individuals adopted healthy lifestyle habits, including heart-healthy exercise on a regular basis.

Chronic Obstructive Pulmonary Disease

COPD, also known as *chronic obstructive lung disease* and *chronic obstructive airway disease*, is the fourth leading cause of death and is expected to be the third leading cause of death by 2020.[24] Primarily resulting from smoking, the condition is associated with *emphysema* (damaged lung alveoli or air sacs become enlarged as they lose elasticity for ventilation), *chronic bronchitis* (excess mucus in large airways), and *obstructive bronchitis* (small airway obstruction, inflammation, and fibrosis). The early stages of COPD are asymptomatic, but severe cases can lead to death. In addition to smoking, risk factors for COPD include genetic predisposition, premature birth, deficiency of antioxidants (vitamins A, C, and E) in the diet, exposure to vehicle fumes, industrial pollution, and bacterial or viral infection in young children. "Indoor air pollution—generated largely by inefficient and poorly ventilated stoves burning biomass fuels such as wood, crop waste and dung, or coal—is responsible for the deaths of an estimated 1.6 million people annually."[25] The same risk factors contribute to lung cancer and emphysema.

Generally, individuals with COPD are not seen until they are symptomatic, with changes in chest shape to increase lung efficiency (ie, a barrel-shaped chest evolves over time), dyspnea or difficulty breathing (shortness of breath), and coughing. As the disease progresses, chronic coughing may develop and the individual may become *cyanotic* (ie, bluish coloring, especially of the skin, lips, and nailbeds, as the body copes with lung inefficiency). Health care professionals should alert their clients to see a physician for changes in chronic coughing or a new cough. In addition, individuals should be encouraged to change lifestyle habits incompatible with their health, including smoking and working in areas filled with vehicle fumes or other industrial pollutants.

Patients with COPD frequently exhibit physiologic and psychological impairments, such as dyspnea, peripheral muscle weakness, exercise intolerance, decreased health-related quality of life, and emotional distress. Aerobic exercise, such as walking, should be strongly advocated for improving health and quality of life. In one study, patients with COPD using a bronchodilator in combination with pulmonary rehabilitation improved treadmill walking endurance and health status.[26] Improved ventilation from *bronchodilation* (opening of the airways) enhanced the individuals' ability to perform ambulation and increase exercise tolerance. Improvements with the bronchodilation medication were sustained for 3 months following pulmonary rehabilitation completion. Individuals engaged in a rehabilitation program increased their scores on the 6-minute walk distance and their quality of life measures.[26]

Pneumonia

Pneumonia, an inflammation or infection of the lung, is commonly caused by lung infection or aspiration of food into the lung and often develops as a secondary complication in individuals who have restrictive or obstructive lung diseases and difficulties with pulmonary hygiene. Ideally, infectious pneumonia is prevented through proper infection control with individuals infected with pneumonia and with others at risk for infection, such as immunosuppressed and elderly patients. The health care professional may recommend extra-vigilant behaviors to the client with COPD to avoid community-acquired pneumonia. Pneumonia may present as a high fever, shaking chills, and a cough with sputum production or gradually with a worsening cough, headaches, and muscle aches.

Table 14-4. Examples of Common Pulmonary Pathologies and Risk Factors

LIFESPAN	PATHOLOGY	MODIFIABLE RISK FACTORS	PREVENTION
Infancy	Sudden infant death syndrome	Positioning prone, loose bedding	Using prone position for play rather than sleep
Childhood	Asthma	Environmental triggers, emotional stress, infections	Removal of triggers, stress management, infection control
Adulthood and older adulthood	Sleep apnea	Obesity, sleeping on back, antihistamines for colds and allergies	Weight loss, sleeping on side, decongestants for colds and allergies
	Lung cancer	Smoking, occupational exposure	Smoking cessation, protective gear to reduce inhalation of toxins
	Chronic obstructive pulmonary diseases (bronchitis, emphysema)	Smoking	Smoking cessation
	Pneumonia, tuberculosis	Exposure to infection	Infection control

Tuberculosis

Pulmonary tuberculosis (TB) is a contagious bacterial infection caused by inhaling droplets sprayed into the air from a cough or sneeze by an infected person. TB is a preventable disease, even in those who have been exposed to an infected person. Skin testing for TB is used in high-risk populations or in individuals who may have been exposed to TB, such as health care workers.[27] Pulmonary impairments associated with TB include localized pulmonary signs (eg, coughing up phlegm or blood, wheezing, chest pain, and difficulty breathing) and systemic signs (eg, fever, fatigue, excessive sweating at night, and weight loss).

As with all infectious conditions, infection control is the most appropriate method of preventing the spread of disease. The Centers for Disease Control and Prevention website lists the infectious diseases that may be transmitted and/or acquired in health care settings at http://www.cdc.gov/hai/progress-report/index.html.[28]

Table 14-4 provides examples of common pulmonary pathologies that occur across the lifespan, listing risk factors for each age group.

Additional information about common cardiopulmonary conditions can be found at the websites for the Centers for Disease Control and Prevention (www.cdc.gov), the AHA (www.heart.org), and the American Lung Association (www.lung.org).

Summary

Health care professionals play a key role in identifying risk factors for persons with cardiopulmonary conditions and disease states. It is incumbent on health care professionals to employ strategies to promote health and wellness and prevent secondary complications from cardiopulmonary conditions through screenings that adequately assess cardiovascular and pulmonary risk factors, health education about risk factors and infection control, and promoting healthy lifestyle behaviors, particularly regular physical activity, smoking cessation, and heart-healthy foods.

References

1. Heart attack and angina statistics. American Heart Association. http://www.heart.org/. Accessed January 1, 2013.
2. Chronic obstructive pulmonary disease among adults—United States, 2011. Centers for Disease Control and Prevention. http://www.cdc.gov/mmwr/preview/mmwrhtml/mm6146a2.htm. Accessed January 1, 2013.
3. American Physical Therapy Association. *Guide to Physical Therapist Practice*. Alexandria, VA: American Physical Therapy Association; 2001.
4. International Classification of Functioning, Disability and Health (ICF). World Health Organization. http://www.who.int/classifications/icf/en/. Accessed May 20, 2014.
5. Sinclair D, Dangerfield P. *Human Growth After Birth*. 6th ed. London, UK: Oxford Publishers; 1998.
6. Pimentel AE, Gentile CL, Tanaka H, Seals DR, Gates PE. Greater rate of decline in maximal aerobic capacity with age in endurance-trained than in sedentary men. *J Appl Physiol*. 2003;94(6):2406-2413.
7. Anand SS, Yusuf S. Risk factors for cardiovascular disease in Canadians of South Asian and European origin: a pilot study of the Study of Heart Assessment and Risk in Ethnic Groups (SHARE). *Clin Invest Med*. 1997;20(4):204-210.
8. Facts about heart disease and women: are you at risk? NIH Publication No. 98-3654. National Institutes of Health. http://permanent.access.gpo.gov/lps3589/hdw_risk.pdf. Accessed January 1, 2013.
9. Blumenthal J, Sherwood A, Babyak M, et al. Effects of exercise and stress management training on markers of cardiovascular risk in patients with ischemic heart disease. *JAMA*. 2005;293:1626-1634.
10. High blood pressure (hypertension). Mayo Clinic. http://www.mayoclinic.org/diseases-conditions/high-blood-pressure/basics/tests-diagnosis/con-20019580. Accessed May 20, 2014.
11. Hedley A, Ogden C, Johnson C, Carroll M, Curtin L, Flegal K. Prevalence of overweight and obesity among US children, adolescents, and adults, 1999-2002. *JAMA*. 2004;291(23):2847-2850.
12. Censori B, Agostinis C, Partziguian T, Guagliumi G, Bonaldi G, Poloni M. Spontaneous dissection of carotid and coronary arteries. *Neurology*. 2004;63:1122-1123.
13. Hyperlipidemia. Merck Manual. http://www.merckmanuals.com/professional/endocrine_and_metabolic_disorders/lipid_disorders/dyslipidemia.html. Accessed May 20, 2014.
14. Committee on Fetus and Newborn. American Academy of Pediatrics. Apnea, sudden infant death syndrome, and home monitoring. *Pediatrics*. 2003;111(4 Pt 1):914-917.
15. Lalonde L, Gray-Donald K, Lowensteyn I, et al. Comparing the benefits of diet and exercise in the treatment of dyslipidemia. *Prev Med*. 2002;35(1):16-24.
16. Henzen C. Risk factors for arteriosclerosis. *Schweiz Rundsch Med Prax*. 2001;25;90(4):91-95.
17. Peripheral vascular disease. American Heart Association. http://www.americanheart.org/presenter.jhtml?identifier=4692. Accessed January 1, 2013.
18. Task Force on Sudden Infant Death Syndrome. The changing concept of Sudden Infant Death Syndrome: diagnostic coding shifts, controversies regarding the sleeping environment, and new variables to consider in reducing risk. *Pediatrics*. 2005;116(5):1245-1255.
19. Child asthma attack prevention. The Ad Council. http://www.adcouncil.org/issues/Childhood_Asthma/. Accessed January 1, 2013.
20. Holloway E, Ram F. Breathing exercises for asthma. *Cochrane Database of Syst Rev*. 2005;2:1-2.
21. Spruit M, Troosters T, Trappenburg J, Decramer M, Gosselink R. Exercise training during rehabilitation of patients with COPD: a current perspective. *Patient Educ Counsel*. 2004;52:243-248.
22. Sleep apnea prevention. WebMD. http://www.webmd.com/hw/sleep_disorders/hw49354.asp. Accessed January 1, 2013.
23. Facts and stats. National Sleep Foundation. http://www.sleepfoundation.org/hottopics/index.php?secid=10&id=226. Accessed January 1, 2013.

24. Deaths and mortality. Centers for Disease Control and Prevention. http://www.cdc.gov/nchs/fastats/deaths.htm. Accessed May 20, 2014.
25. Indoor air pollution and household energy. World Health Organization. http://www.who.int/heli/risks/indoorair/indoorair/en/. Accessed May 20, 2014.
26. Treatment of advanced disease. National Lung Health Education Program. http://www.nlhep.org/resources/erly-rec-mng-copd/treatment-6.html. Accessed January 1, 2013.
27. Centers for Disease Control and Prevention. Treatment of tuberculosis. *MMWR Recomm Rep.* 2003;52(RR-11):1-77.
28. Healthcare-associated infections (HAI) progress report. Centers for Disease Control and Prevention. http://www.cdc.gov/hai/progress-report/index.html. Accessed May 20, 2014.

15

Prevention Practice for Neurological Conditions

Mike Studer, PT, MHS, NCS, CEEAA, CWT and Catherine Rush Thompson, PT, PhD, MS

"*The chief function of the body is to carry the brain around.*"—Thomas A. Edison, "Edison in His Laboratory," *Harper's Monthly*, September 1932.

NEUROLOGICAL DISORDERS

A *neurological disorder* is any problem with the body's nervous system affecting the brain, the spinal cord, or the peripheral nerves. Although subtle neurological problems may be unperceivable to others, they can profoundly affect an individual's life. Neurological disorders range from memory loss to life-altering traumatic head injuries that render individuals unconscious and completely dependent. Primary prevention can reduce the risk of neurological accidents and pathologies, whereas secondary and tertiary prevention helps those afflicted with neurological impairments to live longer and healthier lives while adjusting to the changes induced by chronic neurological conditions.

The World Health Organization (WHO) International Classification of Functioning and Disability (ICF) model helps health care professionals identify an individual's neurological impairments and activity limitations or skills affected by these impairments, as well as physical and psychosocial barriers to a person's ability to participate fully in life roles. Once issues are identified, health care professionals can provide both environmental supports and resources designed to help the individual and family cope with life-altering neurological conditions. The optimal outcome for improved health and wellness is enabling each individual with a neurological condition to fully participate in purposeful activities that give meaning to life.

Normal neural function is dependent on the nervous system being anatomically and physiologically intact. The healthy nervous system is well protected by a blood-brain barrier and meninges; its function relies on sufficient nutrients to provide essential neural activity. Trauma, infections, cardiovascular disruption, physiological imbalance, systemic pathology, tumors, and neurotoxins can all disrupt neural function. Many adult neurological disorders are caused by

Thompson CR.
Prevention Practice and Health Promotion: A Health Care Professional's Guide to Health, Fitness, and Wellness, Second Edition (pp 241-265).

multiple etiological factors involving genetic predisposition to illness, combined with nutritional deficiencies, exposure to infective agents, cardiovascular dysfunction, or other agents infiltrating the nervous system.

Primary prevention is directed toward identifying and reducing risk factors through screening, education, and promoting healthy lifestyles. Secondary and tertiary prevention practice attempts to reduce sequelae from pathology to optimize an individual's quality of life, regardless of neurological impairment.

Memory Loss

In *The Importance of Being Earnest*, Oscar Wilde wrote, "Memory...is the diary that we all carry about with us."[1] A person's memories may be treasured or suppressed, but it is the body's only means of carrying a mental record of life's experiences through time. The brain's complex memory function is essential for retaining and recalling experiences, people, thoughts, feelings, perceptions, ideas, and knowledge.

Memory decline is anticipated with aging and may be noticed as early as the fourth decade of life.[2,3] Memory loss may be episodic, such as when a person experiences extreme stress, or it may be symptomatic of a serious health condition. *Amnesia* (or the *amnestic syndrome*) affects an individual's ability to remember facts, events, experiences, and personal information. More specifically, *anterograde amnesia* impairs storage and recall of memories from the recent past, whereas *retrograde amnesia* affects memories prior to a traumatic incident.[2]

Dementia is a condition that interferes with a person's ability to perform everyday tasks requiring memory, judgment, and awareness. Dementia affects approximately 1 in 1000 people younger than 65 years. In people older than 65 years, the rate is approximately 1 in 20.[2-5] One in 5 people older than 80 years has dementia.[2-5] Causes of dementia range from irreversible, organic brain disorders to reversible side effects of medications.

Although memory loss is relatively common, there are hundreds of causes of memory loss that must be assessed when considering its prevention and management, including the following[2-5]:

- Medications affecting memory (eg, antidepressants, antihistamines, antianxiety medications, muscle relaxants, tranquilizers, sleeping pills, and pain medications given after surgery)
- Alcohol, tobacco, and drug use
- Sleep deprivation
- Depression
- Stress
- Nutritional problems (eg, hypercalcemia, hypocalcemia, thiamine or vitamin B12 deficiency, adverse food reactions)
- Neurological conditions (eg, Down syndrome, head trauma, brain tumors, dementia, stroke, Parkinson's disease, thyroid dysfunction, and Alzheimer's disease)
- Brain infections (eg, meningitis and encephalitis)
- Select medical interventions for depression (eg, electroconvulsive or electroshock therapy)

Memory loss may be screened through an interview process incorporating questions related to orientation (current year, month, date, day of the week, and time of day), repetition of word lists using 3 common nouns (eg, apple, table, and penny), and recalling 10 names within a given category (eg, animals or vegetables) in 1 minute. Failure to perform these simple tasks suggests possible memory loss, but hearing loss should be ruled out before referral for more extensive testing. Medical testing for organic causes of memory loss may include blood and urine tests, nerve tests, and neuroimaging tests (eg, axial computed tomography scans or magnetic resonance imaging).

Memory loss can be delayed, averted, or ameliorated by maintaining a healthy lifestyle and by using strategies to boost memory. Table 15-1 provides a list of lifestyle habits and strategies that have been shown to improve memory and potentially avert memory loss typically associated with aging.[2-5]

Alzheimer's Disease

Alzheimer's disease, the most common form of dementia, is a degenerative brain disease characterized by a relatively rapid, progressive impairment in memory, judgment, decision-making, performing routine tasks, orientation to time and physical surroundings, and language. According to the Alzheimer's Association, "More than 5 million Americans are believed to have Alzheimer's disease and by 2050, as the US population ages, this number could increase to more than 15 million. The emotional and financial costs of Alzheimer's disease and dementia are enormous."[6] Health care professionals should be familiar with the following 10 signs identified by the Alzheimer's Association for early detection of this condition[6]:

1. Memory loss disrupts daily life
2. Challenges in planning or solving problems
3. Difficulty completing familiar tasks at home, at work, or during leisure activities
4. Confusion with time or place
5. Trouble understanding visual images or spatial relationships
6. New problems with words when speaking or writing
7. Misplacing things and losing the ability to retrace steps
8. Decreased or poor judgment
9. Withdrawal from work or social activities
10. Changes in mood or personality

Risk factors for Alzheimer's disease include aging, a family history of the disease, and high-risk genes (eg, APOE-e4). Genetic variations directly involved in the progression of Alzheimer's disease coding are 3 proteins: amyloid precursor protein (APP), presenilin-1 (PS-1), and presenilin-2 (PS-2). Genetic testing can be performed for diagnosis along with other medical tests to exclude other possible causes of mental decline.

The same strategies that control memory loss can be used to manage the onset of Alzheimer's disease. At present, there is no known cure for Alzheimer's disease, although there are medications that may slow its progression, including drugs that inhibit the degradation of acetylcholine within synapses. Cholinesterase inhibitors and memantine have been shown to delay the worsening of symptoms up to 12 months for some individuals.[6]

Table 15-2 includes the stages of Alzheimer's disease and the roles of the health care professional dealing with each progressive stage of the disease. The primary focus for health care professionals is helping the family and caregivers manage progressive impairments and providing referrals to resources for education, support, and counseling related to Alzheimer's disease. Caring for a person with Alzheimer's disease is extremely demanding on the caregiver, so respite care and psychosocial support for the caregiver are often necessary. The Bright Focus Foundation provides helpful resources for living with the condition for patients and caregivers alike, including legal and financial matters (http://www.brightfocus.org/).[7]

TABLE 15-1. STRATEGIES TO MAINTAIN AND IMPROVE MEMORY	
HEALTHY LIFESTYLE HABIT	**EFFECT ON MEMORY**
Exercise	Vigorous aerobic exercise increases oxygenation of the brain and increases the level of neurotrophins, substances that nourish brain cells and help protect them against damage from stroke and other injuries.
Nutrition	A healthy and balanced diet is rich in nutrition and filled with fruits and vegetables that contain brain-preserving antioxidants.
Mental stimulation	Level of education correlated most strongly with good mental functioning in old age.
Smoking	Smoking increases the risk for stroke and hypertension, 2 other causes of memory impairment.
Sleep	Sleeping 6 to 8 hours a night allows time for memories to register in the brain without distraction.
Social support	Positive social support that builds self-confidence is associated with maintaining good memory.
Memory problems	Strategies to improve memory
Names	When meeting someone for the first time, use his or her name in conversation.
	Think about the name and whether it is familiar (eg, others have the same name)
	Think of people who have the same name.
	Associate the name with an image, if one comes to mind. For example, link the name Sandy with the image of a beach.
	Write the person's name down in a memory notebook, personal organizer, or address book.
Where things are located	Always put things items used frequently in the same place (eg, keys, glasses, cellphone).
	For other objects, repeat aloud where items are put.
	For objects put down, consciously note where the item was placed.
	Write down where objects that are used infrequently in a memory notebook or personal organizer.
What people say	Ask the person to repeat what he or she just said.
	Ask the person to speak slowly to allow better concentration.
	Repeat what the person said and think about its meaning.
	If the information is lengthy or complicated (such as advice from your doctor), use a small cassette recorder or take notes while the person is talking.

(continued)

Table 15-1 (continued). Strategies to Maintain and Improve Memory	
HEALTHY LIFESTYLE HABIT	**EFFECT ON MEMORY**
Appointments	Write them down in an appointment book, calendar, or personal organizer.
	Write a to-do list in a personal organizer or calendar.
	Write a note and leave it in a place where it will be regularly seen (eg, on the kitchen table, on a cell phone notepad, or by the front door).
	Ask others for reminders, as appropriate (eg, follow up phone conversations with an e-mail summarizing an action plan).
	Leave an object associated with the task in a prominent place at home (eg, leave invitations and bills in a visible location).
	Set an alarm or a reminder on a calendar for appointments.

Epilepsy

Epilepsy is a common brain disorder characterized by repeated seizures that range from short lapses in attention to severe, frequent convulsions. The seizures can occur several times a day or once every few months and are due to bouts of excessive electrical activity in the brain. Usually, the brain region involved in the seizure remains the same from one seizure to the next, so an individual's seizure presentation is relatively predictable, although there can be dramatic differences between individuals. The Epilepsy Foundation (www.epilepsyfoundation.org) offers extensive information, including causes of epilepsy, types of seizures, health risks, treatment, syndromes, diagnosis, and first aid. Table 15-3 lists the common seizure triggers and their management.

The Centers for Disease Control and Prevention estimates that approximately 2.3 million adults[2] and 467,711 children (aged 0 to 17 years)[3] in the United States have epilepsy. Nearly 150,000 Americans develop the condition each year.[4,5] New cases of epilepsy are most common among children and older adults. Causes of epilepsy include oxygen deprivation, brain infections, traumatic brain injury or head injury, stroke, brain tumors, other diseases, or genetic conditions affecting the brain. Some factors contributing to epilepsy are preventable, including (1) proper prenatal care to avoid oxygen deprivation during pregnancy and birth, (2) infection control, and (3) preventing traumatic injuries from accidents, including falls and motor vehicle accidents.[8]

Epilepsy can be diagnosed through a comprehensive neurological examination, electroencephalogram, and brain imaging, such as computed tomography or magnetic resonance imaging. Management of epilepsy includes antiepileptic drugs and, in some cases, surgery. Health care professionals should be mindful of antiepileptic drug side effects (including fogginess, sleepiness, and dizziness) that limit an individual's ability to perform daily tasks.[8] Secondary prevention for individuals with epilepsy should focus on injury prevention when the person is seizing, as well as maintaining or reintegrating the individual into a supportive social network. Protection for those with severe seizures may involve having the person wear a helmet to prevent a head injury or hip protectors to reduce the risk of a fractured hip if a fall were to occur during a seizure. Education for individuals with epilepsy and those living and working with them should include what occurs during a seizure, how to respond to an individual's seizure, and the importance of limiting high-risk activities (eg, driving a motor vehicle), as appropriate.

TABLE 15-2. STAGES OF ALZHEIMER'S DISEASE		
STAGE	**IMPAIRMENT**	**ROLE OF HEALTH CARE PROFESSIONAL**
1	None (normal function) (Preclinical stage)	Screening of cognitive function
2	Very mild cognitive decline, forgetfulness (Mild cognitive impairment)	Detection and management of cognitive decline with patient and caregiver support: • Forgets familiar words • Forgets locations of objects
3	Moderate cognitive decline Noticeable deficits in demanding job situations (Mild or early-stage Alzheimer's disease)	Detection and management of cognitive decline with patient and caregiver support: • Problems recalling correct words or names • Trouble recalling names when introduced to new people • Difficulty performing tasks in social or work settings • Forgets material that one has just read • Loses or misplaces valuable objects • Increasing trouble with planning or organizing
4	Moderate cognitive decline (Mild or early-stage Alzheimer's disease)	Detection and management of cognitive decline with patient and caregiver support: • Forgets recent events • Impaired ability to perform challenging mental arithmetic • Greater difficulty performing complex tasks, such as planning dinner for guests, paying bills, or managing finances • Forgets one's own personal history • Becomes moody or withdrawn, especially socially or mentally • Requires assistance in complicated tasks such as handling finances, planning
5	Moderately severe cognitive decline (Moderate or mid-stage Alzheimer's disease)	Detection and management of cognitive decline with patient and caregiver support: • Unable to recall one's own address or telephone number or the high school or college from which one graduated • Confused about where one is or what day it is • Has trouble with less challenging mental arithmetic, such as counting backward from 40 by 4s or from 20 by 2s • Needs help choosing proper clothing for the season or the occasion • Still remembers significant details about oneself and one's family

(continued)

Table 15-2 (continued). Stages of Alzheimer's Disease		
STAGE	**IMPAIRMENT**	**ROLE OF HEALTH CARE PROFESSIONAL**
6	Severe cognitive decline (Moderately severe or mid-stage Alzheimer's disease)	Detection and management of cognitive and physical decline with patient and caregiver support: • Loses awareness of recent experiences and one's surroundings • Remembers one's own name but has difficulty with one's personal history • Needs help dressing properly and may, without supervision, make mistakes such as putting pajamas over daytime clothes or shoes on the wrong feet • Experiences major changes in sleep patterns (sleeping during the day and becoming restless at night) • Needs help handling details of toileting (flushing the toilet, wiping, or disposing of tissue properly) • Has increasingly frequent trouble controlling one's bladder or bowels • Experiences major personality and behavioral changes, including suspiciousness and delusions (such as believing that one's caregiver is an impostor) or compulsive, repetitive behavior like hand wringing or tissue shredding • Tends to wander or become lost
7	Very severe cognitive decline	Management of behavioral and physical needs with patient and caregiver support: • Needs help with much of one's daily personal care, including eating or using the toilet • Physical decline: deconditioning and muscle tightness • Impaired swallowing • Speech ability declines to approximately a half-dozen intelligible words • Progressively loses abilities to walk, sit up, smile, and hold head up; frequently there is no speech at all, only grunting • Incontinent of urine; requires assistance toileting and feeding; loses basic psychomotor skills (eg, walking, sitting, and head control)
Adapted from Seven stages of Alzheimer's disease. Alzheimer's Association. http://www.alz.org/alzheimers_disease_stages_of_alzheimers.asp. Accessed May 20, 2014; and Dementia care practice recommendations for professionals working in a home setting. Alzheimer's Association. http://www.alz.org/national/documents/phase_4_home_care_recs.pdf. Accessed May 20, 2014.		

TABLE 15-3. TRIGGERS FOR SEIZURES	
TRIGGER	**MANAGEMENT**
Missed medication	Maintain proper schedule for medications
Hormone changes (pregnancy, menstrual cycle)	Medication may be used
Metabolic changes, including low blood sugar	Monitor and manage metabolic needs
Sleep deprivation	Encourage sleep; melatonin, if warranted
Alcohol	Avoid use of alcohol
Emotional stress (worry, anxiety, anger)	Stress management
Flashing or strobe lights	Avoid exposure to flashing lights
Photosensitivity	Wear sunglasses; avoid bright lights; consider risk of playing electronic screen games
Tapping or light touch	Avoid trigger
Thinking about certain situations (eg, eating)	Time management; redirect thoughts
Excessive caffeine	Avoid use of excessive caffeine

STROKE

Stroke, a loss of blood flow to the central nervous system, is the most common and possibly the most preventable neuromuscular condition. According to the American Heart Association, stroke is a leading cause of disability, cognitive impairment, and death in the United States, accounting for 1.7% of national health expenditures.[9] "Overall, total annual costs of stroke are projected to increase to $240.67 billion by 2030."[9] Up to 80% of strokes can be eliminated with an emphasis on implementing effective preventive practice.[10]

Although strokes usually occur in the cerebral hemispheres (a cerebral vascular accident [CVA]), they can occur anywhere in the nervous system, including the brainstem and spinal cord. *Ischemic strokes* (or mini-strokes) account for 87% of strokes and occur when a supplying artery is occluded. In an ischemic stroke, the blood vessel is rapidly occluded by an embolus (often arising from the heart) or more slowly by a thrombosis (often arising from atherosclerosis).[11,12] Another type, the *hemorrhagic stroke*, occurs when an artery ruptures, causing a major brain bleed and potentially significant pressure on the brain.[11] The extent of injury or damage from either type of stroke depends on the timeliness of recognizing the signs and symptoms, as well as instituting appropriate intervention.

Primary prevention of stroke requires knowledge of risk factors in different populations, including unmodifiable risk factors (eg, age, ethnicity, sex, and genetic predisposition). Stroke risk increases with age, sex (more common in males), ethnicity (substantially higher in minorities based on multiple factors including access to health care, beliefs, and socioeconomic status),[6] and medical history. For example, *transient ischemic attacks* (TIAs) are strokes that resolve within 24 hours without apparent deficit or functional loss; however, there is a 10% risk of stroke in the 3 months following a TIA.[11] With such a high stroke risk, a person who experiences a TIA should expediently address and be particularly vigilant in addressing the modifiable stroke risk factors. Modifiable risk factors for stroke include diabetes, hypertension (a systolic pressure of 160 mm Hg

TABLE 15-4. RISK FACTORS FOR STROKE	
HEREDITY	• Family history: A family history of stroke increases the chance of stroke. • Age and sex: The risk of stroke increases with age. For ages 65 and older, men are at greater risk than women to have a stroke.[1] • Race and ethnicity: Blacks, Hispanics, and American Indian/Alaska Natives have a greater chance of having a stroke than do non-Hispanic Whites or Asians.
MEDICAL CONDITIONS	• Hypertension: Hypertension from poor lifestyle behaviors (eg, smoking, poor nutrition, and alcohol) can greatly increase your risk for stroke. • High blood cholesterol: Diet, exercise, and family history affect blood cholesterol levels. • Heart disease: Common heart disorders such as coronary artery disease, heart valve defects, irregular heartbeat (including atrial fibrillation), and enlarged heart chambers can cause a stroke. • Diabetes: Having diabetes can increase your risk of stroke and can make the outcome of strokes worse. • Overweight and obesity: Being overweight or obese can raise total cholesterol levels, increase blood pressure, and promote the development of diabetes. • Previous stroke or TIA: There is a greater risk with prior TIAs. • Sickle cell disease: Approximately 10% of children with sickle cell disease will have a stroke.
UNHEALTHY BEHAVIOR	• Tobacco use: Smoking injures blood vessels and speeds up the hardening of the arteries. The carbon monoxide in cigarette smoke reduces the amount of oxygen that your blood can carry. Secondhand smoke can increase the risk of stroke for nonsmokers. • Alcohol use: Excessive drinking can raise blood pressure and increase levels of triglycerides, a form of cholesterol, resulting in increased stroke risk. • Physical inactivity: Limited physical activity can lead to increased blood pressure and cholesterol levels and creates an additional risk factor for diabetes.

or higher and/or diastolic pressure of 95 mm Hg or higher), smoking (more than 40 cigarettes per day quadruples risk, although cessation can reduce risk to baseline values over 5 years),[5] carotid artery disease, cardiac dysfunction, blood disorders that increase clot formation, high low-density lipoprotein (LDL) cholesterol levels and low high-density lipoprotein (HDL) cholesterol levels, obesity, excessive alcohol intake (more than one drink per day and binge drinking), illegal drug use (intravenous drug abuse carries a high risk of stroke), and use of oral contraceptives.[12] Table 15-4 lists the risk factors for stroke.

The Division for Heart Disease and Stroke Prevention offers a toolkit to help health care professionals deliver preventive services to the community at http://www.cdc.gov/dhdsp/pubs/

docs/toolkit.pdf, including a checklist for key resources for stroke prevention, including blood pressure control, lipid management, tobacco cessation, nutrition/dietary intake, weight management, physical activity, diabetes management, cardiac and stroke rehabilitation, and depression management.[13]

Health care professionals should also caution their clients about signs indicating that a stroke may be occurring because emergent medical treatment can minimize a stroke's damage. The signs of stroke include the following[11]:

- Sudden weakness or numbness of the face, arm, or leg, especially on one side of the body
- Sudden confusion or trouble speaking or understanding
- Sudden trouble seeing in one eye or both eyes
- Sudden trouble walking, dizziness, or loss of balance or coordination
- Sudden, severe headaches with no known cause

Secondary prevention should address prevention of stroke recurrence and death. "At least 1 in 4 (25% to 35%) of the 795,000 Americans who have a stroke each year will have another stroke within their lifetime. Recurrent strokes often have a higher rate of death and disability because parts of the brain already injured by the original stroke may not be as resilient. Within 5 years of a stroke, 24% of women and 42% of men will experience a recurrent stroke."[10] Thus, a first stroke may foreshadow future strokes, resulting in significant disability unless aggressive secondary prevention is implemented. Secondary prevention primarily addresses the factors that increase stroke risk (see Table 15-4). Physical activity reduces stroke risk in a dose-dependent manner; the greater the level of physical activity, the greater the reduction in stroke risk (Table 15-5).[14] A specialist in exercise, such as a physical therapist, is best qualified to develop an exercise program that optimizes cardiovascular endurance without increasing risk of health problems.

The most common disabilities apparent poststroke include *hemiparesis* (weakness on one side of the body), depression and other mental health issues, gait dysfunction, problems performing activities of daily living, incontinence and urinary tract problems, and communication problems. Determining a person's secondary prevention needs poststroke requires knowledge of the stroke's vascular etiology, the function of the affected brain region, preexisting and poststroke comorbidities, and the individual's residual capabilities and remaining debilities. Sensorimotor function is commonly limited by muscle weakness, fatigue, poor coordination, *hypertonicity* (increased muscle tone), *spasticity* (velocity-dependent, increased resistance to passive muscle stretch), or *dyskinesia* (abnormal movement). These impairments are further confounded by the following:

- Pain
- Soft tissue or articular contractures (ie, abnormal joint movement limitation)
- Sensory dysfunction (eg, *anesthesia* [loss of sensation], *hyperesthesia* [increased sensory sensitivity], *dysesthesia* [abnormal, disagreeable sensory feelings], *paresthesia* [burning or prickling sensations], *hemineglect* [lacking awareness of one side of the body], *hemianopsia* [loss of half of the visual field], and *pusher syndrome* [a tendency to push out of postural alignment])
- Altered nonsensory/motor functions (eg, fatigue, inattention, and lack of safety awareness)
- Sexual dysfunction[12-15]

Health care professionals need to monitor their clients poststroke to ensure that these problems are addressed.

When developing a prevention program for stroke survivors, health care professionals should keep in mind that these individuals are usually physically deconditioned prestroke, at increased risk for additional strokes and cardiovascular disease, and often taking antihypertensive, cardiovascular, and/or anticonvulsant medications. Due to motor paralysis, sensory loss, and/or cognitive impairments, certain activities may not be possible and may need to be adapted to meet individualized needs.

Table 15-5. Summary of Exercise Programming Recommendations for Stroke Survivors

MODE OF EXERCISE	GOALS OF EXERCISE	INTENSITY	FREQUENCY	DURATION
Aerobic exercise (Large-muscle activities [eg, walking, treadmill, stationary cycle, combined arm-leg ergometry, arm ergometry, seated stepper])	• Increase independence in activities of daily living • Increase walking speed and efficiency • Improve tolerance for prolonged physical activity • Reduce risk of cardiovascular disease	40% to 70% peak oxygen uptake; 40% to 70% heart rate reserve; 50% to 80% maximal heart rate; rate of perceived exertion 11 to 14 (6 to 20 scale)	3 to 7 d/wk	20 to 60 min/session (or multiple 10-min sessions)
Strength (Circuit training, weight machines, free weights, isometric exercise)	• Increase independence in activities of daily living	1 to 3 sets of 10 to 15 repetitions of 8 to 10 exercises involving the major muscle groups	2 to 3 d/wk	
Flexibility (Stretching)	• Increase range of motion of involved extremities • Prevent contractures		2 to 3 d/wk (before or after aerobic or strength training)	Hold each stretch for 10 to 30 s
Neuromuscular (Coordination and balance activities)	• Improve level of safety during activities of daily living		2 to 3 d/wk (consider performing on same day as strength activities)	

Recommended intensity, frequency, and duration of exercise depend on each patient's level of fitness. Intermittent training sessions may be indicated during the initial weeks of rehabilitation.

Adapted from Gordon NF, Gulanick M, Costa F, et al. Physical activity and exercise recommendations for stroke survivors: an American Heart Association scientific statement from the Council on Clinical Cardiology, Subcommittee on Exercise, Cardiac Rehabilitation, and Prevention; the Council on Cardiovascular Nursing; the Council on Nutrition, Physical Activity, and Metabolism; and the Stroke Council. *Circulation.* 2004;109(16):2031-2041.

Spinal Cord Injury

The spinal cord is the pathway for communication between the brain and the body. It is protected by meninges and a flexible vertebral column cushioned by cartilaginous disks. *Spinal cord injury* (SCI) can result from traumatic injuries (eg, falls, motor vehicle accidents, sport injuries, and gunshot wounds); infections; edema; a blocked blood supply; and compression by a displaced disk, fractured bone, tumor, abscess, or narrowing of the spinal column.[15] All of these problems can result in temporary or permanent muscle weakness or paralysis, sensory abnormalities or loss, and, in some cases, loss of bladder and bowel control, depending on the extent and duration of injury. If only the lower extremities are involved, the paralysis is called *paraplegia* (loss of strength in the legs). *Tetraplegia* (weakness in all 4 limbs) refers to loss of function in both upper and lower extremities. The injury is incomplete if any sensory or motor function is preserved below the injury level. The American Spinal Injury Association Impairment Scale (AIS) is used to classify SCI[16]:

A. "Complete" SCI is defined by the absence of deep anal sensation and voluntary anal contraction. Sacral sensation is defined as light touch and pinprick at S4-S5, or deep anal pressure.

B. "Sensory Incomplete" SCI is defined by the presence of anal sensation. Other preserved sensation may be present below the injury level. No motor function is preserved more than 3 levels below the motor level on either side of the body.

C. "Motor Incomplete" SCI is defined by the presence of anal sensation or voluntary sphincter contraction and some voluntary motor activity that is less than 50% of the summed motor score below the injury level. More than half of key muscle functions below the single neurological level of injury (NLI) have a muscle grade of less than 3 (grades 0 to 2). The standards at this time allow even non-key muscle functions more than 3 levels below the motor level to be used in determining motor incomplete status (AIS B vs C). A classification of C requires voluntary anal contraction or sacral sensory sparing with sparing of motor function more than 3 levels below the motor level for that side of the body.

D. "Motor Incomplete" SCI is defined by the presence of anal sensation or voluntary anal sphincter contraction and motor activity that is greater than or equal to 50% of the motor score below the injury level. The definition requires voluntary anal contraction or sparing of motor function more than 3 levels below the motor level for that side of the body.

E. "Normal" SCI is defined by normal motor and sensory scores, as well as anal sensation and sphincter contraction. To receive this classification, the patient had prior deficits, so someone without an initial SCI does not receive an AIS grade.

It is estimated that the annual incidence of SCI in the United States, not including those who die at the scene of the accident, is approximately 40 cases per million population, or approximately 12,000 new cases each year. Working to improve the physical and mental health and wellness of individuals who have a SCI presents unique challenges for the clinician. Health care providers and patients alike can be inspired by the words of Christopher Reeve, founder of The Christopher and Dana Reeve Foundation: "Once you choose hope, anything's possible."[17]

Management of SCI involves a team approach to addressing problems associated with weakness and risk for contractures, sensory loss in certain parts of the body, pain with musculoskeletal repetitive trauma of intact muscles, pressure sores, urinary and bowel problems, altered sexuality, risk for scoliosis, and risk for pneumonia for those with high-level lesions affecting breathing and blot clots, which are typically managed by anticoagulant drugs. The presence of these conditions is closely related to these individuals' psychosocial function with resultant social isolation, depression, and substance abuse.[18] Mobility and perceived health appear to be the consistent predictors of life satisfaction 2 years post-SCI.[18]

Rehabilitation helps people recover as much function as possible. The best care is provided by a team that includes nurses, physical and occupational therapists, a social worker, a nutritionist, a psychologist, and a counselor, as well as the individual and family members. Team members need to encourage a healthy diet, provide options for appropriate physical activity (possibly augmented by functional electrical stimulation), educate regarding skin care to prevent pressure sores, monitor for cardiovascular and pulmonary complications (eg, deep vein thrombosis, pulmonary embolism, pneumonia), encourage healthy stress management habits (eg, avoid smoking and drugs), provide respiratory hygiene for those with high-level lesions, monitor the autonomic system for dysfunction (blood pressure changes in lesions above T6 during physical activity), prevent urinary tract infections, and monitor to prevent bowel problems.

A wide variety of problems and complications are associated with the neurological and musculoskeletal systems of individuals with SCI, including pain caused by the lesion itself; *myelopathy* (spinal cord disease); weakness; spasticity; *heterotopic ossification* (new bone formation in the connective tissue or muscle surrounding the major joints); musculoskeletal pain from tendon, bursa, or joint inflammation; peripheral neuropathy; autonomic dysfunction; joint contracture; degenerative joint disease; and osteoporotic fracture.[15] Pain and impaired function increase with time. The overused shoulder from wheelchair propulsion and transfers is the most common painful joint, including tendonitis, bursitis, impingement syndrome, and possible rotator cuff tears and joint degeneration. These conditions can be severely disabling for persons with SCI who depend on their arms for mobility and manual tasks. Health care professionals need to educate individuals with SCI about the prevention of secondary complications and facilitate connections with resources and environmental supports to maximize participation at work, at home, and in recreational settings.

Traumatic Brain Injury

Traumatic brain injury (TBI), also known as *acquired brain injury*, results from either intentional or unintentional trauma to the brain. Although a direct traumatic impact causes some brain injury, the major impairments and functional limitations result from vascular hemorrhage and *diffuse axonal injury* (tearing of nerves located throughout the brain).[19] Although a TBI can occur in a single traumatic event, such as a motor vehicle accident, repetitive microtrauma from activities such as boxing or heading the ball in soccer can impair cognitive and motor functions.

Males are almost twice as likely as females to sustain a TBI, and African Americans have the highest death rate from TBI.[20] There are 2 high-risk age groups: those aged 15 to 24 years and those older than 75.[20] The younger group is prone to sustain TBI in a motor vehicle accident or in a fall while participating in a high-risk activity.[20] Alcohol or drugs are often involved. The older age group often acquires a brain injury in a slip/fall accident.[20] The risk of sustaining another head injury increases with each subsequent injury. Due to their commonalities in causality, TBI and SCI commonly occur together.

A TBI can be *mild*, resulting in a brief concussion, or *severe*, leading to death or a *persistent vegetative state* (a condition characterized by the inability to speak, follow simple commands, or respond in a meaningful way).[20] Although each person's presentation is unique, there are general classification schemes for categorizing individuals who have a TBI. The Glasgow Coma Scale is used for recovery from a coma, and the revised Ranchos Los Amigos Levels of Cognitive Functioning[21] assesses functional limitations and general behavior through stages of recovery.

The most devastating problems following a TBI are cognitive deficits. Cognitive deficits are further complicated by motor and sensory dysfunction, such as a *hemiparesis* (weakness in one half of the body), *apraxia* (inability to plan voluntary movement), *dystonia* (abnormal muscle tone), and *ataxia* (inability to coordinate movement resulting in errors of accuracy and force). The types of complications that arise are dependent on the severity of the injury, the neural functions involved, the concurrent injuries, and comorbid conditions.[22] A major concern following a TBI is the person's increased risk of sustaining another TBI. This risk needs to be actively addressed by use of protective gear when engaged in sports and avoiding high-risk activities. An additional complication of TBI, as well as SCI, is *heterotopic ossification* (the formation of bone in an abnormal location).[22] Treatment for heterotopic ossification is maintaining as much movement as possible at the joints without further tissue damage or surgery to remove affected bone. In addition to these risks, the person with a TBI faces myriad challenges. Neurological dysfunction includes movement disorders, seizures, headaches, visual deficits, and sleep disorders. Non-neurological problems include pulmonary, metabolic, nutritional, gastrointestinal, musculoskeletal, and dermatologic dysfunction.[22] Behaviorally, the person may exhibit verbal and physical aggression, agitation, learning difficulties, shallow self-awareness, altered sexual functioning, impulsivity, social disinhibition, mood disorders, personality changes, altered emotional control, and depression. Socially, the person with a TBI is at increased risk for suicide, divorce, chronic unemployment, economic strain, and substance abuse.[22] Health care professionals need to work collaboratively and make appropriate referrals to address the multiple complications and risk factors facing an individual post-TBI.

Concussion

A concussion is a *mild traumatic brain injury* (mTBI) resulting from a blow or a jolt to the brain or a penetrating head injury.[23] Concussions may occur from a variety of injuries sustained in sports (eg, football, boxing, soccer, and other contact sports), in accidents (eg, falls, bicycling, or motor vehicle accidents), on the battlefield (eg, blasts, fragments, bullets, motor vehicle accidents, and falls during battle), or from other causes.[24] Because these injuries are often mild, they are commonly unreported. Without an immediate screening for neurological function, the person with a concussion may lack the needed brain function to escape further injury.[23]

The US military diagnosis of concussion or mTBI is based on one or more of the following criteria: (1) loss of consciousness for less than 30 minutes, (2) loss of memory for events before or after the injury resolving within 24 hours, or (3) alteration of consciousness or mental state (confusion, disorientation, or dazed feeling) resolving within 24 hours.[23] Imaging of the brain typically shows no changes, and scores on the Glasgow Coma Scale (top score is 15) typically range from 13 to 15 within the first 24 hours.[23]

Clinical manifestations of concussion may include physical symptoms (eg, headache, dizziness, balance disorder, nausea, fatigue, sleep disturbance, blurred vision, light sensitivity, hearing loss, noise sensitivity, seizures, transient neurological abnormalities, numbness, and tingling), cognitive symptoms (attention, memory, concentration, processing speed, judgment, and emotional control), or behavioral or emotional symptoms (depression, anxiety, agitation irritability, impulsivity, and aggression).[23]

On one hand, the signs and symptoms may be subtle, depending on the extent of injury. A person may simply report feeling "foggy" or not feeling well. On the other hand, a concussion may be more obvious with significant brain trauma, leading to more severe symptoms, including, but not limited to, worsening headaches, repeated vomiting, weakness, numbness, and incoordination. Individuals experiencing a concussion should be taken to the emergency department if they have (1) slurred speech, (2) one or both pupils dilated, (3) convulsions, (4) increasing confusion, (5) increasing agitation, (6) increasing restlessness, or (7) lethargy.[23] Although many of these symptoms may be temporary (lasting only minutes), they may last for days to weeks. The Epworth Sleepiness Scale is a helpful measure for screening for sleep problems that may persist post-mTBI.[25]

Other conditions presenting with similar findings include posttraumatic stress disorder, substance use disorders, and mental health conditions, so a medical referral is needed for confirmation of the medical diagnosis if problems persist.[23] Physical therapists play an important role in managing headaches, dizziness and disequilibrium, and coordination problems. Management of other symptoms includes pharmacologic management, cognitive rehabilitation, patient education regarding resources for recovery and living a healthy lifestyle, referral for evaluation for driver rehabilitation training and education (as needed), and monitoring for persistent problems.

Many organizations support the prevention of concussion; the US government has a website dedicated to its prevention, identification, and management (www.cdc.gov/concussion). This site provides the Heads Up program for health care professionals, coaches, parents, and athletes. The

Acute Concussion Evaluation is in the Heads Up toolkit and outlines key questions to ask a person who has suffered a recent concussion. These questions include the injury characteristics, symptoms (physical, thinking, emotional, and sleep), risk factors, red flags, diagnosis, and follow-up plan for the individual.

Parkinson's Disease

Many movement disorders arise from subcortical, cerebellar, and brainstem damage resulting from genetic abnormalities, metabolic dysfunction, stroke, toxins, infections, and oxidative stress. These causes include, but are not limited to, an adverse reaction to prescription drugs, use of illegal drugs, exposure to environmental toxins, stroke, thyroid and parathyroid disorders, repeated head trauma (eg, the trauma associated with boxing), brain tumor, hydrocephalus, and encephalitis.[26] *Parkinson's disease* (PD) is the most common movement disorder, with impairments arising primarily due to damage to the substantia nigra's dopanergic neurons.[26] It is likely caused by a combination of genetic and environmental factors, including viral infection or exposure to environmental toxins such as pesticides, carbon monoxide, or the metal manganese, although the exact cause is unknown.[23]

The initial diagnosis of persons with PD typically relies on clinical observations of its cardinal signs: (1) *resting or postural tremor* (small movements at rest), (2) *bradykinesia* (slow movement), (3) *rigidity* (increased resistance to the passive movement of a limb), and (4) postural instability.[26] These motor signs may present as *micrographia* (small handwriting), *masked facies* (a "reptilian stare"), a stooped shuffling gait with decreased arm swing, difficulty in mobility and performing daily activities, and *hypophonic* (low-volume) speech. Nonmotor signs may include autonomic dysfunction, slowed gastric and intestinal motility, urinary dysfunction, sexual dysfunction, pain, cognitive changes, sleep dysfunction (acting out dreams), speech problems, and swallowing dysfunction.[27] Although more difficult for the clinician to observe, the nonmotor signs may change a person's health and wellness more than the motor signs. Dementia can occur in up to one-third of persons with PD. Depression occurs in approximately half of these individuals and arises from the neurological impairment, rather than as a secondary symptom.[27] Aspiration pneumonia is a major cause of morbidity and mortality in persons with PD. Health care professionals must address these complications and caution these individuals of risks associated with motor and nonmotor impairments that can influence functional abilities.

Medications currently are the best conservative treatment for persons with PD. Pharmacological treatment can frequently change, so they must be monitored continuously by a qualified health care professional, usually a neurologist.[27] Overmedication can lead to problems with hallucinations, *dyskinesias* (uncontrolled movements), insomnia, nausea, reduced appetite, weight loss, and *dystonia* (abnormal muscle tone).[27]

Because PD is a progressive condition, there is increasing interest in discovering ways to slow the progression rate. A most promising avenue is the effect of exercise on slowing the progression of PD.[28,29] Many of the signs and symptoms of PD may respond to nonpharmacological treatments. Nonpharmacologic and pharmacologic treatments for persons with PD often give transient results, producing an effect only while the person is using or engaged in the treatment. Therefore, adherence to the intervention program should be encouraged. Problems that may be managed with nonpharmacologic interventions include the following[29]:

- Difficulties with motor control, balance, posture, gait, and mobility
- Difficulties with activities of daily living and instrumental activities of daily living (IADL; skills that enable a person to live independently, such as shopping, managing money, and using technology)
- Problems with speech and swallowing

- Issues with proper nutrition
- Sleep dysfunction
- Pain
- Constipation
- Sexual dysfunction
- Psychosocial issues, including depression

Physical therapy can address the motor problems in an effort to maintain or increase activity levels, decrease rigidity and bradykinesia, optimize gait, and improve balance and motor coordination. Features of a physical therapy program that are shown to be effective may include the following[30]:

- Regular exercise, such as walking, swimming, dancing, and bicycle ergometry (providing both physical and psychological benefits)
- Stretching
- Strengthening
- Providing mobility aids as needed
- Training in transfer techniques
- Training in techniques to improve posture and walking
- Fall prevention, including balance activities such as t'ai chi

Referrals to occupational therapists, dietitians, and speech and language pathologists who specialize in oromotor training and management of swallowing problems are often appropriate. Health care professionals should be alerted to sexual problems that can arise with PD, including erectile dysfunction in men, vaginal dryness in women, loss of libido, and hypersexuality from use of dopaminergic drugs.[31] Because this condition is progressive, a strong social support network is helpful for the individual and caregiver.

Multiple Sclerosis

Multiple sclerosis (MS) is a neuropathology that damages the myelin surrounding axons in the central nervous system, resulting in *sclerosis* (scarring) and neurological dysfunction.[32]

The most common initial symptoms are paresthesias or sensory disturbances in one or more extremities, in the trunk, or on one side of the face; weakness or clumsiness of a leg or hand; visual disturbances (eg, partial loss of vision and pain in one eye or double vision); and subtle mood swings.[32] Table 15-6 lists the common clinical manifestations of MS.

Because the demyelination process is variable in each individual, clinical manifestations may be subtle and may go undetected initially, often leading to a delayed diagnosis of MS. MS has variable courses or patterns of progression, including the following[32]:

- A *relapsing-remitting pattern* with *exacerbations* (increased intensity and frequency) and *remissions* (reduced intensity and frequency) lasting for months or years
- A *primary progressive pattern* with a gradual progression without remission
- A *secondary progressive pattern* that begins with relapses and remissions, then gradually progresses
- A *progressive relapsing pattern* that progresses with sudden relapses

The cause of MS is unknown; however, environmental and genetic factors appear to interact to cause an autoimmune dysfunction. This condition most commonly affects young adults between

Table 15-6. Impairments Associated With Multiple Sclerosis

SENSORY IMPAIRMENTS	MOTOR IMPAIRMENTS	PSYCHOLOGICAL IMPAIRMENTS
• Abnormal sensations, such as numbness, tingling, pain, burning, and itching • Visual disturbances, including double vision, partial blindness and pain in one eye, dim or blurred vision, and loss of central vision • Difficulty in reaching orgasm, lack of sensation in the vagina, and sexual impotence in men • Dizziness or vertigo	• Weakness and clumsiness • Difficulty walking or maintaining balance • Tremor • Uncoordinated eye movements • Problems with control of urination and bowel movements • Constipation • Stiffness, unsteadiness, and unusual fatigue	• Mood swings • Inappropriate elation or giddiness • Depression • Inability to control emotions (eg, crying or laughing without reason) • Subtle or obvious mental impairment

the ages of 20 and 40 years, with women affected twice as often as men in those with a Northern European genetic history.[32] Risk factors include living before age 15 years in a temperate climate, lower levels of vitamin D (possibly due to less sun exposure in temperate climates), and cigarette smoking.

Treatment includes corticosteroids for acute exacerbations, immunomodulatory drugs to prevent exacerbations, and supportive measures.[32] During an exacerbation, the individual should not engage in strenuous physical activity because fatigue can be debilitating, limiting function for hours to days. Also, individuals with MS should exercise caution in the heat, including hot tubs and warm baths because this environmental factor can significantly impair a person's movement.[33,34] Additional management may include antispasmodic drugs to manage spasticity, therapy for sensory dysfunction, and prevention of secondary complications related to limited physical activity, including contracture formation, skin breakdown, urinary tract infections, and pneumonia.[33,34] Regular physical activity (eg, walking, aerobic activity, resistance training, balance and postural control activities, and range of motion exercises) in socially supportive environments combined with time management to accomplish important daily tasks and other stress reduction techniques can help an individual with MS achieve balance and control in life amidst the unpredictable progression of the disease.[34-36] Recognizing the restrictions imposed by fatigue, health care providers need to facilitate participation in meaningful activities that have a positive effect on both the physical and mental well-being of the individual with MS.

Peripheral Neuropathy

Peripheral neuropathy refers to a dysfunction or disease in a peripheral nerve, and a *polyneuropathy* involves multiple nerves. Causes of peripheral neuropathy range from systemic pathology (eg, Guillain-Barré syndrome and diabetes) to localized nerve compression (eg, *carpal tunnel*) and nerve root damage (eg, *lumbar radiculopathy*). There are many causes of neuropathies, including diabetes, alcoholism, vitamin deficiency, and certain types of chemotherapy. The neuropathy, whether caused by nerve entrapment, inflammation, trauma, or metabolic dysfunction, disrupts a peripheral nerve's sensory, motor, and/or autonomic nervous system components.

Generally, the clinical signs and symptoms include muscle paralysis or weakness and/or sensory dysfunction (eg, anesthesia, paresthesias, and dysesthesias). If motor function is disrupted, there will be flaccid paralysis of the muscles innervated by the nerve(s). Secondary prevention must address the complications that can arise from limited movement (contractures and deformities), as well as education to reduce the risk of injury from sensory loss and sensory impairments influencing movement. Because the etiology and clinical presentation of patients with neuropathy is greatly varied, it is unwarranted to make broad generalizations about neuropathy as a whole, with the exception of the following:

- In all patients with neuropathy, secondary prevention should include activities to strengthen the remaining unaffected body parts and capacities as able (core strength, muscular endurance) because individuals will rely on compensatory movements and stability to function.
- Progressive neuropathies, especially Charcot-Marie-Tooth disease, should be given consideration for future skin and joint protection. Bracing may be considered for early ankle preservation.
- Balance training is essential. Forcing the brain to adapt to a loss of sensory input from the lower extremities, processing alternate sensory signals can help greatly with fall prevention.

Table 15-7 provides an overview of the key features of neurological conditions and associated wellness concerns.

Table 15-8 provides a range of physical activities that can prove beneficial for individuals with neurological conditions and can be supervised by physical therapists or health care professionals with expertise in exercise and chronic conditions.

Tension Headache

A *headache* is a complaint of pain related to any part of the head, including the scalp, face (including the orbitotemporal area), and interior of the head, and is one of the most common reasons patients seek medical attention.[36] Headaches result from activation of pain-sensitive structures in or around the brain, skull, face, sinuses, or teeth and may be related to extracranial problems (eg, temporomandibular joint dysfunction), intracranial disorders (eg, brain tumors), systemic conditions (eg, viral infections), or drugs and toxins (eg, caffeine withdrawal).[36] Interview questions that can be used to screen for referral include those listed in Table 15-9.

Red flags that indicate the need for an immediate medical referral include the following[36]:

- Neurologic symptoms or signs (eg, altered mental status, weakness, diplopia, papilledema, focal neurologic deficits)
- Suspected immunosuppression or cancer
- Meningismus
- Onset of headache after age 50
- Thunderclap headache (severe headache that peaks within a few seconds)
- Symptoms of giant cell arteritis (eg, visual disturbances, jaw claudication, fever, weight loss, temporal artery tenderness, proximal myalgias)
- Systemic symptoms (eg, fever, weight loss)
- Progressively worsening headache
- Red eye and halos around lights

Table 15-7. Characteristics of Chronic Neurological Impairment and Associated Wellness Concerns

KEY FEATURES OF THE MEDICAL CONDITION	ASSOCIATED WELLNESS CONCERN
Age of onset • Pediatric or young adult onset (eg, SCI, head injury) • Intermediate onset (eg, peripheral neuropathies) • Older adult (eg, stroke, Alzheimer's disease, PD)	• Address the individual's age-appropriate biological and developmental tasks. • Consider changes in body structure that can result from motor dysfunction.
Speed of onset • Rapid (eg, SCI, stroke) • Progressive (eg, MS) • Insidious (eg, Alzheimer's disease, PD)	• Consider whether the symptoms are sudden or insidious throughout the screening process. A rapid onset usually results in a clearly delineated injury.
Progression • Relatively static (eg, SCI) • Variable (eg, MS, peripheral neuropathies) • Progressive (eg, PD, Alzheimer's disease)	• Consider how the progression of the pathology affects the person's coping mechanisms and ability to anticipate future needs. • Consider how chronic conditions may burden caregivers and family members.
Etiology • Inborn mechanism of injury (eg, arteriovenous malformation, Huntington's chorea) • Interaction with genetics and lifestyle (eg, possibly MS) • Acquired through lifestyle choices (eg, SCI, ischemic stroke)	• Consider how lifestyle behaviors can prevent initial injuries and subsequent injuries. • Educate these individuals about genetic predisposition to disease when family histories are positive.
Lifestyle behaviors • High-risk activities (eg, SCI, TBI) • Long-term lifestyle habits (eg, atherosclerosis leading to stroke)	• Educate these individuals about healthy lifestyle choices to reduce the risk of chronic pathology.
Cognitive impairment • No cognitive impairment (eg, peripheral neuropathies) • Cognitive impairment (eg, TBI, Alzheimer's disease)	• Consider how a cognitive impairment may impair the person's ability to comprehend and implement the treatment.

(continued)

Table 15-7 (continued). Characteristics of Chronic Neurological Impairment and Associated Wellness Concerns

KEY FEATURES OF THE MEDICAL CONDITION	ASSOCIATED WELLNESS CONCERN
Sensory changes • Changes (eg, diabetic peripheral neuropathy) • No change (eg, poliomyelitis)	• Provide precautions regarding the risk of self-injury.
Perceptual changes • Probable change (eg, right parietal stroke) • Minimal changes (eg, SCI)	• Consider that these individuals may have altered perceptions of reality.
Communication changes • Profound changes (eg, TBI with aphasia) • No changes (eg, SCI with paraparesis)	• Consider how difficulty with communication can affect interventions. • Offer various options for communication and refer to speech pathology as appropriate.
Respiratory involvement • Minimal (eg, paraparetic SCI) • Variable (eg, PD) • Significant impairment (eg, tetraparesis)	• Consider how impaired respiration predisposes individuals to pneumonia and reduces their exercise tolerance.

Headache types are described as primary or secondary; 90% of people present with primary headaches, including migraine, tension-type, and cluster headaches. Although generally harmless, recurrent headaches that began at a young age in patients with a normal examination may return periodically. Episodic headaches are characterized by mild-to-moderate tightening on both temples (not aggravated by physical activity, nausea, or vomiting) and possible sensitivity to light or sound. People with chronic tension-type headaches have an average headache frequency of 15 days per month or 180 days per year for 6 months and must also meet the criteria for episodic tension-type headache.[36] In addition, people with chronic tension-type headaches must not have another disorder, as shown by physical and neurological examination.

Studies show that some people with primary headache disorders respond to medications that specifically target and influence serotonin, whereas others respond to electromyographic biofeedback training, cognitive behavioral training, and progressive muscle relaxation therapy for tension headaches.[37] As with all health conditions, healthy lifestyle habits and a supportive social environment may help prevent tension headaches and help the individual cope with the chronic pain and anxiety of recurrent headaches.[38]

Psychological Disorders

Common psychological disorders in adulthood include bipolar affective disorder, schizophrenia, and substance abuse. Substance abuse, specifically drug abuse, plagues all ethnic groups and

Table 15-8. Activities for Secondary Prevention of Neurological Disorders

	STROKE	TBI	SCI	PERIPHERAL NEUROPATHIES	PD	MS	ALZHEIMER'S DISEASE
Mental imagery	X	X	X	X	X	X	
Relaxation exercises	X	X	X	X	X	X	X
Walking programs	X	X	X	X	X	X	X
Aquatic programs	X	X	X	X	X	X	
Balance exercise	X	X	X	X	X	X	X
Resistance exercises	X	X	X	X	X	X	X
Tái chi	X	X	X	X	X	X	
Yoga	X	X	X	X	X	X	
Pilates	X	X	X	X	X	X	
Biofeedback	X	X	X	X	X	X	
Physical activity	X	X	X	X	X	X	X
Circuit training	X	X	X	X	X	X	
Sports activities	X	X	X	X	X	X	X

social classes worldwide and is a top priority of the US Surgeon General, as outlined in the Healthy People 2020 goals for the nation. *Drug or substance abuse* is defined as an intense desire to obtain increasing amounts of a particular substance or substances to the exclusion of all other activities.[39] *Drug dependence* is the body's physical need, or addiction, to a specific agent.[39] Over the long term, this dependence results in physical harm, behavior problems, and association with people who also abuse drugs. Stopping the use of the drug can result in a specific withdrawal syndrome.

> Common risk factors for drug abuse include: family history of substance abuse, a mental or behavioral health condition, such as depression, anxiety or attention-deficit/hyperactivity disorder (ADHD), aggressive or impulsive behavior, a history of traumatic events (such as experiencing a car accident or being a victim of abuse), low self-esteem or poor social coping skills, feelings of social rejection, anxiety, depression, peer pressure, lack of nurturing by parents or caregivers, academic failure, relationships with peers who abuse drugs, drug availability, belief that drug abuse is okay, or taking a highly addictive drug after it is needed for a medical condition.[39]

Vital sign readings can be increased, decreased, or absent completely. Sleepiness, confusion, and coma are common. Because of this decline in alertness, the drug abuser is at risk for assault or rape,

Table 15-9. Screening for Headaches
The following questions are suggestive of a migraine headache: • Are you disabled by your headaches? • Are you nauseated with your headaches? • Are you sensitive to light with your headaches? Diagnostic criteria for migraine include multiple headache attacks with the following features: • Headaches last from a few hours to a few days • Headaches have at least 2 of the following characteristics: ○ Moderate or severe intensity ○ Worsening with physical activity ○ Unilateral location ○ Pulsating pain Headaches are associated with at least one of the following characteristics: • Nausea or vomiting • Aversion to noise and light • No other cause for headache is evident on history taking or physical examination
Adapted from Headache diagnosis and testing. American Headache Society. http://www.americanheadache-society.org/assets/1/7/NAP_for_Web_-_Headache_Diagnosis___Testing.pdf. Accessed May 20, 2014.

robbery, and accidental death. Skin can be cool and sweaty or hot and dry. Chest pain is possible and can be caused by heart or lung damage from drug abuse.[40] Individuals who are alcoholics are sometimes difficult to identify because alcohol can influence people differently. Certain behaviors suggest that someone may have a problem with alcohol, including alcohol on the breath, insomnia, frequent falls, bruises of different ages, blackouts, chronic depression, anxiety, irritability, tardiness or absence at work or school, employment loss, divorce or separation, financial difficulties, frequent intoxicated appearance or behavior, weight loss, or frequent automobile collisions.[40] A health care professional should consult a physician or psychologist whenever any of these signs or symptoms are observed or reported during a client screening.

Vestibular Disorders

The vestibular system has sensors in the inner ear delivering information that is processed in the brain for balance and coordination needed to align the head, eyes, and body during movement. Serious pathologies of this system can render a person motionless. According to the Vestibular Disorders Association, as many as 35% of adults aged 40 years or older in the United States—approximately 69 million Americans—have experienced some form of vestibular dysfunction.[41] The system may be impaired by disease, aging, or injury, resulting in a range of clinical manifestations, including, but not limited to: *vertigo* (spinning or whirling sensation or an illusion of movement of self or the world), dizziness (lightheaded, floating, or rocking sensation), imbalance and spatial disorientation (sensation of being heavily weighted or pulled in one direction), imbalance, stumbling, difficulty walking straight or turning a corner, clumsiness or difficulty with coordination, difficulty maintaining straight posture, a tendency to look downward to confirm the location of the ground, holding the head in a tilted position, a tendency to touch or hold onto something when standing or to touch or hold the head while seated, a sensitivity to changes in walking surfaces or footwear, muscle and joint pain (due to struggling with balance), difficulty finding stability in crowds or in large open spaces, visual disturbances (trouble with visual tracking, light sensitivity, poor depth perception, and problems with focus), hearing changes (*tinnitus* [ringing in the ear], hearing loss, sensitivity to sounds), and cognitive and/or psychological changes (anxiety and loss of self-reliance and self-confidence). Symptoms of chronic dizziness or imbalance can have a significant effect on the ability of a disabled person to perform one or more activities of daily living, such as bathing, dressing, or simply getting around inside the home. These issues affect 11.5% of adults with chronic dizziness and 33.4% of adults with chronic imbalance.[42]

The Dizziness Handicap Inventory is a helpful questionnaire for screening for the effect of dizziness on the individual, including *functional* (eg, "Does your problem interfere with your household responsibilities?"), *physical* (eg, "Do quick movements of your head increase your problem?"), and *emotional* (eg, "Because of your problem, are you depressed?").[43]

A wide range of tests are used to detect vestibular dysfunction, including electronystagmography and videonystagmography (tests that measure eye movements), rotation tests (tests that evaluate how well the eyes and inner ear work together during head movement), vestibular-evoked myogenic potential (evaluates inner ear function), computerized dynamic posturography and posturography (tests postural stability), and hearing tests.[42]

Management of vestibular disorders relies on experts in the field of vestibular dysfunction. Referrals should be made to clinicians with training in vestibular rehabilitation therapy (eg, canalith repositioning maneuvers such as the Epley maneuver that includes specific head, body, and eye exercises to retrain the vestibular system), clinicians who may prescribe medications to address etiological factors, and surgeons, if repair of inner ear function is required. Psychological counseling is advised for vestibular disorders that result in anxiety, depression, or altered self-esteem.

Summary

Medical conditions affecting the nervous system may be transient or chronic depending on the etiology, the part of the nervous system affected, and the lifestyle habits of the individual at risk for further injury. Health care professionals play an essential role in identifying risk factors for neurological conditions that can irreversibly alter the lives of those with acute and chronic medical conditions affecting the brain, spinal cord, and peripheral nervous system. By promoting healthy lifestyle habits and identifying risk factors for neuropathology, health care professionals can substantially reduce the costly loss of neurological function for those at greatest risk and decrease the number of sequelae that often accompany both temporary and chronic neurological conditions.

References

1. Wilde O. *The Importance of Being Earnest.* New York, NY: Pearson Longman; 2006.
2. Memory problems. HealthCommunities.com. http://www.healthcommunities.com/memory-problems/overview-of-memory-loss.shtml. Accessed June 1, 2013.
3. Memory loss. Right Diagnosis. http://www.rightdiagnosis.com/sym/memory_loss.htm#intro. Accessed June 1, 2013.
4. Simple tests for dementia. John's Hopkins Medicine Health Alerts. http://www.johnshopkinshealthalerts.com/reports/memory/138-1.html. Accessed June 1, 2013.
5. Preventing memory loss. Harvard Medical School. http://www.health.harvard.edu/newsweek/Preventing_memory_loss.htm. Accessed June 1, 2013.
6. Know the 10 signs. Alzheimer's' Association. http://www.alz.org/alzheimers_disease_know_the_10_signs.asp. Accessed June 1, 2013.
7. Living with Alzheimer's. Bright Focus Foundation. http://www.brightfocus.org/. Accessed June 1, 2013.

8. Epilepsy: increasing awareness and improving care. Centers for Disease Control and Prevention. http://www.cdc.gov/Epilepsy/. Accessed June 1, 2013.
9. Forecasting the future of stroke in the United States: a policy statement from the American Heart Association and American Stroke Association. American Heart Association. http://stroke.ahajournals.org/content/early/2013/05/22/STR.0b013e31829734f2. Accessed June 1, 2013.
10. Stroke prevention. National Stroke Association. http://www.stroke.org/site/PageServer?pagename=prevent. Accessed June 1, 2013.
11. Stroke. Centers for Disease Control and Prevention. http://www.cdc.gov/stroke/. Accessed June 1, 2013.
12. Leary, MC, Saver JL. Annual incidence of first silent stroke in the United States: a preliminary estimate. *Cerebrovasc Dis.* 2003;16:280-285.
13. Successful business strategies to prevent heart disease and stroke. US Department of Health and Human Services. http://www.cdc.gov/dhdsp/pubs/docs/toolkit.pdf. Accessed June 1, 2013.
14. Gordon N, Cochair M, Gulanick M, et al. An American Heart Association Scientific Statement from the Council on Clinical Cardiology, Subcommittee on Exercise, Cardiac Rehabilitation, and Prevention; the Council on Cardiovascular Nursing; the Council on Nutrition, Physical Activity, and Metabolism; and the Stroke Council. *Circulation.* 2004;109:2031-2041.
15. Overview of spinal cord injuries. Merck Manual. http://www.merckmanuals.com/home/print/brain_spinal_cord_and_nerve_disorders/spinal_cord_disorders/overview_of_spinal_cord_disorders.html. Accessed June 1, 2013.
16. Young W. An update of the ASIA/ISCOS SCI classification system. Care Cure Community. http://sci.rutgers.edu/forum/showthread.php?t=175519. Accessed May 8, 2013.
17. Reeve C. *Still Me.* Toronto, Canada: Random House; 1999.
18. Putzke JD, Richards JS, Hicken BL, DeVivo MJ. Predictors of life satisfaction: a spinal cord injury cohort study. *Arch Phys Med Rehabil.* 2002;83(4):555-561.
19. Centers for Disease Control and Prevention (CDC). Traumatic brain injury—Colorado, Missouri, Oklahoma, and Utah, 1990-1993. *MMWR.* 1997b;46(01):8-11.
20. Thurman D, Alverson C, Dunn K, Guerrero J, Sniezek J. Traumatic brain injury in the United States: a public health perspective. *J Head Trauma Rehabil.* 1999;14(6):602-615.
21. The Rancho Levels of Cognitive Functioning. Ranchos Los Amigos National Rehabilitation Center. http://www.rancho.org/Research_RanchoLevels.aspx. Accessed May 8, 2013.
22. Classification and complications of traumatic brain injury. Medscape. http://emedicine.medscape.com/article/326643-overview#aw2aab6b5. Accessed May 8, 2013.
23. Mild traumatic brain injury pocket guide. Defense Center of Excellence for Psychological Health and Traumatic Brain Injury and Veterans Brain Injury Center. http://www.publichealth.va.gov/docs/exposures/TBI-pocketcard.pdf. Accessed May 8, 2013.
24. Facts about concussion and brain injury. Centers for Disease Control and Prevention. http://www.brainline.org/landing_pages/Basics.html. Accessed October 11, 2013.
25. Johns MW. A new method for measuring daytime sleepiness: the Epworth Sleepiness Scale. *Sleep.* 1991;14(6):540-545.
26. Parkinson's disease. WebMD. http://www.webmd.com/parkinsons-disease/default.htm. Accessed May 8, 2013.
27. Overview of spinal cord disorders. Merck Manual. http://www.merckmanuals.com/professional/neurologic_disorders/spinal_cord_disorders/overview_of_spinal_cord_disorders.html. Accessed May 20, 2014.
28. Tillerson JL, Caudle WM, Reveron ME, Miller GW. Exercise induces behavioral recovery and attenuates neurochemical deficits in rodent models of Parkinson's disease. *Neuroscience.* 2003;119(3):899-911.
29. Butler RN, Davis R, Lewis CB, Nelson ME, Strauss E. Physical fitness: benefits of exercise for the older patient. *Geriatrics.* 1998;53(10):46, 49-52, 61-62.
30. Canning CG, Alison JA, Allen NE, Groeller H. Parkinson's disease: an investigation of exercise capacity, respiratory function, and gait. *Arch Phys Med Rehabil.* 1997;78(2):199-207.
31. Klos KJ, Bower JH, Josephs KA, Matsumoto JY, Ahlskog JE. Pathological hypersexuality predominantly linked to adjuvant dopamine agonist therapy in Parkinson's disease and multiple system atrophy. *Parkinsonism Relat Disord.* 2005;11(6):381-386.
32. Multiple sclerosis. Merck Manual. http://www.merckmanuals.com/professional/neurologic_disorders/demyelinating_disorders/multiple_sclerosis_ms.html. Accessed May 20, 2013.
33. Schwid SR, Covington M, Segal BM, Goodman AD. Fatigue in multiple sclerosis: current understanding and future directions. *J Rehabil Res Dev.* 2002;39(2):211-224.
34. Rietberg MB, Brooks D, Uitdehaag BMJ, Kwakkel G. Exercise therapy for multiple sclerosis. *Cochrane Database Syst Rev.* 2005;(1):CD003980.
35. Gutierrez GM, Chow JW, Tillman MD, McCoy SC, Castellano V, White LJ. Resistance training improves gait kinematics in persons with multiple sclerosis. *Arch Phys Med Rehabil.* 2005;86(9):1824-1829.
36. Approach to the patient with headache. Merck Manual. http://www.merckmanuals.com/professional/neurologic_disorders/headache/approach_to_the_patient_with_headache.html?qt=headaches&alt=sh. Accessed May 30, 2013.

37. Arena JG, Bruno GM, Hannah SL. A comparison of frontal electromyographic biofeedback training, trapezius electromyographic biofeedback training, and progressive muscle relaxation therapy in the treatment of tension headache. *Headache*. 1995;35(7):411-419.
38. Headaches: prevention. Mayo Clinic. http://www.mayoclinic.com/health/tension-headache/DS00304/DSECTION=prevention. Accessed May 6, 2013.
39. Substance abuse. HealthyPeople.gov. http://www.healthypeople.gov/2020/topicsobjectives2020/overview.aspx?topicid=40. Accessed May 6, 2013.
40. Drug addiction. Mayo Clinic. http://www.mayoclinic.com/health/drug-addiction/DS00183/DSECTION=risk-factors. Accessed May 6, 2013.
41. Understanding vestibular disorders. Vestibular Disorders Association. http://vestibular.org/understanding-vestibular-disorder. Accessed May 6, 2013.
42. Ko C, Hoffman HJ, Sklare DA. Chronic imbalance or dizziness and falling: results from the 1994 Disability Supplement to the National Health Interview Survey and the Second Supplement on Aging Study. Vestibular Disorders Association. http://vestibular.org/understanding-vestibular-disorder#sthash.3jjENkfQ.dpuf. Accessed May 6, 2013.
43. Jacobson GP, Newman CW. The development of the Dizziness Handicap Inventory. *Arch Otolaryngol Head Neck Surg*. 1990;116: 424-427.

16

Preventive Care for Chronic Conditions

Amy Foley, DPT, PT and Catherine Rush Thompson, PT, PhD, MS

"Illness is the night side of life, a more onerous citizenship. Everyone who is born holds dual citizenship, in the kingdom of the well and in the kingdom of the sick. Although we all prefer to use the good passport, sooner or later each of us is obliged, at least for a spell, to identify ourselves as citizens of that other place."—Susan Sontag, *Illness as Metaphor*

Health is the restoration of wholeness, despite illness or injury. Those with chronic illness or injury causing permanent disability have had a part of their lives inextricably broken. Health care professionals must use their care and compassion to reconstruct a new wholeness, restoring quality of life for those with chronic pathology and those who become their caretakers.

Chronic conditions are health conditions or diseases that persist or result in long-lasting effects. The term *chronic* is typically applied when the course of the disease lasts for more than 3 months. Nearly 50% of Americans between the ages of 18 and 64 have at least one chronic medical condition, and that percentage increases to 90% for seniors.[1,2] For most people, chronic conditions unnecessarily limit participation in daily activities and social roles. Previous chapters discussed chronic conditions related to multiple body systems, including the musculoskeletal system (eg, osteoarthritis), the cardiopulmonary system (eg, congestive obstructive pulmonary disease), and neurological system (eg, Parkinson's disease). This chapter discusses common concerns shared by many with chronic conditions and how they can be averted by preventive care.

Chronic illness can be progressive but can often be stabilized if managed through healthy lifestyle habits and appropriate medical care. However, the knowledge that an illness is *chronic* vs *acute* elicits emotions that must be recognized by health care professionals. Chronic illness can affect every aspect of a person's life and the lives of those surrounding him or her. This chapter covers psychological and physical aspects of chronic illnesses.

Psychological Effect of Chronic Illness

Psychological stress occurs when a loss or change cannot be met by an individual's time, energy, money, or support system. Chronic illness results in ongoing psychological stress related to the

Thompson CR.
Prevention Practice and Health Promotion: A Health Care Professional's Guide to Health, Fitness, and Wellness, Second Edition (pp 267-280).

loss of health and the need for lifestyle adaptations. Typically, these adaptations require additional time, money, and assistance. The range of psychological stressors experienced by an individual with chronic illness can be alarming:

- Body structures may function less effectively, leading to debilitation.
- Activities may be more difficult to perform.
- Frustration may develop with failed attempts to do activities that were once perfunctory.
- Fatigue may become an additional barrier to accomplishing daily tasks.
- Embarrassment may result from loss of bowel and bladder control.
- Friends and family may pity, overprotect, control, or avoid the person.
- Strangers may express intolerance, impatience, or frustration or fearfully stare at a person with visible impairments.
- Coworkers may resent the additional workload caused by the person's inability to perform efficiently and/or effectively.
- Environmental barriers may limit access to participation in social events.
- Motivation to participate in the community may dwindle.
- Depression may settle into a person's daily existence and lead to social isolation.
- Finances related to medical bills and job loss may become a burden.
- Feelings of self-worth and self-esteem may plummet.
- Family members may feel despair with their inability to manage additional roles.

As with all aspects of life, change is inevitable and adaptation is necessary. Health care professionals can help usher those with chronic illness through the maze of life changes, including physical challenges that are often treatable and psychological stressors that require additional coping skills. Helping those with disabilities learn new skills can help alleviate the stress of lost function.

The following emotions are commonly experienced by patients with chronic illness[3]:

- *Helplessness* resulting from reliance on others due to functional limitations
- *Frustration* with reduced functional abilities and persistent symptoms
- *Hopelessness* based on uncertainty about their future
- *Sadness* for what was lost
- *Resentment* toward others who have no limitations
- *Anxiety* about the future
- *Irritability* related to the illness and its sequelae
- *Tension* due to the multiple ongoing challenges that aggravate the illness
- *Stress* related to external and internal stressors that accompany illness
- *Anger* at themselves for being ill, at others for not "fixing" things, or at a higher power for punishing them

Grieving the Loss of Health

The diagnosis of a chronic illness begins a grieving process commonly seen when experiencing the loss of one's health. This process of grieving typically follows stages outlined by Elizabeth Kubler-Ross; however, these stages are not linear and may not all be experienced by those dealing with chronic illness.[4]

- Stage 1 is *denial*. The mind and body are numb as the patient tries to make meaning of a medical diagnosis. This stage is thought to help an individual cope with the shock of lost health and to allow time to face the stress induced by uncertainty. Patients at this stage may not be able to appreciate educational information, use medication as prescribed, or seek support from others.
- Stage 2 is *anger*. Anger is matched by the feelings of pain from the injustice of being afflicted with the chronic illness. This anger may be felt by a patient's family and friends as well. Why did this happen to them? It is helpful to let those close to the patient, including family, friends, caregivers, and other health care professionals, know that they will likely be the ones who will have anger directed toward them.
- Stage 3 is *bargaining*. Those with chronic illness may believe that they can bargain their illness away: "[Higher power], if I promise to be good, will you heal me of this illness?" They may even bargain with their health care professionals in hopes of a magical cure.
- Stage 4 is *grieving*. At this point, the individual with chronic illness is beginning to feel regret, sadness, fear, and uncertainty, indicating a realization of the loss his or her chronic condition might impose. Individuals with chronic illness are at increased risk for suicide. This risk is increased for youth and young adults who feel profound loss of opportunities during the prime of their lives.
- Stage 5 is *acceptance*. In this final stage, the individual with chronic illness develops a more objective view of the condition, sometimes before family members and friends. The person begins to develop coping strategies and consider alternatives for managing the chronic illness. Health care professionals can be sensitive to the grieving process and offer support whenever those with chronic illness and their families are open to it.

Everyone working with an individual with chronic conditions should be aware of additional emotional reactions that a person might use to handle anxiety. These emotional reactions may include *projection* (taking own unacceptable qualities or feelings and ascribing them to other people), *displacement* (taking out frustrations, feelings, and impulses on people or objects that are less threatening), and *introjection* (picking up traits or behaviors from others), as well as depression, *overdependency* (overreliance on others), and nonadherence to a prescribed regimen.[5,6] A referral to a psychologist will help all through this natural process while members of the health care team offer resources, such as the following:

- Age-appropriate education to provide knowledge about the condition and resources for its management
- Meaningful activities that help the individual build self-efficacy
- Support groups where individuals can share their experience and build a sense of community
- Individual counseling and family counseling for personal needs
- Physical therapy to help manage mobility needs (transfers, equipment, walking, gross motor skills) and adaptive physical activity and exercise
- Occupational therapy to help adapt daily living activities
- An environment with positive inspirational sayings, family pictures, etc.
- A registered dietician for guidance in healthy nutrition and cooking ideas for restricted diets
- Nursing care to help manage medications and hygiene issues
- Information about community resources, such as health promotion programs serving those with chronic conditions

Health care professionals must interact effectively with individuals experiencing these emotions to avoid aggravating the individual's dependency needs (a secondary gain) and preoccupation with the illness.[5,6]

Depression in Chronic Illness

Although depression is commonly experienced by those with chronic illness within the first 2 years of diagnosis, it is not necessarily caused by the pathology and should always be addressed. "Depression can aggravate many chronic conditions, intensifying pain, causing fatigue, and triggering or worsening a sense of isolation. In worst-case scenarios, depression associated with chronic illness can even result in suicide."[3]

As discussed in Chapter 10, prolonged stress from chronic illness is a significant health risk. Interventions that address depression in patients with chronic illness have been shown to improve both psychological and physical conditions, enhancing their quality of life. Suggestions that can help individuals cope with chronic illness and hopefully reduce the risk of depression include the following[7]:

- Teaching them to *live effectively with their physical symptoms* and associated treatments by giving them an understanding of the pathology and its long-term management
- Reminding them to *communicate clearly and honestly* with health care professionals
- Teaching them to *maintain emotional balance*
- Encouraging them and help them *maintain a positive attitude*
- Doing meaningful activities to help them *feel good about themselves* and improve their self-image and self-esteem
- Giving them information and *expose them to ideas, people, and places that will help build hope*
- Encouraging them to *get help* when it is medically or psychologically indicated

Helping those with chronic illness cope enables them to remain engaged in the activities that make their lives purposeful. While addressing psychological concerns, health care professionals also need to monitor the development of secondary complications commonly encountered with each disease.

Physical Complications of Chronic Illness

Health care professionals can help their clients cope with chronic illness by offering specific and accurate information about the anticipated physical complications of their conditions. Secondary and tertiary prevention involves a concerted effort by the health care team to offer consistent, accurate, and evidence-based information to families, deferring to the expertise of those best qualified to discuss specific issues. For example, the patient's doctor is the one person who delivers a medical diagnosis. Educating clients with chronic conditions and their families about common preventable physical complications reduces stress by shifting responsibility for decision making to those most affected by the chronic condition. Common secondary complications arise from the malaise, fatigue, irritability, and anxiety that many feel with chronic illness or complications arising from its management. The following section discusses preventable problems arising from limited physical activity and options for dealing with the side effects of medications.

General Deconditioning

Bedrest and immobility are restricted levels of activity often necessitated by chronic or acute illness, resulting in potentially adverse effects on body systems and on psychological equilibrium.

Considerable knowledge has accumulated in recent decades concerning the significance of physical activity to retard the deleterious effects of bedrest and chronic illness.[8] Health care professionals need to recognize the multiple body systems affected by immobility and be prepared to educate on and select the most efficacious interventions. General effects of immobility and their contribution to deconditioning[9] affect all body systems.

Cardiopulmonary Issues From Inactivity

Bedrest, or physical inactivity, leads to hypotension due to decreased neurovascular vessel control, increased workload on the heart for all activity, abnormal thrombus formation, decreased basal metabolism, and poor chest expansion from limited muscle power. Increased secretions with ineffective airway clearance leading to pneumonia and poor ventilation and gas exchange are all effects on the cardiopulmonary system.[8,9] Even positioning the client upright periodically can help the body adapt to hypotensive tendencies and elicit metabolism.

Musculoskeletal Issues From Inactivity

The muscles, joints, bones, and posture are all affected by disuse atrophy, loss of muscle power and length, reduction in weight bearing leading to bone demineralization, and decreased joint and capsule nutrition. Chronic bed positioning can lead to kyphosis if multiple pillows are used. Encouraging physical activity and good posture (eliminating pillows that increase neck flexion) can help reduce postural deformity and prevent the effects of deconditioning.

Genitourinary and Gastrointestinal Issues With Immobility

The general effects from immobility and deconditioning are difficulty with *micturition* (urination) related to an inability to relax pelvic floor muscles; *calculi formation* (stone formation in the kidney) from *urinary stasis* (reduced or halted flow of urine), increased minerals and salts excreted from protein breakdown and bone demineralization; and continual protein breakdown leading to a *catabolic state* (metabolic breakdown) and *negative nitrogen balance* (a marker in urine analysis indicating wasting).[10-15]

Hydration with physical activity promotes healthy urination. Many chronic diseases have multiple system involvement and origins. In the genitourinary system, water metabolism or hydration is quantitatively the more important nutrient.[10] A sufficient intake of fluids is one of the most important preventive measures for urinary stone recurrence or *urolithiasis* (calcifications or stones in the urinary system). In a prospective, randomized study of 199 patients with a first episode of idiopathic urolithiasis, the intervention group was instructed to increase fluid intake, whereas the remaining patients received no therapy. During the 5-year follow-up period, patients in the intervention group displayed a significantly higher urine volume, a 50% lower recurrence rate of urolithiasis, and a longer period before the first recurrence.[11] Similarly, a prospective study of 25 patients with urolithiasis showed that an increased fluid intake and limited intake of salt and protein resulted in an increased urine volume and a decreased number of stones. From 2001 to 2004, there were 13 epidemiological reports, 11 of which showed a significant association between a favorable hydration status and a lower stone recurrence rate.[12]

No definitive evidence has been found to show that a susceptibility to urinary tract infection (UTI) is influenced by fluid intake.[13] Prospective studies in girls from 2001 to 2004 showed recurrent UTI was associated with infrequent urine voiding and poor fluid intake.[13] A study in adults with urinary catheters showed that low urine output was significantly related to UTI. Health care professionals should recommend a high fluid intake in patients with UTI and in particular those with an indwelling urinary catheter.

The findings of epidemiological studies investigating the relationship between fluid intake and bladder or colon cancer are inconsistent.[14] A prospective study of fluid intake in 267 patients with superficial bladder cancer at risk for recurrence found no association between fluid intake and tumor recurrence. There is some evidence to suggest mineral water consumption and frequency of urination were identified as protective factors against bladder cancer.[14]

Additionally, the lack of movement leads to problems with bowel movement, resulting in chronic constipation. Constipation is a secondary and common sequelae to chronic disease. Health care professionals should educate the client on prevention by discussing causes and interventions. Poor nutrition and lack of physical exercise (causing muscle atrophy and loss of tone to the gastrointestinal smooth muscle and sphincter muscles) are the 2 most frequent causes.[9] Fluid restriction is another common cause of constipation. The beneficial effect of increased fluid intake may perhaps be limited to patients with dehydration because fluid overload in *euhydrated* patients (those with a normal state of body water content) may not improve stool consistency.[16] In a prospective, randomized study of 21 patients with *functional dyspepsia* (indigestion) and secondary constipation, the constipation score was decreased after drinking carbonated water but not after drinking tap water.

Fiber, as well as hydration with water, benefits those experiencing constipation. Fiber exerts its effects by accelerating gut transit time, leading to increased stool frequency. Because fiber has few side effects, its use should be considered first-line in constipation prevention.[16] Upright posture and regular movement can also aid the digestive process.[16]

General Metabolic Issues With Immobility

Metabolic effects associated with bedrest and inactivity include decreased metabolic rate, pronounced tissue *atrophy* (wasting), *protein catabolism* (breakdown of protein), and bone demineralization. Homeostasis of body temperature is difficult to regulate, leading to fluid and electrolyte loss. Physical activity increases the metabolic rate.

Integumentary Issues With Immobility

The integumentary system contains the largest organ of the body: the skin. This system also includes *subcutaneous* tissues (responsible for storing energy and absorbing trauma), the nails, the hair, and the structures immediately under the superficial skin layer. The most important function of the integumentary system is protection. In addition to serving as a barrier against infection and injury, the skin helps to regulate body temperature, removes waste products from the body, protects internal structures (to some extent) from ultraviolet radiation, and produces vitamin D, an essential nutrient for maintaining normal blood levels of calcium and phosphorus needed to form and maintain strong bones. When the skin is compromised from overexposure to radiation, infectious agents, toxins, allergens, insect bites, and other types of injurious agents, the entire body becomes vulnerable. Maintaining skin integrity is essential for health and wellness. Simply observing someone's skin provides some clues about the overall health of that person.

With aging and exposure to UV radiation, toxins, and other damaging agents, the skin tends to lose its elasticity, vascularity, thickness, strength, and thermoregulation properties. In older adults, the overall function of the skin is compromised with the graying of hair and the physiological changes underlying changes in physical appearance, including tissue dehydration and impaired wound healing. Primary practice includes health education about maintaining skin hydration and avoiding the various risk factors leading to premature aging and pathology.

Bedrest, immobility, or confinement to a wheelchair for extended periods of time without weight shifting leads to extended pressure on the skin at bony prominences (eg, ischial bones in the buttocks when seated). This can lead to skin breakdown, commonly known as a *pressure sores* or *decubitus ulcers*. The health care team should be alerted when treating clients at risk for skin breakdown, including clients with periods of immobility, prolonged pressure on bony prominences, poor nutrition, incontinence of bowel or bladder, lowered mental alertness, history of pressure sores or open wounds, or lack of sensation.

The National Pressure Ulcer Advisory Panel (NPUAP) recommends that a pressure ulcer risk assessment be performed on a patient's admission to a health care facility and on an ongoing basis as the patient's condition changes.[17] This assessment should include follow-up by a health care professional with expertise in managing pressure ulcers, as well as a review of environmental (eg, at home) and personal factors contributing to the pressure sore, especially if the patient has any disability.

In 1996, the American Medical Directors Association (AMDA), a professional association of medical directors and physicians practicing in the long-term care continuum, developed clinical practice guidelines on pressure ulcers, highlighting the following additional responsibilities of the health care team in the prevention of pressure sores[18]:

- Identify and manage underlying medical risk factors, including disease states, nutritional compromise, skin disorders, and drugs that affect skin, such as corticosteroids
- Identify and treat modifiable causes of decreased alertness, incontinence, and immobility
- Identify and manage acute changes in condition that may increase the risk of skin breakdown, such as delirium
- Identify subacute changes that increase risk, such as weight loss or progression of dementia
- Clarify overall condition, prognosis, and realistic goals, if appropriate to the patient's situation

The Agency for Health care Policy and Research (AHCPR; now the Agency for Health care Research and Quality) recommended the Braden Scale and the Norton Scale as appropriate tools for assessing a patient's risk for pressure ulcers.[19] The primary objective of these scales is to predict pressure sore occurrence of clients in inpatient and outpatient settings. Because the scores are determined by direct observation, health care providers can individualize interventions needed for clients with pressure ulcers and those who are at risk.

The Braden Scale (Table 16-1) is a risk assessment that incorporates 6 subscales: (1) sensory perception, (2) skin moisture, (3) activity, (4) mobility, (5) nutritional status, and (6) friction and shear factors. Each subscale is delineated by a status level with a weighted value, ranging from 1 to 4. For example, in the category of activity, a score of 1 is assigned to a patient who is bedfast, and a score of 4 indicates an individual who walks frequently. Total scores, ranging from 6 to 23, are based on subscale scores and determine an individual's level of risk for developing pressure ulcers. Predictive validity has been established for scores of 16 or less. Reported sensitivity for the tool ranges from 83% to 100%, and specificity ranges from 64% to 90%.[19]

Often, the older adult patient is seen by the health care professional for an unrelated condition, and will present with a unique risk for skin breakdown. These clients are commonly seen in long-term care facilities but can just as easily be seen in acute care environments. Berlowitz et al[19] collected clinical information on large numbers of nursing home residents while researching the development and assessment of pressure sores. Using the Minimum Data Set from 1997, they developed a risk-adjustment model for pressure ulcer development, a tool that could be used to assess the quality of nursing home care. The study involved 14,607 nursing home residents without blistered skin and tissue damage or larger pressure ulcer on initial assessment (stage 2). Pressure ulcer status was determined 90 days later, and the researchers identified potential predictors of pressure ulcer development. A total of 17 resident characteristics were associated with pressure ulcer development, including dependence in mobility and transferring (eg, from bed to wheelchair), diabetes mellitus, peripheral vascular disease, urinary incontinence, lower body mass index, and end-stage disease. The researchers developed the risk-adjustment model based on these characteristics and validated it in 13,457 nursing home residents. They used patients' risk of developing pressure ulcers to calculate expected rates of pressure ulcer development for 108 nursing

Table 16-1. Braden Scale for Predicting Pressure Sore Risk

PATIENT'S NAME:		EVALUATOR'S NAME:		DATE:	SCORE
Sensory perception (Ability to respond meaningfully to pressure-related discomfort)	1. Completely limited: Unresponsive (does not moan, flinch, or grasp) to painful stimuli, due to diminished level of consciousness or sedation. OR Limited ability to feel pain over most of body surface.	2. Very limited: Responds only to painful stimuli. Cannot communicate discomfort except by moaning or restlessness. OR Has a sensory impairment that limits the ability to feel pain or discomfort over half of body.	3. Slightly limited: Responds to verbal commands but cannot always communicate discomfort or need to be turned. OR Has some sensory impairment that limits ability to feel pain or discomfort in 1 or 2 extremities.	4. No impairment: Responds to verbal commands. Has no sensory deficit that would limit ability to feel or voice pain or discomfort.	
Moisture (Degree to which skin is exposed to moisture)	1. Constantly moist: Skin is kept moist almost constantly by perspiration, urine, etc. Dampness is detected every time patient is moved or turned.	2. Moist: Skin is often but not always moist. Linen must be changed at least once a shift.	3. Occasionally moist: Skin is occasionally moist, requiring an extra linen change approximately once a day.	4. Rarely moist: Skin is usually dry; linen requires changing only at routine intervals.	
Activity (Degree of physical activity)	1. Bedfast: Confined to bed.	2. Chairfast: Ability to walk severely limited or nonexistent. Cannot bear own weight and/or must be assisted into chair or wheelchair.	3. Walks occasionally: Walks occasionally during day but for very short distances, with or without assistance. Spends majority of each shift in bed or chair.	4. Walks frequently: Walks outside the room at least twice a day and inside room at least once every 2 hours during waking hours.	
Mobility (Ability to change and control body position)	1. Completely immobile: Does not make even slight changes in body or extremity position without assistance.	2. Very limited: Makes occasional slight changes in body or extremity position but unable to make frequent or significant changes independently.	3. Slightly limited: Makes frequent though slight changes in body extremity position independently.	4. No limitations: Makes major and frequent changes in position without assistance.	

(continued)

Table 16-1 (continued). Braden Scale for Predicting Pressure Sore Risk

PATIENT'S NAME:		EVALUATOR'S NAME:		DATE:	SCORE
Nutrition (Usual food intake pattern)	1. Very poor: Never eats a complete meal. Rarely eats more than one-third of any food offered. Eats 2 servings or less of protein (meat or dairy products) per day. Takes fluids poorly. Does not take a liquid dietary supplement. OR Is NPO and/or maintained on clear liquids or IV for more than 5 days.	2. Probably Inadequate: Rarely eats a complete meal and generally eats only about half of any food offered. Protein intake includes only 3 servings of meat or dairy products per day. Occasionally will take a dietary supplement. OR Receives less than optimum amount of liquid diet or tube feeding.	3. Adequate: Eats over half of most meals. Eats a total of 4 servings of protein (meat, dairy products) each day. Occasionally will refuse a meal but will usually take a supplement if offered. OR Is on a tube feeding or TPN regimen, which probably meets most of nutritional needs.	4. Excellent: Eats most of every meal. Never refuses a meal. Usually eats a total of 4 or more servings of meat and dairy products. Occasionally eats between meals. Does not require supplementation.	
Friction and shear	1. Problem: Requires moderate to maximum assistance in moving. Complete lifting without sliding against sheets is impossible. Frequent slides down in bed or chair, requiring frequent repositioning with maximum assistance. Spasticity, contractures, or agitation leads to almost constant friction.	2. Potential problem: Moves feebly or requires minimum assistance. During a move, skin probably slides to some extent against sheets, chair, restraints, or other devices. Maintains relatively good position in chair or bed most of the time but occasionally slides down.	3. No apparent problem: Moves in bed and in chair independently and has sufficient muscle strength to lift up completely during move. Maintains good position in bed or chair at all times.		
ADOPTED 1997				TOTAL SCORE:	

Abbreviations: IV, intravenous; NPO, nothing by mouth; TPN, total parenteral nutrition.
Reprinted with permission from Prevention Plus, LLC.

homes; expected rates ranged from 1.1% to 3.2% and observed rates ranged from 0% to 12.1%, demonstrating the model's effectiveness.[19]

Attention should also be given to the potential complications associated with pressure ulcers once they have occurred. Complications such as *endocarditis* (heart infection), *heterotopic bone formation* (bone formation in soft tissue), maggot infestation, *osteomyelitis* (bone infection), *bacteremia* (blood infection), *fistulas* (abnormal openings between organs), *septic arthritis* (infection of inflamed joints), sinus tract or abscess, and systemic complications of topical treatment (such as iodine toxicity and hearing loss after topical neomycin and systemic gentamicin), are not uncommon and can result from poor hygiene and exposure to infectious agents.[20] Health care professionals need to be cognizant of the potential secondary complication of pressure sores in their patients, measures to prevent these from occurring, and appropriate care of pressure sores once integumentary integrity is compromised. Simply relieving pressure at these sites periodically (every 15 minutes) can reduce the incidence of pressure sores.

Following are suggestions for appropriate exercises and physical activities for various chronic conditions to reduce the risks of deconditioning.[20] In all cases, physical activity should be integrated into a regular routine that enables each individual to enjoy movement and participate as much as possible in daily activities. The severity of any chronic condition necessitates an expert, such as a physical therapist, to safely prescribe the needed dosage for exercise (FITTE; see Chapter 4). Also, the use of medications and supplements, as well as the environment (physical and psychosocial), need to be taken into account when prescribing activities designed to become part of an individual's healthy lifestyle behaviors.

- Asthma: Aerobic exercise in a nonpolluted environment
- Chronic obstructive lung disease: Endurance activities to tolerance in nonpolluted environments, monitor dyspnea
- Coronary heart disease: Frequent endurance activities (eg, walking, swimming, cycling) at lower intensity and shorter duration
- Depression: Low- to moderate-intensity activity that is enjoyable
- Heart failure: Frequent endurance activities (eg, walking, swimming, cycling) at lower intensity and shorter duration
- Hypertension: Endurance activities at low intensity
- Low back pain: Endurance activities with no physical contact (eg, avoid recreational sports as well as sitting or overhead reaching)
- Osteoarthritis: Strength and endurance training with attention to pain
- Rheumatoid arthritis: Strengthening and endurance (eg, aquatic therapy)
- Type 2 diabetes: Endurance and strength training (eg, resistance muscle training)

Helping individuals with chronic conditions practice safe physical activity can prevent secondary impairments and improve the quality of life for the patient and family.

Sensory Loss Leading to Injury

The skin is protected by sensory receptors that contribute to the perception of touch and pressure. The skin is commonly affected by other pathologies, such as amputation, congestive heart failure, diabetes, malnutrition, neuromuscular dysfunction, obesity, peripheral nerve involvement, spinal cord dysfunction, and vascular disease. Any clients with impairments limiting levels of activity, reducing sensation, or causing edema, inflammation, pain, or ischemia are at increased risk for integumentary problems and need to be monitored carefully by health care professionals.

Individuals, particularly those with frail skin or those with type 1 or type 2 diabetes causing sensory loss, should be educated about skin protection, including the following: (1) keeping nails trimmed, (2) avoiding scratching the skin, (3) bathing in nonfragranced warm water rather than hot water, and (4) avoiding rubbing or touching rough or hot surfaces.

The Lower Extremity Amputation Prevention (LEAP) organization advocates routine and frequent screening of skin for risk factors associated with diabetes. These risk factors include prominence of metatarsal heads, dry skin, callus formation, and inability to perceive 10-g force (5.07 Simmes-Weinstein filament). Decreased thermal and vibration sensation tends to dry the skin.[21]

Other risk factors for integumentary problems include allergens and skin irritants (eg, fabric softeners, perfumed soaps, and household cleansers). For those engaged in aquatic activities, bathing is essential following swimming to remove pool chemicals. Protection from the sun can be achieved by avoiding peak sunshine (10 AM to 4 PM) and limiting unnecessary sun exposure through protective clothing and sunscreen. Over-the-counter topical ointments (such as topical steroids) can be used to manage minor skin irritations and to reduce skin infections when there is skin injury. However, any patient presenting with chronic skin inflammation, pruritis, or suspicious skin lesions should be more thoroughly examined by a dermatologist.

Side Effects of Medications

The majority of clients receive some form of adjunctive or primary pharmacological care to assist in the management of their chronic medical conditions. The most common medications encountered in the management of acute conditions include analgesics, anti-inflammatory agents, and muscle relaxants. Health care professionals need to be aware of adverse drug reactions associated with these medications. Adverse drug events are the leading cause of medical injury in hospitalized clients in the United States.[22] The number of persons affected is roughly *4 times* the total number killed in automobile accidents every year. Adverse drug events account for an estimated one-fifth of the total 1 million hospitalized clients who are injured each year. Analgesics and antibiotics cause the majority of allergic reactions.[23] Health care professionals should regularly monitor vital signs and current medical records to ensure their clients keep updated lists of their medications, are aware of known side effects, and take their medications as prescribed. In addition, all clients should include any supplements and agents they use on this list as an extra precaution. The use of alcohol can seriously affect the use of medications and should be avoided unless allowed by the client's physician.

Integumentary Side Effects of Medications

In general, cutaneous drug reactions are the most common adverse responses to drugs, although not the only adverse reaction. *Urticaria* (itchy, swollen red bumps or patches on the skin) is the most common drug reaction; however, there are many different types of reactions, and some are life-threatening.

Aspirin and *nonsteroidal anti-inflammatory drugs* (NSAIDs) can cause *angioedema* (swelling beneath the skin) and urticaria. The prevalence of aspirin-induced angioedema and urticaria is approximately 5% in the general population but only approximately 1.5% in patients with aspirin-induced asthma.[24] Use of aspirin over time will effectively prevent aspirin-induced bronchospasm but few data support its effectiveness for reducing urticaria or angioedema. Instead, affected clients should be given analgesics with minimal cyclooxygenase inhibition. NSAIDs can cause common cutaneous reactions, such as *pruritus* (itching), *morbilliform rash* (measles-like rash), urticaria, and photosensitivity. Urticaria is most frequent in salicylate-sensitive patients. Other skin reactions are unusual, although *purpura* (bruise-like coloration) and *cutaneous vasculitis* (an allergic-inflammatory reaction of vessels) have been attributed to NSAIDs.[24]

Acetaminophen was once thought to be a safe alternative to aspirin, and NSAIDs were thought to be safe for clients with aspirin sensitivity. However, more recent data suggest that high doses of acetaminophen inhibit cyclooxygenase and can exacerbate asthma in aspirin-sensitive patients. Settipane et al[24] studied cross-sensitivity to acetaminophen doses up to 1500 mg in asthmatic clients with aspirin sensitivity. The probability of acetaminophen tolerance could be predicted by the degree of aspirin sensitivity. Aspirin-desensitized clients were able to tolerate acetaminophen at higher doses. The study also suggested that high doses of acetaminophen (more than 1000 mg) may cause sufficient cyclooxygenase inhibition to induce bronchospasm.

Skeletal muscle relaxants are commonly prescribed to relieve the stiffness, pain, and discomfort caused by strains, sprains, or other injury to muscles treated in physical therapy. The common cutaneous reactions to this drug classification are large, hive-like swellings on the face (eyelids, mouth, lips, and/or tongue), itching, and redness. Additional cutaneous reactions include tenderness, swelling over a blood vessel, pinpoint red spots on the skin, sores/ulcers/white spots on the lips or in the mouth, and unusual bruising or bleeding.[25] All of these reactions should be reported to the patient's physician.

Neurological Side Effects of Medications

The neurological side effects of drugs range from confusion, headaches, sensory disturbances, and dizziness to seizures, hallucinations, and visible *dyskinesias* (movement disorders). Health care professionals should be alert to changes in behavior, problems sleeping, movement disorders (tremors, erratic movements, or decreased movement), or sensory disturbances that might arise from a client's medication. These signs and symptoms suggest *neurotoxicity* (toxicity to the nervous system). The physician should be contacted if these clinical manifestations are evident.

Immunological Side Effects of Medications

Many drugs are designed to reduce the body's response to outside agents by the immunological system. These drugs are typically for chronic conditions suspected to be autoimmune disorders that require immunosuppression. Although these medications may reduce the body's reaction to the pathological antigen, they are not selective and may suppress the body's natural defense mechanisms against minor bacterial or viral infections. Health care professionals need to remind others of protecting individuals on immunosuppressant medications from infection and ensure medical attention if risk of infection is suspected.

Hepatic Side Effects of Medications

The liver, the vital organ in the hepatic system, serves multiple bodily functions, including bile production, glycogen storage, decomposition of red blood cells, plasma protein synthesis, hormone production, and blood detoxification, clearing medications and toxins from the body. In the case of an overdose or poisoning, the liver can be injured, leading to *hepatotoxicity* (chemical-driven liver damage). Factors influencing the development of hepatotoxicity include age, ethnicity and race, sex, nutritional status, underlying liver disease, renal function, pregnancy duration and dosage of drug, enzyme induction, alcohol ingestion, and drug-to-drug interaction.

More than 900 drugs have been implicated in causing liver injury, and health care professionals need to be alert to the signs and symptoms of hematoxicity. A person complaining of fatigue, weakness, weight loss, poor appetite, nausea, fever, and abdominal pain may be suspected of liver problems and should see a doctor as soon as possible. Additional clinical manifestations suggesting hepatotoxicity include, but are not limited to *jaundice* (yellowing of the skin and whites of the eyes), *hepatomegaly* (liver enlargement), *ascites* (accumulation of fluid within the abdomen, sometimes causing the abdomen to swell), *hepatic encephalopathy* (confusion caused by deterioration of brain function due to buildup of toxic substances in the blood, which are normally removed by the liver), gastrointestinal bleeding (bleeding in the esophagus and/or stomach), varicose veins, *portal hypertension* (abnormally high blood pressure in the veins that bring blood from the intestine to the liver), red palms, bright red complexion, itching, a tendency to bleed, lightheadedness, missing menstrual periods (women), erectile dysfunction (men), and hypotension.

Summary

The advent of direct access has increased the responsibility of all health care professionals to closely screen clients for a variety of medical conditions, differentially diagnose those needing specialized care, appropriately refer clients to other health care professionals, and recognize secondary complications of chronic conditions needing medical management. Psychological and physical issues are common, so health care providers, individuals with chronic conditions, their caretakers, and their family members need to be alert to these preventable secondary complications.

Health education about the condition, helping the client gain control of its management, and monitoring the body systems for possible side effects of medications, along with encouraging appropriate physical activity and adherence to prescribed interventions and promoting healthy lifestyle habits, optimize health and wellness. Health care providers can work as a team along with clients and their families to face the challenges of chronic illness and to pursue resources that enable a desirable quality of life unfettered by preventable problems.

References

1. Chronic conditions: making the case for ongoing care. Robert Wood Johnson Foundation and the Partnership for Solutions. Johns Hopkins University. http://www.improvingchroniccare.org/. Accessed May 5, 2013.
2. Anderson G, Horvath J. The growing burden of chronic disease in America. *Public Health Rep.* 2004;119(3):263-270.
3. Chronic illness. American Psychological Association. http://www.apa.org/helpcenter/chronic.aspx. Accessed June 1, 2013.
4. Elizabeth Kubler-Ross Foundation. Based on the Grief Cycle model first published in *On Death & Dying.* Interpretation by Alan Chapman 2006-2009. http://www.ekrfoundation.org/five-stages-of-grief/. Accessed June 1, 2013.
5. Abram H. The psychology of chronic illness. *J Chronic Dis.* 1972;25(12):659-664.
6. Simon GE. Treating depression in patients with chronic disease: recognition and treatment are crucial; depression worsens the course of a chronic illness. *West J Med.* 2001;175(5):292-293.
7. Drummond N. The psychology of chronic illness. American Psychological Association. http://www.apa.org/helpcenter. Accessed June 1, 2013.
8. Pedersen B, Saltin B. Evidence for prescribing exercise as therapy in chronic disease. *Scand J Med Sci Sports.* 2006;16(Suppl 1):3-63.
9. Morof Lubkin I, Larsen PD. *Chronic Illness: Impact and Interventions.* 6th ed. Burlington, MA: Jones & Bartlett Publishers; 2005.
10. Siener R, Hesse A. Fluid intake and epidemiology of urolithiasis. *Eur J Clin Nutr.* 2003;57(Suppl 2):S47-S51.
11. Borghi L, Meschi T, Amato F, Briganti A, Novarini A, Giannini A. Urinary volume, water and recurrence in idiopathic calcium nephrolithiasis: a 5-year randomized prospective study. *J Urology.* 1996;155:839-843.
12. Carvalho M, Ferrari AC, Renner LO, Vieira MA, Riella MC. Quantification of the stone clinic effect in patients with nephrolithiasis. *Rev Assoc Méd Bras.* 2004;50:79-82.
13. Beetz R. Mild dehydration: a risk factor of urinary tract infection? *Eur J Clin Nutr.* 2003;57(Suppl 2):S52-S58.
14. Wilde MH, Carrigan MJ. A chart audit of factors related to urine flow and urine tract infection. *J Adv Nurs.* 2003;43:254-262.
15. Altieri A, La Vecchia C, Negri E. Fluid intake and risk of bladder and other cancers. *Eur J Clin Nutr.* 2003;57(Suppl 2):S59-S68.
16. Suares NC, Ford AC. Prevalence of, and risk factors for, chronic idiopathic constipation in the community: systematic review and meta-analysis. *Am J Gastroenterol.* 2011;106:1582-1591.

17. National Pressure Ulcer Advisory Panel, European Pressure Ulcer Advisory Panel. Pressure ulcer prevention recommendations. In: *Prevention and Treatment of Pressure Ulcers: Clinical Practice Guideline.* Washington, DC: National Pressure Ulcer Advisory Panel; 2009:21-50.
18. Clinical practice guidelines on pressure ulcers. American Medical Directors Association. https://www.amda.com/tools/guidelines.cfm#pressureulcer. Accessed March 14, 2014.
19. Berlowitz DR, Brandeis GH, Anderson JJ, et al. Evaluation of a risk-adjustment model for pressure ulcer development using the minimum data set. *J Am Geriatr Soc.* 2001;49(7):872-876.
20. Kujala UM. Evidence for exercise therapy in the treatment of chronic disease based on at least three randomized controlled trials—summary of published systematic reviews. *Scand J Med Sci Sports.* 2004;14(6):339-345.
21. Bates DW, Cullen DJ, Laird N, et al. Incidence of adverse drug events and potential adverse drug events: implications for prevention. ADE Prevention Study Group. *JAMA.* 1995;274(1):29-34.
22. Stevenson DD. Diagnosis, prevention, and treatment of adverse reactions to aspirin and nonsteroidal anti-inflammatory drugs. *J Allergy Clin Immunol.* 1984;74(4 Pt 2):617-622.
23. Roujeau JC. Clinical aspects of skin reactions to NSAIDs. *Scand J Rheumatol.* 1987;65:131-134.
24. Settipane RA, Schrank PJ, Simon RA, et al. Prevalence of cross-sensitivity with acetaminophen in aspirin-sensitive asthmatic subjects. *J Allergy Clin Immunol.* 1995;96(4):480-485.
25. Friedman SE, Grendell JH, McQuaid KR. *Current Diagnosis & Treatment in Gastroenterology.* New York, NY: Lang Medical Books/McGraw-Hill; 2003.

17

Prevention Practice for Individuals With Developmental Disabilities

Catherine Rush Thompson, PT, PhD, MS

"A person's health has a dramatic effect on their quality of life and ability to reach their full potential of independence, participation in family and social activities, educational achievements and vocational contributions.... Ensuring people with developmental disabilities have access to timely assessment and treatment by qualified health care providers ultimately leads to better health outcomes, greater quality of life, fuller participation in society and reduced costs."—Louisiana Developmental Disabilities Council Position on Health Care for People with Developmental Disabilities

Definitions of Developmental Disability

Developmental disability is defined as "a cognitive, emotional, or physical impairment, especially one related to abnormal sensory or motor development, appearing in infancy or childhood and involving a failure or delay in progressing through the normal developmental stages of childhood."[1] This definition focuses on the onset of impairments during childhood that alter normal child development. The Department of Health and Human Services gives the following criteria for developmental disability[2]:

- Is attributable to a mental or physical impairment or combination of mental and physical impairments
- Is manifested before the person attains age 22, unless the disability is caused by a traumatic head injury and is manifested after age 22
- Is likely to continue indefinitely
- Results in substantial functional limitations in 3 or more of the following areas of major life activity: self-care, receptive and expressive language, capacity for independent living, learning, mobility, self-direction, and economic self-sufficiency

Thompson CR.
Prevention Practice and Health Promotion: A Health Care Professional's Guide to Health, Fitness, and Wellness, Second Edition (pp 281-295).

- Reflects the person's need for a combination and sequence of special interdisciplinary or generic care, treatment, or other services that are of a lifelong or extended duration and are individually planned and coordinated

Examples of diagnoses include congenital conditions affecting physical or mental abilities, arising before adulthood, and usually lasting throughout life, such as cerebral palsy and Down syndrome. Although developmental disabilities are considered one category of individuals with disabilities, the range of physical impairments, functional limitations, and disabilities is too great to discuss as one population. Medical diagnoses often included in the category of developmental disabilities include, but are not limited to, those listed in Table 17-1.

From the viewpoint of health promotion, the majority of individuals with developmental disabilities have impaired neuromotor development and impaired sensory and motor function. The global outcomes for children, youth, and adults with developmental disabilities include the following[3]:

- Mitigating or reducing the effect of the condition as much as possible through education about the pathology and awareness of likely complications
- Limiting impairments, especially those contributing to reduced postural control, limited mobility, health-related fitness, and wellness
- Reducing functional limitations through *habilitation* (developing sufficient ability to perform functional activities), *compensation* (using alternative methods to accomplish a task), or *adaptation* (providing assistive devices as appropriate)
- Reducing health risks and preventing complications associated with the pathology (using secondary prevention measures, such as protecting the skin, preventing musculoskeletal limitations, and reducing exposure to infections)
- Promoting health, fitness, and wellness
- Providing appropriate resources
- Ensuring family and child satisfaction

When providing health, fitness, and wellness resources to individuals with developmental disabilities, health care providers must be cognizant of the medical diagnosis, clinical manifestations, and secondary complications, as well as the various physical and psychosocial environments each individual will encounter across the lifespan. For example, a young child with a congenital condition has opportunities to spend time at home, in day care, at preschool, at a playground, at recreational facilities, and in other settings with family and friends. This chapter discusses the most common types of developmental disabilities and provides suggestions for preventive practice to enhance health, fitness, and wellness, building on the roles of health care professionals discussed in previous chapters.

Misconceptions About Individuals With Disabilities

The authors of the earlier version of Healthy People 2020, Healthy People 2010,[4] list 4 main misconceptions about individuals with disabilities that interfere with implementation of the national agenda: (1) all individuals with disabilities are in poor health, (2) the focus of public health should only be on preventing disabling conditions, (3) a standard definition of "disability" or "people with disabilities" is not needed, and (4) the environment does not play a role in the disabling process. The first step in promoting health is eliminating these misconceptions.

TABLE 17-1. DEVELOPMENTAL DISABILITIES

- Adrenoleukodystrophy (a genetic disorder affecting boys, characterized by abnormal development of the adrenal gland and the brain's white matter)
- Ataxia telangiectasia (syndrome characterized by movement disorders and slowly progressing mental deterioration)
- Attention deficit disorders (disorders characterized by severe difficulty in focusing and maintaining attention)
- Autism spectrum disorders and pervasive developmental disorders (neurological disorders affecting behavior and sensorimotor function)
- Barth syndrome (a genetic disorder affecting multiple body systems and resulting in delayed growth and motor skills)
- Behavioral disorders (including self-injurious behavior disorders)
- Birth defects
- Brain injuries
- Brain malformations
- Brain tumors
- Cerebral palsy (a neurological disorder usually caused by brain damage in the fetus or infant)
- CHARGE syndrome (an acronym referring to children with a specific pattern of birth defects including the eyes, heart, ears, and genitourinary system)
- Communication, speech, and language disorders
- Down syndrome (a combination of birth defects caused by the presence of an extra 21st chromosome)
- Duchenne muscular dystrophy (a progressive pathology affecting muscle strength)
- Encephalopathy (brain dysfunction secondary to infection)
- Epilepsy (seizure disorder)
- Fetal alcohol syndrome (a combination of birth defects caused by the mother's consumption of alcohol during pregnancy)
- Fragile X syndrome (genetic disorder that is the most common form of inherited mental retardation)
- Hearing impairment
- Holoprosencephaly (a relatively common birth defect of the brain, which often also affects facial features, causing closely spaced eyes, small head size, and sometimes clefts of the lip and roof of the mouth)
- Lead poisoning (typically causing brain damage)
- Learning disorders (academic difficulties experienced by individuals of average to above-average intelligence)
- Mental retardation (characterized by intellectual functioning at least 2 standard deviations below the norm)
- Metabolic disorders

(continued)

Table 17-1 (continued). Developmental Disabilities
• Mitochondrial disorders (disorders affecting the energy functions of the cell)
• Movement disorders
• Neurodegenerative disorders (progressive neurological orders than worsen with age)
• Neurological disorders
• Osteogenesis imperfecta (an autosomal-dominant disorder of connective tissue characterized by brittle bones that fracture easily)
• Prematurity (any infant born before 37 weeks' gestation)
• Psychiatric disorders
• Rett syndrome (disorder of the nervous system that leads to regression in development, especially in the areas of expressive language)
• Skeletal disorders
• Nonrespiratory sleep disorders
• Smith-Lemli-Opitz syndrome (an autosomal recessive disorder characterized by multiple congenital anomalies)
• Spina bifida (a birth defect in which the neural tube fails to close during fetal development and a portion of the spinal cord and nerves fail to develop properly)
• Spinal cord injury and paralysis

Misconception 1: Disability Equals Poor Health

It is inaccurate to say that all individuals with disabilities are in poor health. Often, these individuals are at an increased risk of illness, but with proper care, they can be as healthy as individuals without disabilities, depending on their medical diagnoses. The same health education and prevention/protection strategies offered to the general public should be offered to all individuals with disabilities. Health care professionals need to be advocates, ensuring multiple health and fitness options for all populations served, and should tailor health education and protection/prevention strategies to the unique needs of individuals with developmental disabilities.

Misconception 2: Disability Is the Focus

To eliminate another misconception, the focus of public health should be on health, fitness, and wellness for all individuals, rather than on disability prevention. For individuals with disabilities, appropriate accommodations should be made to ensure equal access to health promotion.

Misconception 3: Standard Definition of Disability

One of the greatest barriers to achieving equitable care is the variance in definitions for the term *disability*. There needs to be a universal definition of disability encompassing the educational, medical, legal, social, and economic issues that can be addressed through teamwork and advocacy.

Misconception 4: Environment Is Not Important

Not surprisingly, the environment plays a key role in the disabling process. The environment includes not only the physical environment, but also the psychosocial environment created by the attitudes people share about individuals with disabilities. Although it is possible to remove many physical, legal, and civic barriers through time and effort, it takes more time, effort, and vigilance to change people's attitudes about disabilities. Negative attitudes can profoundly affect the health, wellness, and perspectives of life of those with developmental disabilities. People with disabilities encounter many different forms of attitudinal barriers, including pity, intolerance, impatience, ignorance, and those generated by stereotypes projected through the media. Health care professionals must first assess their own attitudes toward individuals with disabilities to ensure a positive psychosocial environment for their clients. Once they explore their own prejudices or attitudes, then they can help others, including family members and educators, deal more effectively with individuals who are developmentally disabled. Health care professionals can help change the psychosocial environment by educating others about how to interact effectively with people with disabilities, including the use of "people first" language. For example, a child with Down syndrome should not be referred to as a "Down syndrome child."

Assessing Health, Fitness, and Wellness

Many of the screening tools and tests discussed earlier in this book can be used for determining the special needs of a client with developmental disabilities. Tests and measures should be conducted in the appropriate physical environments to ensure the individual's safety and full attention. Although standardized testing may be valuable for metabolic fitness measures, more creative criterion-referenced tests that examine the individual's function can yield valuable information for creating customized health, fitness, and wellness programs.

After completing the examination with all necessary history and current information, health care providers can determine the special needs of the individual and others engaged in the person's life who are seeking resources for health, fitness, and wellness.

It is important to examine both the structure and function of each individual to determine whether any habitual behaviors have resulted in problems with body structure. For example, children may assume a variety of postures to accommodate their muscle tone or instability in sitting. Some children prefer W-sitting when sitting on the floor. This posture is characterized by sitting with both hips flexed, externally rotated, and adducted; both knees flexed; and both ankles plantarflexed, creating a "W" with their legs. Children who W-sit for prolonged periods put additional stress on bones, joints, and soft tissue, potentially altering normal growth. If this habit is chronic, it can lead to subsequent postural problems. Examining each individual's body structures and functions, activity limitations and functional skills, environmental barriers and facilitators, personal factors (lifestyle behaviors and motivation) and, most importantly, desire to participate in society (noting participation restriction), provides a baseline for the development of an individualized health and wellness program, focusing on the needs of the individual.

Metabolic Fitness

Metabolic fitness, as described in Chapter 3, involves tests of bodily functions at rest, including vital signs and blood tests. Often, individuals with developmental disabilities have stable vital signs and negative blood tests; nevertheless, determining healthy baseline measures enables the health care professional to either progress to health-related fitness activities or to consult with other professionals to procure necessary information. Individuals with developmental disabilities should have a preparticipation screening conducted by a physician to reveal medical issues that need monitoring during physical activity.

Health-Related Fitness

Individuals with disabilities are at a higher risk than the general population for developing medical problems due to limited activity, psychosocial problems, and reduced lifespans. The benefits of exercise extend beyond physical fitness to include physical wellness, social wellness, psychological wellness, and emotional wellness, as described in Chapter 1. Overall, the healthy individual develops *salutogenesis* (a complete physical, mental, and social well-being) and not merely the absence of disease. Allowing individuals with disabilities to choose their own options for health promotion is conducive to long-term involvement in healthy activities. Those with developmental disabilities may need specialized adaptations for their activities and to their environments for flexibility, posture, muscular strength, muscular endurance, cardiorespiratory fitness, and body composition. For example, toddlers with limited postural control would benefit from a floor device for postural support during floor play with peers.

Flexibility

The majority of children with developmental disabilities have atypical sensory or motor development contributing to abnormal growth patterns of the body. Children who do not begin walking by the age of 2 years may not experience the normal stresses of weight bearing to develop fully. Children with developmental disabilities must be encouraged to bear weight in appropriate positions to promote bone growth without developing musculoskeletal deformities. Physical therapists can recommend assistive devices for walking, as needed. Children who are at risk for delayed motor development and reduced growth include those with *cerebral palsy* (most commonly those with *spastic quadriparesis* that limits voluntary movement of the head, neck, trunk, and limbs), *spina bifida* (especially those with spinal cord lesions that compromise muscle strength and muscle balance), and *Down syndrome* (a condition often affecting both physical and cognitive development).[5] In many children with developmental disabilities, delays in motor development result in range of motion limitations that can last a lifetime. Providing flexibility exercises, either active exercise performed by the individual or assisted/passive range of motion exercise, is essential for health-related fitness for this population. Health care professionals with expertise in caring for children with developmental disabilities can monitor range of motion of all at-risk joints to ensure that growth spurts and functional habits do not affect the individual's flexibility.

Posture

Postural Control

Postural control provides the base of support for the performance of motor skills, such as walking, feeding, and handwriting. Smooth transitions from one posture to another require the fine muscle adjustments of larger muscle groups evidenced with postural control. Postural control provides the individual with *antigravity stability* in postures, *automatic reactions with unexpected perturbations*, and postural adjustments when reaching for objects or preparing to catch a ball (ie, *anticipatory postural control*). Many children with developmental disabilities have difficulty with controlling their bodies in sitting and standing postures. For example, individuals with cerebral palsy who have spastic quadriparesis (involving reduced motor control of the entire body) often have problems with feeding, swallowing, and speech secondary to poor control of the head, neck, trunk, mouth, and jaw. Working with these children on holding the correct postural alignment in sitting, or working in other developmental postures, helps to provide a more stable base for muscles to function effectively. Consultation with physical therapy, occupational therapy, and speech therapy can guide appropriate interventions to facilitate function and enable children to participate in a wide range of activities while managing postural problems.

Therapeutic Positioning

When individuals lack postural control in sitting, they are often positioned by their caretakers in *prone* (on the stomach), *supine* (on the back), or lying on one side. A number of studies have associated the prone sleeping position in infants with an increased risk of sudden infant death syndrome (SIDS), so pediatricians and nurseries have encouraged parents to position children in other positions, such as supine, as part of the Back to Sleep campaign, as discussed in Chapter 12.[6] In many parts of the country, this Back to Sleep campaign is successful based on the significantly increased proportion of infants sleeping supine and the reduced incidence of SIDS. Although reducing SIDS by positioning children supine is important, this change in positioning coincides with an increase in infant cranial deformity.[7] "Abnormalities of the occipital cranial suture in infancy can cause significant posterior cranial asymmetry, malposition of the ears, distortion of the cranial base, deformation of the forehead, and facial asymmetry."[7] These cranial abnormalities can be prevented by frequent changes of position and the use of alternate positions, such as sidelying. The role of health care professionals is to clarify that prone positioning for play is not a risk factor for SIDS and that it is desirable for infants to spend supervised wakeful time in the prone position, especially for children with developmental disabilities and poor postural control.

For those individuals who do not develop independent sitting, the physical therapist or occupational therapist may prescribe therapeutic positioning to support the child, youth, or adult for antigravity activities, such as sitting. The Seated Postural Control Measure, which offers 22 seating postural alignment items and 12 functional movement items, each scored on a 4-point criterion referenced scale, can be used for seating assessment.[8] *Adaptive seating devices* (ASDs) are commonly used in the treatment of individuals with developmental disabilities. In one longitudinal study, 19 individuals with multiple handicaps and developmental disabilities (aged 1 to 6 years) were evaluated through direct observation and parent-guardian assessment pre- and postpositioning for 6 months. Activities observed included head control, controlled sitting posture, visual tracking, reach, and grasp. Over the 6 months of intervention, sitting posture, head control, and grasp improved significantly. Parents were freed from handling their children and allowed to engage in other activities with the children and around the home.[9]

Children with Down syndrome need guidance in proper sitting and transitional movements to and from sitting because they tend to have excessive hip external rotation and hip abduction, excessive hip mobility in sitting and transitions to and from sitting, and a wide-based gait. For these children, physical therapy intervention should focus on developing strength in hip muscles, providing support (such as a stretch garment that restricts hip abduction and external rotation), and incorporating body rotation in transitional movement from prone to supine and from sitting to all fours.[10]

Children with spastic cerebral palsy have a tendency to adduct and internally rotate their hips if they are not seated with proper support. In looking at bilateral hand skills, the recommended posture for improving fine motor function is sitting with hip abduction with a straddling device to optimize postural stability by increasing the child's base of support.

Muscular Strength and Endurance

Muscle strength is essential for controlling the body. Simply encouraging normal motor development provides opportunities to strengthen muscles through daily activities. Older individuals with developmental disabilities can benefit from more directed exercises for general body strengthening, using the principles of progression, overload, periodization, individualization, and specificity described in Chapter 4. For many individuals, fitness training can be accomplished through standard exercise; however, for individuals with decreased muscle tone, movement is more challenging and spasticity management must be addressed along with efforts to strengthen muscles. Although some have thought that maximal efforts to contract muscles could increase spasticity, research suggests otherwise.[11] Using prolonged stretching exercises (including serial casting and positioning in a prone stander), antispasmodic medications (including botulinum toxin A or baclofen), coactivation of antagonistic muscles, and electrical stimulation have been used to reduce spasticity, aiding the development of greater muscle strength and endurance.[11] Studies have consistently shown that children engaged in muscle strengthening have improved motor function.[12]

Individuals with low tone also benefit from muscle-strengthening activities. Adults with Down syndrome demonstrated significant gains in muscle strength, muscle endurance, and cardiovascular endurance (in addition to slight but significant reduction in body weight) after engaging in a 12-week exercise program (3 days a week for 45 minutes per session) consisting of cardiovascular and strengthening exercises. "Greater effort must be made to promote increases in physical activity participation among persons with Down syndrome and developmental disabilities in order to reduce the potential health risks associated with low fitness and sedentary behavior."[13] Simply engaging in more antigravity activity can increase muscle strength and endurance. In one study comparing the muscle activation of individuals with normal vs delayed motor development, results indicated that children with slower motor development had greater muscle activity in their legs.[13]

Equipment for strengthening can be inexpensive and low risk. Resistance bands are lightweight materials that can be easily adjusted in length and resistance by folding the band, increasing or reducing the slack, or placing them around the extremities to work arms and legs simultaneously. One precaution is that some children are allergic to the materials used to fabricate these bands. It is best to use latex-free materials.

Improving Cardiorespiratory Fitness

Cardiorespiratory endurance is another key component of fitness training. The running and jumping subtests of the Gross Motor Function Measure are helpful in determining a child's level of anaerobic fitness of the legs; however, it is not a suitable tool for determining aerobic capacity of the body or the anaerobic capacity of the arms.[14] Another method of measuring cardiorespiratory endurance is the arm ergometer. In a study using arm ergometry and comparing the oxygen consumption (VO_2), heart rate (HR), and physical working capacity (PWC) of able-bodied individuals with those of individuals with cerebral palsy, individuals with cerebral palsy had comparable measures in all except PWC, or the ability to perform maximal work at equal intensities and durations.[14,15] In practice, aerobic work capacity (VO_2 max) is the capacity most often considered. Children and adolescents with cerebral palsy have lower maximal oxygen consumption (VO_2 max) and subnormal values for peak anaerobic power and muscular endurance of the upper and lower limbs when compared with their able-bodied peers.[16]

Gait abnormalities in children with cerebral palsy have been shown to increase submaximal walking energy expenditure almost three-fold when compared with healthy children. A study examining the energy costs of gait concluded that "a certain level of muscle co-contraction is necessary for achieving joint stability during locomotion, particularly at the ankle and knee. There appears, however, to be a co-contraction threshold beyond which there are associated elevated metabolic costs during locomotion in children with CP [cerebral palsy]."[17] In studies using wheelchair ergometry, measures of maximum oxygen uptake (VO_2 max) can be used as a helpful tool for evaluating the cardiorespiratory fitness of individuals who are nonambulatory.[16] When considering an individual's physiologic demands for increasing cardiorespiratory fitness, it is important to note that these demands are increased for individuals with neurologic and orthopedic disabilities.[16] Furthermore, individuals with intellectual disabilities need supervised treadmill training programs to provide needed cardiorespiratory exercises for endurance and prevention of heart-related diseases.[16]

Continuous exercise, such as walking, cycling, or swimming at slower speeds, is generally less demanding both mentally and physically than interval exercise (exercise with rest breaks). Continuous exercise is effective for cardiovascular fitness and is less likely to produce injury. Interval exercise enables the individual to work at higher intensities for shorter periods of time, pushing the individual's performance to higher levels for competition.

Body Composition

Individuals who tend to be more sedentary are likely to become overweight. Physical activity is known to have a positive influence on body composition, decreasing body fat and increasing muscle mass. One study examining the effectiveness of a 45-minute exercise program for individuals with Down syndrome found that those with regular activity (consisting of cardiovascular and strength activities) reduced body weight and potential health risks associated with sedentary behavior.[18] In a similar study examining the effects of a 9-month sports program for children with spastic cerebral palsy, researchers found that children with higher intensity programming (4 sessions vs 2 sessions per week) had relatively reduced fat mass and increased peak aerobic power (VO_2 max).[19] These studies suggest that children with abnormal muscle tone, sensorimotor impairments, and cognitive impairments can benefit from cardiovascular and strength training, provided they have no conditions precluding such activities.

A nutritional diet is recommended for all children, regardless of their disabilities; however, children with developmental disabilities require specialized diets and adaptive equipment for feeding. For example, a child with cerebral palsy might require additional thickening of liquid and soft-textured foods because of possible oromotor problems, including difficulties with chewing, swallowing, and mouth closure. Other issues include abnormal muscle tone, poor head control, and gastroesophageal reflux. Occupational therapists can provide helpful counsel regarding adaptive equipment for feeding, including weighted utensils, nonslip placemats, and dishes with guards. Before providing food or beverages as part of a program, screen each child for food allergies and dietary needs. A registered dietician can provide valuable consultation for healthy meals to satisfy the needs of special populations.

One final caution: children who have limited mobility also typically do not expend as much energy as those who are physically active. Additional empty-calorie foods should not be offered for any reason, especially to those at risk for obesity due to inactivity.

Promoting Health for Individuals With Developmental Disabilities

Individuals with developmental disabilities are at a higher risk of developing both physical and psychosocial problems due to limited physical activity. These problems include obesity, hypertension, circulatory problems, reduced muscle strength, reduced flexibility, osteoporosis, scoliosis, skin breakdown, reduced endurance, social isolation, and depression. Proper exercise in an inclusive setting reduces the risk of disease and promotes both physical and mental wellness. Exercise prescription principles for persons with developmental disabilities should be designed to enhance physical fitness, promote health by reducing the risk for chronic disease, and ensure safety during exercise participation. The focus of the exercise prescription should be on each individual's interests, health

TABLE 17-2. IMPROVEMENTS ASSOCIATED WITH PARTICIPATION IN SPECIAL OLYMPICS	
DECREASED	**INCREASED**
Weight	Overall fitness and strength
Body fat	Aerobic capacity
Stereotypic, self-stimulatory behaviors	Athletic achievement
Inappropriate vocalizations	Cardiovascular fitness
Off-task behaviors	Appropriate or correct academic responding
Aggression	On-task behavior at work or school
Hyperactivity	Task completion at work or school
	Self-esteem
	Social competence
	Peer relationships

Adapted from Dykens E, Rosner B, Butterbaugh G. Exercise and sports in children and adolescents with developmental disabilities. *Sports Psychiatry.* 1998;7(4):757-768.

needs, and clinical status. Often, the exercise mode, intensity, frequency, and duration are modified according to the individual's clinical condition and can be prescribed by a physical therapist.

Sometimes, caretakers are hesitant to initiate physical fitness programs for fear they might exacerbate any conditions these individuals might have. Encouraging athletic performance through adaptive physical education and Special Olympics can increase engagement in regular activity (Table 17-2). Participation in sports is important for the physical and emotional health of all individuals. Sports can improve strength, endurance, and cardiopulmonary fitness while providing companionship, a sense of achievement, and heightened self-esteem.[20] Improved physical and psychosocial functioning are found in studies of both children and adults with mental retardation, as well as in research on athletes enrolled in Special Olympics International, the largest recreational sport program in the world for persons with developmental disabilities.[21] Health care professionals should educate families about the need for a preparticipation screening by a physician, appropriate athletic options, specialized equipment, and risks associated with specific sports.

BARRIERS TO HEALTH PROMOTION OPPORTUNITIES

A disparity exists between what individuals with developmental disabilities seek for fitness and health promotion options and what is available for their use. Proper exercise in an inclusive setting promotes both physical and mental wellness. Participation in community activities, specifically community-based fitness opportunities, depends on the restrictions, barriers, and facilitators influencing a given environment or social situation. Adaptations of activities, assistive devices/technology, and specialized training often enable individuals with impairments to function in daily activities (mobility, communication, personal care, domestic activities, simple movements, learning, and appropriate behavior). Assuming that accommodations are made to meet the individual's needs (modifying or reducing functional limitations for exercise), social restrictions, physical barriers, and facilitators could either limit or enhance an individual's participation in fitness activities. Lack of time, money, staffing, transportation, knowledge about specific disabilities, and motivation, along with negative attitudes, are barriers that could limit participation in community-based activities. Identification of these barriers provides a mechanism for matching resources to areas of need.

Resources to Enhance Participation in Health Promotion and Fitness Opportunities

Experts in special adaptations for individuals with physical impairments include physical therapists, occupational therapists, and recreational therapists. These professionals can serve as facilitators, addressing concerns and removing barriers to inclusive health promotion opportunities. Lack of self-motivation to exercise is one of the most confounding factors to overcome. Extrinsic motivators for participation in health promotion activities include the following:

- Offering T-shirts as clients reach specific goals
- Creating charts listing progress toward fitness goals (eg, walking across the state)
- Writing news stories featuring active clients in facility's newsletter
- Providing awards or special recognition to clients (eg, Client of the Month)
- Providing coupons/tickets for local activities or events to clients who meet fitness goals
- Emphasizing socialization as part of fitness programs (create exercise groups)
- Developing a bulletin board that lists activities and regular participants

Local libraries (public, college and university, medical centers and hospitals) and Internet searches provide an array of fitness information for those with special needs.

Public law mandates the removal of physical barriers to public facilities, making them accessible to individuals of all ability levels. Educating the private sector about an untapped consumer base of individuals with disabilities could encourage private sector facilities to become more accessible to individuals with impairments.

Many of the negative stereotypes and inappropriate behaviors that restrict socializing can be reduced by regular participation in structured activities. Rather than isolate individuals with developmental disabilities from the community at large, efforts should be made to encourage continuous interaction in leisure activities.

Additional Considerations for Health Promotion Programs

- *Medical release form*: An annual medical release form listing the client's health problems and special needs (including medications and side effects) should be signed by a physician. A list of recommended activities and special care techniques would also prove useful. A new release form should be signed whenever the individual's health condition changes.
- *Availability of medical staff for clients with significant health needs*: In addition to providing helpful information for specific clients, medical staff can help to maintain records of body height and weight and heart rate and blood pressure at rest and during exercise.
- *Posted information to encourage self-directed fitness monitoring*: Exercise areas should be equipped with charts and illustrations identifying target heart rates for fitness and how to measure them, muscles of the body, proper body mechanics, proper use of all equipment, and normal height/weight charts.
- *Community integration*: The best way to accomplish social integration is to schedule activities open to the entire community; develop relationships with other facilities in the community that offer additional amenities; share expertise about health, fitness, and wellness; and encourage sports.
- *Use available resources*: Many camps offer specialized health and fitness programs for children and adults with developmental disabilities. Checking with local park departments, recreational facilities, special education programs, and health agencies can help identify these programs.

Table 17-3. Key Categories for Improved Quality of Life for Individuals With Developmental Disabilities

BEING	BELONGING	BECOMING
Being healthy: • Looking after physical health • Eating a balanced diet • Hygiene and body care	Belonging in a place: • Having a place of residence • Having space for privacy • Living in a neighborhood	Becoming more independent: • Learning at work, school, or program • Learning how to take care of the home • Taking responsibility for self and others
Being in control of thoughts and feelings: • Demonstrating self-control • Having a clear self-concept • Feeling free of anxiety	Belonging to social circles: • Having a spouse or special person • Having a connection with family • Having friends	Becoming healthy, fit, and well: • Visiting and socializing • Engaging in leisure activities/hobbies • Participating in fitness activities
Being aware of beliefs and values: • Understanding right and wrong • Attaching meaning to life • Celebrating life	Belonging to the community: • Having access to meaningful work • Having access to community places • Having access to education	Becoming capable of handling changes in life: • Learning more about oneself and the world • Attaining new independent-living skills • Adjusting to life changes

Quality of Life Indicators

Quality of life (QOL) involves being healthy, being in control of thoughts and feelings, and being aware of beliefs and values. It also involves belonging in a place, within a social circle, and to a community. Finally, QOL enables individuals to become more independent, healthy, fit, and well, while handling inevitable changes in life (Table 17-3). A good QOL is essential for individuals with developmental disabilities.

According to a survey examining the QOL of individuals with developmental disabilities,[22] people with higher QOL scores were associated with the following characteristics:

- Living in community settings
- Having verbal skills
- Having higher functional abilities
- Not seeing a psychiatrist or taking psychotropic medications
- Not having complex medical needs

For nonverbal individuals, higher QOL[22] was associated with:

- Having some type of occupational activity
- Having community-based recreational and leisure-time opportunities
- Having decision-making opportunities
- Increasing levels of independence for continued development
- Receiving practical and emotional support from others
- Not having marked behavior problems

The role of health care providers is to provide support in whichever areas of life positively impact QOL for individuals with disabilities. "To improve QOL for individuals or groups of individuals, services need to consider all areas of a person's life, and to focus on environments that can enhance life—at the policy level (laws and broad principles), and in culture (values, attitudes and behavior of others), as well as the service level (specific supports)."[22] Health care providers can help their clients with developmental disabilities by connecting these individuals with social support systems in the community, increasing acceptance by the general public (including advocating for policies and laws discouraging disparities in health care and discrimination in access to health, fitness, and wellness opportunities), and supporting efforts to increase financial resources that ensure a reasonable standard of living for adults with developmental disabilities. When developing a program for individuals with developmental disabilities, it is important to consider that high-quality support services for people with disabilities are[22]:

- Designed with input of all involved individuals, including those with disabilities
- Considered acceptable by people without disabilities
- Integrated into the community
- Individualized and relevant to each individual's needs
- Changed, as needed, to meet the needs of the dynamic individual
- Adequately funded
- Designed to maximize independence
- Developed with respect for the dignity and privacy of individuals (see Table 17-3)

Wellness

Good health is crucial for all individuals, particularly those with developmental disabilities. Every effort should be made to provide persons with developmental disabilities with access to fitness and health promotion opportunities. The World Health Organization's International Classification of Functioning, Disability and Health (ICF) model provides an outline for addressing factors that contribute to limited participation in life activities. Although impairments and functional limitations can be modified on an individualized basis, participation in community-based fitness programs requires a concerted effort by individuals with developmental disabilities, parents, professionals, and local organizations to provide their varying perspectives and to identify the restrictions and barriers to inclusion. Once these limitations are identified, resources in the community (eg, information, professionals, community organizations) can serve as facilitators to enhance community opportunities for health promotion and fitness.

Summary

The health-related needs of individuals with disabilities are broad in scope, yet health care professionals working in a network of consultants or as direct-access providers have the knowledge to help these individuals, their families, and their caretakers provide optimal health, fitness, and wellness opportunities. The prevalence of childhood disability is on the rise, yet life expectancies are improving, and it is not uncommon for children with severe disabilities to live well into adulthood. The paradigm shift to focus on health and function rather than impairment and disability fits well with the national initiative to promote health for all. The management of individuals with disabilities from childhood throughout adulthood demands continual monitoring and adaptation to deal with disability-related problems. Just as individuals without disabilities must transition into healthy lifestyle habits, individuals with developmental disabilities must be counseled about their perceptions and values, social networks, a sense of personal control, and a readiness to change attitudes toward changing lifestyles.

Preventive measures for the management of this population are essential for the individual, the community, and society at large. Optimal management involves teamwork and coordination of services between medical, health, and social agencies for measures such as health education, nutrition, psychological and family support, and funding sources for adaptive equipment and health-related services.

References

1. *The American Heritage Stedman's Medical Dictionary.* New York, NY: Houghton Mifflin Company; 2005.
2. Developmental disabilities. NC Division of Mental Health, Developmental Disabilities, and Substance Abuse Services. http://www.ncdhhs.gov/mhddsas/providers/developmentaldisabilities/index.htm. Accessed June 1, 2013.
3. *Guide to Physical Therapist Practice.* 2nd ed. http://guidetoptpractice.apta.org/. Alexandria, VA: American Physical Therapy Association; 2003.
4. Disability and secondary conditions. Healthy People 2010. http://www.healthypeople.gov/Document/HTML/Volume1/06Disability.htm. Accessed May 30, 2006.
5. Duff SV, Charles J. Enhancing prehension in infants and children: fostering neuromotor strategies. *Phys Occup Ther Pediatr.* 2004;24(1-2):129-172.
6. HCCA Back to Sleep Campaign. American Academy of Pediatrics. http://www.healthychildcare.org/sids.html. Accessed May 30, 2006.
7. Persing J, James H, Swanson J, et al. Prevention and management of positional skull deformities in infants. American Academy of Pediatrics Committee on Practice and Ambulatory Medicine, Section on Plastic Surgery and Section on Neurological Surgery. *Pediatrics.* 2003;112(1 Pt 1):199-202.
8. Seated postural control measure. BC Children's Hospital. http://www.bcchildrens.ca/Services/SunnyHillHealthCtr/Research/Seatedposturalcontrolmeasure.htm. Accessed May 30, 2006.
9. Fife SE, Roxborough LA, Armstrong RW, Harris SR, Gregson JL, Field D. Development of a clinical measure of postural control for assessment of adaptive seating in children with neuromotor disabilities. *Phys Ther.* 1991;71(12):981-993.
10. Lydic JS, Steele C. Assessment of the quality of sitting and gait patterns in children with Down syndrome. *Phys Ther.* 1979;59(12):1489-1494.
11. Almeida GL, Campbell SK, Girolami GL, Penn RD, Corcos DM. Multidimensional assessment of motor function in a child with cerebral palsy following intrathecal administration of baclofen. *Phys Ther.* 1997;77(7):751-764.
12. Fowler EG, Ho TW, Nwigwe AI, Dorey FJ. The effect of quadriceps femoris muscle strengthening exercises on spasticity in children with cerebral palsy. *Phys Ther.* 2001;81(6):1215-1223.
13. Pitetti K, Rimmer J, Fernall B. Physical fitness and adults with mental retardation. *Sports Med.* 1993;16(1):23-56.
14. Parker DF, Carriere L, Hebestreit H, Salsberg A, Bar-Or O. Muscle performance and gross motor function of children with spastic cerebral palsy. *Dev Med Child Neurol.* 1993;35(1):17-23.
15. Wei S, Su-Juan W, Yuan-Gui L, Hong Y, Xiu-Juan X, Xiao-Mei S. Reliability and validity of the GMFM-66 in 0- to 3-year-old children with cerebral palsy. *Am J Phys Med Rehabil.* 2006;85(2):141-147.
16. Tobimatsu Y, Nakamura R, Kusano S, Iwasaki Y. Cardiorespiratory endurance in people with cerebral palsy measured using an arm ergometer. *Arch Phys Med Rehabil.* 1998;79(8):991-993.

17. Waters RL, Mulroy S. The energy expenditure of normal and pathologic gait. *Gait Posture.* 1999;9(3):207-231.
18. Lotan M, Isakov E, Kessel S, Merrick J. Physical fitness and functional ability of children with intellectual disability: effects of a short-term daily treadmill intervention. *Scientific World Journal.* 2004;4:449-457.
19. Van den Berg-Emons RJ, Van Baak MA, Speth L, Saris WH. Physical training of school children with spastic cerebral palsy: effects on daily activity, fat mass and fitness. *Int J Rehabil Res.* 1998;21(2):179-194.
20. Durstine JL, Painter P, Franklin BA, Morgan D, Pitetti KH, Roberts SO. Physical activity for the chronically ill and disabled. *Sports Med.* 2001:31(8):627.
21. Quality of life indicators. Ontario Adult Autism Research and Support Network. http://www.ont-autism.uoguelph.ca/STRATEGIES4.shtml. Accessed May 30, 2013.
22. Quality of life indicators. Ontario Adult Autism Research and Support Network. http://www.ont-autism.uoguelph.ca/STRATEGIES4.shtml. Accessed May 20, 2014.

18

Advocacy for Preventive Care

Catherine Rush Thompson, PT, PhD, MS

"He who has health has hope; and he who has hope has everything."—Arabian Proverb

Advocacy

As health care professionals, we can influence outcomes for others and our professions; this is *advocacy*. Advocacy can directly affect the lives of millions through public policy and resource allocation without governmental, economic, and social systems. Advocacy requires evaluating a current reality, determining the critical issues that have been ignored or overlooked, and bringing to light a new vision that incorporates the needs of those who are disenfranchised. The key to advocacy is using this vision to bring about social justice. Although some individuals have the knowledge, the will, and the strength to single-handedly make dynamic changes in institutions and social structures, others may require teamwork and organization to influence the attitudes of those unfamiliar with important needs of others and to enact changes to accomplish their visions. As health care providers, we should be asking "what if?" and transforming what is into what should be. Advocacy for others protects human rights—whether they are social, political, or economic—and promotes human dignity.

Even self-advocacy, a skill that should be practiced by health care professionals and clients alike, can remove barriers to quality health care and improve the lives of others. Advocacy gives those without power some hope of realizing that their needs are being recognized. Health care professionals can be powerful advocates for the needs of their clients and the greater community, as well as promoters of self-advocacy.

Key Health Care Issues

Advocacy is empowerment of consumers who may be denied access to services. It is also enabling health care providers to best meet the needs of intended consumers of their services. In many respects, advocacy is one individual acting in the interests of another to help that individual gain a certain degree of power to pursue those interests.

Thompson CR.
Prevention Practice and Health Promotion: A Health Care Professional's Guide to Health, Fitness, and Wellness, Second Edition (pp 297-308).

As health care professionals, it is important to identify significant health issues, to recognize the populations at greatest risk for health problems, and to determine what cost-effective sources of support can be offered for those specific populations. Some communities, such as a university setting, may need to focus health promotion efforts on the needs of younger adults. For example, health issues for young adults on college campuses may include the following:

- Infectious diseases, including sexually transmitted diseases
- Obesity
- Substance abuse
- Lack of access to health care
- Depression
- Rape

Older adults have different risk profiles and need advocacy that addresses issues of greater importance to their population, such as the risk for falls, access to health care, affordable health promotion resources, and funding for special health needs.

The Healthy People 2020 initiative provides a wealth of information about these key health issues facing various populations, providing statistics about populations at the greatest risks for problems and current data on the incidence and prevalence of health problems. These data can be obtained at http://www.healthypeople.gov/.

There are various ways to advocate for health care issues. Table 18-1 lists several options for the individual who wants to contact policy makers about health care issues.

The Legislative Process

One of the best ways to affect public policy is to get new legislation introduced; however, only members of Congress can introduce legislation. Legislation includes bills, joint resolutions, concurrent resolutions, and simple resolutions. The official legislative process begins when a bill or resolution is numbered; a House bill is labeled *H.R.* and a Senate bill is labeled *S.* The initial step in the legislative process is the referral of the legislation to committee (generally to standing committees in the Senate or House of Representatives). Once the bill has reached committee, it is reviewed carefully by the committee or a subcommittee to determine its chances for passage. Often, bills referred to subcommittees include a review of testimony (in person or in writing) in support or against the legislation. At this point, health care professionals can affect the opinions of committee members by writing or providing testimony about a specific bill. After subcommittee hearings, the legislation is modified, as needed, to move forward, or the bill dies. The full committee can vote to support recommendations or make additional amendments after reviewing the subcommittee's report on the bill. The full committee then votes on recommendations to the House or Senate.

After the committee votes to have a bill reported, staff prepare a written report on the bill in preparation for presentation to the chamber where it originated. The written report provides information about the intent, scope, and effect of the pending legislation, as well as the views of those who do not support the bill. When the bill comes up for debate, time is allotted to discuss the strengths and benefits of the bill, and the members vote to pass or defeat the bill. If the bill passes, it is referred to the other chamber for the same action. At this point, the legislation may continue to be altered until an agreement is reached between legislators or the bill dies. If agreement is reached, a conference report summarizing the final bill must be approved by both the House and Senate. Finally, after this approval, it is sent to the President for approval. If approved, the bill is signed and becomes law. The President can take no action for 10 days, and it automatically becomes law. If the President opposes the bill, the bill may be vetoed. If there is no action after Congress has adjourned its second session, the legislation dies. Congress may override the President's veto; this

Table 18-1. Tips for Advocates

Always Remember

- If you represent a program, invite program participants. They are in the best position to explain the benefits of your program.
- Keep it positive.
- Be prepared. Practice what you will say in the meeting. Anticipate questions that might be asked and practice answering them.
- Arrive on time and stay in the meeting until the end.
- Take care of business before the meeting starts (eg, bathroom, phone calls, cell phone off, hang up coat).
- Treat staffers and legislators with equal respect.

Before Visiting With Legislators

- Know the status of the budget.
- Know "the ask": how much does your program need and how will you spend it?
- Have a briefing. Provide tip-sheets with key facts and messages to everyone who is going into the meeting.
- Participate in role-playing exercises. More experienced advocates will know what to expect from legislators and their staffs.

How to Dress

- Wear comfortable shoes. If you have several meetings scheduled, you will be doing a lot of walking.
- Dress appropriately for the weather.
- Wear interview attire.
- Dress neat and clean.
- Represent your culture.

When Speaking

- Be polite. Thank the legislator and his or her staff for their time.
- Remember legislators' titles and use them.
- Stick to your key messages.
- Avoid acronyms and program jargon.
- Speak from your heart.
- Give families and participants in your program time to offer their perspective.

What to Tell Legislators

- Who you are and why you are there.
- The purpose of the program you represent and the services it offers.
- The number of families your program serves.
- How the program has benefited the families and communities in your legislator's constituency.

(continued)

Table 18-1 (continued). Tips for Advocates
• Current limitations and expansion requests.
• How important legislators are to the growth of your program.
• The consequences of funding cuts; how many families will lose services if your program loses funding. Example: Child abuse prevention is an investment. Investing in preventing abuse before it happens is much less expensive than intervening and treating the consequences of abuse after it has already occurred. Giving data to support this fact will give this statement more authority.

requires two-thirds of members who are present for a quorum. To be successful, most bills must have broad, preferably bipartisan, support.[1]

Health care professionals need to contact their legislators about legislation affecting preventive care and their profession. Whereas professional lobbyists work with professional organizations to advocate for specific health care issues, many clients and their families are unfamiliar with the legislative process and need advocates for their health care causes.

Direct Advocacy

Health care professionals can play a key role in advocating for all health-related issues but are uniquely qualified to advocate for their clients and their families, populations at risk for injury or disease, and individuals in their local community in need of preventive care. Advocacy can be carried out directly with legislators or may be achieved by contacting others to serve as advocates for desired policy changes. Direct advocacy often involves e-mails, telephone calls, or personal contacts with legislators at the national, regional, state, or local level.

E-mails or Letters

If e-mails or letters are used, it is useful to have a form that summarizes the key issues. All letters or e-mails should be typewritten or written legibly using correct grammar and spelling. If the letter is mailed, include the recipient's name and address on both envelope and letter. Ideally, letters or e-mails should include the following components:

- *Correct Legislative Address and Salutation*

  Honorable [Representative or Senator]

  Address a Senator or Representative as follows:

  The Honorable ______________

  US Senate

  Washington, DC 20510

  Dear Senator ______________:

  OR

  The Honorable ______________

  US House of Representatives

  Washington, DC 20510

  Dear Representative ______________:

- *Statement of the issue* (Use your own words and avoid form letters. Write a brief, specific, and focused statement about why the issue is important to you and the legislator's constituents.)
- *Acknowledgment of the legislator's position* (Include references to the legislator's background and voting record on this or similar issues.)
- *Restating the issue/anticipation of continued support* (Include factual details about the issue/legislation with links to more detailed information about the issue. Enclose applicable editorials or position papers, as appropriate.)
- *Identity* (Provide details about yourself, including your address [constituency], professional credentials, and association with professional, social service, or other organizations.)
- *Thanks* (Express gratitude for the legislator's time and consideration. Ask the policy maker for a response.)
- *Closing* ("Sincerely.")
- It is also helpful to provide a courtesy copy of the letter or e-mail to organizations supporting the same issues. See the sample letter in Table 18-2.

Telephone Contacts

Telephone contacts with national Senators or Representatives can be initiated by calling the United States Capitol Switchboard at (202) 224-3121 and asking for the designated Senator or Representative.

The following suggestions can streamline telephone contacts with legislators[1]:

- *Identify yourself.* State your name, the organization that you represent, and where you live.
- *State your position.* For example, say, "I am calling to support/oppose HB ______________ /SB ______________." Focus on only 1 or 2 points with anecdotal evidence to support your facts. Keep the message succinct and clear. Ask about the legislator's position on the issue. Be prepared to supply additional information about the issue, as needed.
- *Don't assume that your legislator is already an expert on the issue.* Be prepared to educate him or her, using local or personal examples in your explanation.

Be aware that telephone calls to the legislators' offices are often taken by staff members. Ask to speak to the legislator or to the aide who handles health care or preventive care issues. If that individual is not available, leave a message. Note the name and title of the person with whom you spoke and ask that the legislator send you a written response. It is important to be courteous, thanking the person who took the phone call. It is appreciated when an individual's time and effort is recognized.

Personal Contacts

Health care professionals can also meet directly with those in power to effectively advocate for others. The simple steps for meeting with political or health care policy makers involve preparation and planning. The following are suggestions for planning a meeting with politicians or other policy makers[2]:

- Make an appointment.
- State your specific purpose.
- Always introduce yourself. If you are with other representatives, select a primary spokesperson.
- Limit discussion to only 1 or 2 topics.
- Provide illustrations of the effect of policy change.
- Relate any adverse effect.

Table 18-2. Sample Letter Asking for Support for Health Promotion

The Honorable (fill in name of individual Senator or Congressperson)

US (Senate/House of Representatives)

Washington, DC (20510 [senate] / 20515 [house])

Dear (Senator __________ / Representative __________)

I am writing to urge you to support __________ (*specify funding, legislation, or other action*) for (*specify program, agency, program, event, or initiative*). The __________ (*specify name*) provides __________ (*give examples of the benefits provided by the program, etc.*)

The __________ (*specify organization*) is a nonprofit voluntary health organization based in __________ (*specify location*). This organization works with __________ (*populations served*) to __________ (*specify mission of the organization*). I support the mission and goals of this organization.

(Insert your personalized comments here, sharing some of your own experience with the issue or population served through the specific program, etc.)

The program offers __________ (*specify details of program offerings.*) I hope you will support __________ (*program, activity, funding, initiative, or event*) by __________ (*specify request*).

(Provide a brief paragraph with data supporting the program/effort and research supporting the efficacy of the proposed program, initiative, or effort.)

Thank you for consideration of this request. I hope you will contact __________ (*agency, funding source, other*) to express your support for this __________ (*organization, program, event, or initiative*). If you have any additional questions or need more information, feel free to contact __________ (*provide contact information*).

Sincerely,

Name

Address

City, state, zip

Telephone number

- Be flexible and avoid being argumentative.
- Be prepared for questions.
- Offer assistance or further information.

Table 18-3. Sample Thank You Letter
Organization Address Date Name of letter recipient Address First paragraph: *Express appreciation for support of the individual.* Second paragraph: *Indicate 1 or 2 areas discussed in the meeting that are key issues you would like to reinforce. Add additional data or relevant experience to reinforce the issue or to answer questions raised in discussion.* Third paragraph: *Express appreciation for the opportunity, time, and effort to discuss concerns with the individual.* Sincerely, (signature) Typed name

- Provide an accurate, up-to-date fact sheet.
- Thank the person for his or her time and consideration.
- Report back to your organization.
- Call or write with answers or information requested.
- Follow up with a note later (Table 18-3).

It is helpful to become acquainted with legislators to learn about their personal interests and goals, especially if they focus on community health and wellness. The best times to meet legislators are during a campaign, at fund-raising events, and at town meetings. Most state legislative offices maintain websites.

Indirect Advocacy

Health care professionals can indirectly affect public policy by becoming actively involved in a professional organization responsible for developing policy statements that guide lobbying efforts to affect national legislation. Developing a strong coalition can help move issues to the forefront.

In addition, health care professionals should help empower their clients and families to self-advocate. The United Cerebral Palsy Association has long supported families advocating for individuals with disabilities. One parent with a son who has cerebral palsy stresses how critical it is for parents and family members to not only push the system to maximize access to services for their own children or relatives, but also to speak out as a public advocate for all people with disabilities. "Don't be afraid to raise a little hell because, after all, you are your child's best advocate," says the mother of 3 who, besides caring for a family, also has a career with the Institute on Disabilities at Temple University.[3] This mother's experience led her to offer the following information to families of children with disabilities[3]:

- Most importantly, parents and family members are a child's best advocates.
- Get involved in coalitions, parent associations, and support groups.

- Go to public hearings.
- Attend rallies and participate in legislative visit days.
- Get to know the staff in local offices of your Congressional delegation.
- Build on small victories and positions of strength.
- Respond to requests from government agencies for public comment on policy changes.
- Search disability websites; you'll be surprised at what you can learn.
- Be patient and be prepared to hang in there for the long haul.
- Above all, never give up!

In addition to supporting clients and families in their advocacy efforts, health care professionals must share their educated opinions about health care issues.

As advocates, health care professionals must be diplomatic and take a broad view of the multiple factors involved in determining health care policy. The website Making Your Voice Heard by US Federal Legislators, the White House, State Legislators and Governors (https://w2.eff.org/congress/) offers helpful suggestions for contacting Congress. The site helps you identify your legislators and contact them appropriately via phone, fax, postal letters, e-mail, and in person. It also has a helpful link to do's and don'ts when contacting your legislator with an important message. For example, it is important to state that you are a constituent to gain more attention for your message. If you represent an organization or corporation, it is helpful to mention this larger set of constituents supporting legislation. Also, legislation should be referred to by its number and title (eg, "I am writing to urge you to support H.R.# *title*, sponsored by *name of representative*.") Finally, this site offers background information on activism and the legislative process. Polite and meaningful dialogue provides policy makers with needed information to make sound decisions. As advocates, health care professionals should convince their policy makers of the importance of addressing key issues for the benefit of their constituents and society at large.

Advocacy at the National Level

Health care professionals can align themselves with national organizations to gain support for preventive care issues. Many organizations advocate for public health and preventive care, including the American Physical Therapy Association, the American Public Health Association (APHA), the American Academy of Pediatrics, the American Academy of Family Physicians, and numerous other professional and national organizations.

The APHA is the oldest and largest organization of public health professionals in the world, representing more than 50,000 members from over 50 occupations of public health.[4] The APHA is concerned with a broad set of issues affecting personal and environmental health, including federal and state funding for health programs, pollution control, programs and policies related to chronic and infectious diseases, a smoke-free society, and professional education in public health. The APHA has a website listing the congressional record of support for health issues (http://www.apha.org/),[4] as well as fact sheets for major health issues, including ergonomics, health disparities, mental health parity, obesity, the patient's bill of rights, and others. Their website also links to other organizations offering health information, including aging, children's health, diabetes, cancer, autoimmune diseases, chronic conditions and disorders, health policy and advocacy, and related topics.

> [The APHA has] significant concerns about the ongoing changes in the organization and financing of medical care and health services and the impact of these changes on public health. Specific issues of concern include denials of necessary care, underfunding of public health and prevention services, lack of accountability, loss of choice of health care provider, inadequate access to care (especially specialists), lack of comparable and

consumer-friendly information and data about health plans, and abuses in marketing. In addition, APHA is troubled by research findings that raise questions about the effectiveness of managed care organizations in meeting health care needs associated with prevention and with managing chronic conditions.[4]

These issues need to be addressed through advocacy by health care professionals, other health care providers, patients and families receiving care, as well as policy makers.

Working to create a grassroots network for important preventive care issues requires time and effort but affords advocates much-needed support for the passage of legislation that benefits community members with unmet health care needs. Contacting the APHA, American Physical Therapy Association (APTA) special interest groups, health organizations who support health promotion, and other groups affected by health care issues can further develop the needed network for influencing public policy at a national level.

Advocacy at the State Level

Health care professionals can have a major effect on health care by addressing policy makers at the state level. If the legislation is a health care bill, it will fare better with support from the state's professional health care associations, health department, specialty medical organizations, and interested consumer groups. Enlisting support may be as easy as making a phone call or sending an e-mail to an organization's president or a university program. Meeting with a group's board of directors to make a brief presentation can help advocate for a specific issue. Some state legislatures have study committees and task force meetings between legislative sessions. The work these groups do often results in legislative recommendations for the upcoming session. Health care professionals can ask their organization(s) if they can serve on these advisory boards as proponents for preventive care. As advisors, health care professionals can educate policy makers about the cost benefits and societal benefits of health promotion and prevention practice.

Advocacy at the Local Level

Many state allocations for health care are dispersed to local health departments for the dissemination of health-related educational materials, as well as the development and management of health-related programs. Preventive care should be designed to meet the specific needs of a given community. Health care professionals should work in concert with their local health departments to ensure that comprehensive preventive care, including fitness programs, can be accessed by all populations in need.

When attempting to work in partnership with local health departments, it is essential to acknowledge the department's overall mission, as well as the scope of services available. Generally, the mission of the local health department is to promote, preserve, and protect the health of citizens in the particular locality. Programs meeting local health care needs often include communicable disease control programs; community partnerships and chronic disease programs; health education and health communication programs; environmental health programs; and maternal, child, and family health programs. Although health departments attempt to meet the needs of their local community, many citizens are not receiving adequate services. Health care professionals should help address issues of accessibility and affordability through advocacy at national, state, and local levels and partner with local health departments to provide health information and strategies for improving health, fitness, and wellness. Health care professionals are uniquely qualified to address preventive care issues for all segments of the population, especially in the areas of fitness and lifestyle behaviors.

Keys to successful advocacy at the local level include (1) clearly identifying the health issue, (2) describing the effect of the health concern on individual and the community (both positive and negative consequences), and (3) providing cost-effective solutions to the health problem. Offering financial data allows policy makers to consider whether health promotion options are cost-effective. For example, the following fact could be used to secure financing for education about children's preventive care: "Every $1 spent on child safety seats saves $71."[5] Encouraging the purchase of child safety seats as a preventive measure can help reduce the overall costs of injuries acquired in motor vehicle accidents. A small investment in educating the public about child safety seats is a cost-effective measure for ensuring child safety and reducing expenses for health care. Thorough research about an issue, including financial data, can provide the needed information to make a particular issue a priority for legislators at the local, state, and national levels.

Advocacy for World Health

More health care professionals are becoming involved in international causes, providing health care services to third-world countries and advocating for improved health care. This effort requires expanding cultural competency for enhanced communication and program effectiveness.

The World Health Organization (WHO), established in 1948, is the United Nations specialized agency for health, designed to help all peoples reach the highest possible level of health. Health is defined in the World Health Organization's Constitution as "a state of complete physical, mental and social well-being and not merely the absence of disease or infirmity."[6] This organization aims to improve the health of people around the world, especially disadvantaged populations.

> Health promotion strategies are not limited to a specific health problem, nor to a specific set of behaviors. WHO as a whole applies the principles of, and strategies for, health promotion to a variety of population groups, risk factors, diseases, and in various settings. Health promotion, and the associated efforts put into education, community development, policy, legislation and regulation, are equally valid for prevention of communicable diseases, injury and violence, and mental problems, as they are for prevention of non-communicable diseases.[6]

WHO established 8 Millennium Development Goals, which all 191 United Nations member states have agreed to try to achieve by the year 2015. The 8 Millennium Development Goals are the following:

1. To eradicate extreme poverty and hunger
2. To achieve universal primary education
3. To promote gender equality and empower women
4. To reduce child mortality
5. To improve maternal health
6. To combat HIV/AIDS, malaria, and other diseases
7. To ensure environmental sustainability
8. To develop a global partnership for development[6]

Health care professionals should work in collaboration with other national organizations to advocate on an international level for health promotion strategies for a healthy lifestyle, healthy life course, supportive environments, and supporting settings, as outlined above.

Health care professionals can connect with the international community through various means, but the Internet probably is the easiest route. Advocacy for health education, as well as removal of barriers to physical activity, can benefit all communities. The WHO website (www.who.

int) lists information about various countries, including health indicators, health risks, resources/health expenditures, health system organization and regulation (including key legislation), disease prevalence, human resources (doctors, nurses, and other health professionals), and media centers. In addition, national contact information is provided for health care professionals seeking additional information about international advocacy for health promotion.

The World Federation of Public Health Associations (WFPHA)[7] is:

> [A]n international, nongovernmental organization composed of multidisciplinary national public health associations. It is the only worldwide professional society representing and serving the broad field of public health. WFPHA's mission is to promote and protect global public health. It does this throughout the world by supporting the establishment and organizational development of public health associations and societies of public health, through facilitating and supporting the exchange of information, knowledge, and the transfer of skills and resources, and through promoting and undertaking advocacy for public policies, programs and practices that will result in a healthy and productive world.

The WFPHA offers international public health educational information and training. For more information about this organization, go to http://www.wfpha.org/.

Advocacy for Older Adults

The older adult segment of our population is growing rapidly, and policy makers are seeking to implement policies that prevent or delay the onset of disabilities in this population for as long as possible. It is in the public's best interest to help older individuals remain independent and economically active as long as possible. Health care professionals need to advocate for optimal environments that enable older adults to function independently and maintain a good quality of life. Barriers to physical activity and healthy living include limited access to public transport and physical barriers to health care facilities. Policy makers must be encouraged to implement age-friendly environments for optimal health promotion.

In the closing session of the American Geriatric Society in 2004, Jessie C. Gruman, PhD, discussed "Health Promotion for Older Adults: Nice or Necessary?"[8] In her presentation, Dr. Gruman discussed the paradox of our current society:

> In the past century, Americans—through better nutrition, better medical care, and better social policy—have experienced a 56% increase in life expectancy, from 49 years to 77 years, and have earned the means to enjoy it. Overall, older Americans have the lowest poverty rate of any age group. But they also spend far more of the nation's health care dollars per capita than any other group. Almost 30% of Medicare spending is on those who are in the last year of their lives. So, one 'moral values' question we have been asking is how to even things out so that health promotion can reduce unnecessary pain and suffering and thus decrease the need for acute and post-acute medical intervention? This raises another, much tougher question: How much energy are we, in this time of mind-numbing deficits, going to devote to promoting health and preventing disability in older people, when the benefits may be minimal, hard-won, or short-lived? The answers to this last question will be powerfully influenced by the three A's—ageism, affordability, and accommodation.[8]

The barriers to health promotion in older populations include not only physical barriers, but also psychological barriers that limit options. *Ageism*, or prejudice against older adults, affects the amount of research conducted to fully explore options for healthy aging. Affordability of health promotion options is often beyond the means of many older adults: a gym membership can cost over $600 a year, personal trainers charge $40 an hour, good shoes cost $100 a year, and a home treadmill can cost between $700 and $1,700. Dr. Gruman continues:

> [W]hile the economic barriers are formidable, so, too, are the agglomeration of frustrating annoyances faced by older people who just want to get around like they used to do, if only a bit slower and safer. For example, if you do have good shoes and good knees, what use are they to your health if your neighborhood is poorly lit with high crime and broken sidewalks inviting you to fall?... I wish I could foretell a different, more expansive, enthusiastic future for health promotion, but I think that the sage poet, Mick Jagger, nails what I believe should be the new theme song for advocates of health promotion for older adults: You can't always get what you want, but if you try sometimes, you just might find you get what you need.[8]

Health care professionals must be willing to remove barriers that older adults face when trying to access health promotion education and activities, as difficult as this may be. These challenges are not unique to older adults in the United States. Other countries face similar issues as people age and health care costs soar. As advocates, health care professionals play an important role in preparing older adults for later stages of life and encouraging their involvement in social policies that encompass physical, psychological, cultural, religious, spiritual, economic, health, and other factors that will challenge them with aging.

Summary

Health care professionals must serve as advocates for access to health care services and products across the life span and around the world, as all communities benefit from preventive practice and health promotion. Advocacy must penetrate the barriers of ageism, racism, and other discriminatory practices that limit access to health protection, health promotion, and prevention of illness and injury. Health care professionals must be leaders in promoting health and wellness while ensuring that barriers to achieving the overarching goals of Healthy People 2020 are removed. In addition, advocacy must extend beyond national borders to international communities with similar health care challenges. Through organized efforts, such as networking and advocacy, culturally competent health care professionals can restore hope to people in need.

References

1. Advocacy tools. FamiliesUSA. http://familiesusa.org/resources/tools-for-advocates/. Accessed May 21, 2013.
2. Advocacy skills. Brain Injury Association. http://www.headinjury.com/advocacy.htm. Accessed May 23, 2013.
3. Advocacy tools: individual and family advocacy. United Cerebral Palsy. http://www.ucp.org/ucp_generaldoc.cfm/1/8/6602/6602-6628/3163. Accessed January 18, 2006.
4. About APHA. American Public Health Association. http://www.apha.org/about/. Accessed May 23, 2013.
5. National action plan for child injury prevention: an agenda to prevent injuries and promote the safety of children and adolescents in the United States. Centers for Disease Control and Prevention. http://www.cdc.gov/safechild/pdf/National_Action_Plan_for_Child_Injury_Prevention.pdf. Accessed May 20, 2013.
6. About WHO. World Health Organization. http://www.who.int/about/en/. Accessed May 23, 2013.
7. About us. World Federation of Public Health Associations. http://www.wfpha.org/about-us.html. Accessed May 20, 2014.
8. Gruman JC. Health promotion for older adults: nice or necessary? Paper presented at: American Geriatric Society Confronting Ageism and Economics in Promoting Elder Health; November 23, 2004.

19

Marketing Health and Wellness

Steven G. Lesh, PhD, PT, SCS, ATC and
Catherine Rush Thompson, PT, PhD, MS

"Health promotion is the process of enabling people to increase control over their health and its determinants. This is done by strengthening individual skills and capabilities and the capacity of groups to change the many conditions, particularly the social and economic causes,that affect health." —Kwok-Cho Tang, Robert Beaglehole, and Desmond O'Byrne, "Policy and partnership for health promotion action—addressing the determinants of health," World Health Organization

Good health is an asset, and health care providers need to share this message with the public to build a prevention practice. According to the American Marketing Association, marketing health promotion involves creating a unique message that attracts the attention of the general public but also carves out a successful niche to meet the unique needs of individuals with special needs. Marketing involves thoughtful planning and development of health and wellness concepts and promotion through multiple media, including mass media, newsprint, television commercials, social media, and websites. The long-term success of any prevention practice requires sustained efforts to connect with a target market, recognizing that others are similarly wooing clients. Creating a network of reliable referrals, along with marketing successfully to individuals with special needs, requires building a reputation based on trust and success for those seeking health and wellness services. Ideally, marketing should provide valuable health and wellness information that is appreciated by its clients. Above all, health care practitioners should remember 2 essential aspects of marketing: (1) knowing the target audience and (2) building positive relationships with the consumer.[1]

Make It Personal

The best way to market health and wellness is to make it personal. This requires knowing the personal characteristics of those who might benefit from health and wellness services (ie, the target market). Classic marketing is founded at the intersection of the target market and focused strategies designed to meet clients' expectations and needs. Before any marketing plans can be put

Thompson CR.
Prevention Practice and Health Promotion: A Health Care Professional's Guide to Health, Fitness, and Wellness, Second Edition (pp 309-321).

into action or any revenues from converted clients can be counted, a careful understanding and appreciation of the target audience must be conducted.[2]

As health care professionals designing a health promotion and wellness program, it is important to ask the following questions:

- *Who*: Who is the target market seeking health and wellness services? In theory, everyone is interested in personal health and wellness, yet many periodically lapse into unhealthy lifestyle behaviors. Prevention practice demands a healthy lifestyle daily; it requires discipline, dedication, and consistency, especially in a world filled with messages that encourage drinking sugary colas and eating fried foods, as well as watching television or playing on the computer for hours. Considering the transtheoretical model of change, some individuals may not even consider changing poor lifestyle habits; however, health promotion messages can help individuals, especially those at risk for pathology or those with chronic conditions, to focus on and contemplate changes in lifestyle to optimize their health. Programs targeted for special populations, such as those with chronic pathologies, are offered by health care professionals with an expertise in a particular condition. When seeking quality care, those with chronic conditions are especially concerned that their needs are recognized and met.
- *Why*: Why engage in a health promotion program rather than doing it alone? Ample evidence suggests that exercise and diet adherence is enhanced by social support.[2-4] The benefits of a healthy lifestyle can be spelled out in physical and psychological benefits, but often, the reality of costly medical care can motivate engagement in maintained health promotion activities. A structured health and wellness program offers social support that promotes adherence to healthy lifestyle habits.
- *When*: When should clients begin a health and wellness program? Given the various states of health and illness, it is important to provide the benefits of specific services tailored to the various stages of recovery and health maintenance. Many individuals with health conditions are wary of engaging in physical activity for fear of injury or exacerbating their conditions.[5] Outlining comprehensive, safe, and effective health promotion programs with preventive care offers this population a broad spectrum of options that can be personalized for their needs. For example, older adults with arthritis could be involved in a program comprising aquatic therapy, socialization, nutrition seminars, exercise, and support groups designed for secondary prevention.
- *Where*: Where should health care providers connect with clients and referrals alike? Marketing can be achieved through a wide range of options, including newsletters and websites that serve specific populations, blogs featuring updated health news, and educational forums addressing the needs of both clients and referral sources. Connecting avenues include e-mail, social media, health fairs, trade fairs, sporting events, and support groups.
- *Options*: What alternative programs offer the same services? At present, there are limited options for health and wellness programs designed for populations at risk for pathology or who have chronic conditions. Given the scarcity of such programs, it is important to explore available options and to create new offerings with unique programming for a target market in need. Additionally, each community benefits from a network of programs that can offer a wide range of options that meet clients' needs. A collaborative relationship between programs can offer a ready referral source for specialized health promotion for unique populations.

Understanding the answers to these questions will help focus the marketing plan on specific populations. However, marketing health promotion may also be directed to a diverse target market, spanning all ages and levels of functional abilities. The key is to create a message that connects with the target markets by gaining their attention, captivating their interests, appealing to their emotions and desires, and spurring them into action. For example, the eye-catching message, "Your body is worth $45 million—take care of it!" combines the cognitive and affective bases that affect behavior by validating personal value and the need to preserve this key asset.

Diversity in the population needs to be appreciated and addressed through a marketing plan with multiple strategies to reach all elements of the target market. For example, if a wellness organization produces a marketing campaign designed to prevent birth defects through regular prenatal care, will it reach all of the target market if it fails to produce Spanish-language versions of the program? Marketing campaigns must be formulated using input from multiple sources, including data collection using personal interviews, written questionnaires, technology-based interfacing, and the review of current data available on national websites, including Healthy People 2020,[6] the Centers for Disease Control and Prevention,[7] and Health.gov.[8]

Surveys (a method of gathering information in writing or in person from a sample of individuals) are a commonly used tool, followed closely by focus groups.

Focus groups are live samples of members from the desired target market organized to give opinions and reactions to products or marketing campaigns.

Opinion polls are surveys using sampling and are designed to represent the opinions of a population by asking a small number of people a series of questions and then extrapolating the answers to the larger group.

Building a Positive Relationship

The second essential aspect of marketing is building a positive relationship with potential clients and referral sources. A positive relationship can be developed if targeted clients perceive the health, fitness, and wellness services to be reliable, cost-effective, and easily accessed. Individuals with disabilities "face substantial barriers and they fear the costs of participating in health promotion activities will be high. Moreover, if medical providers have said that their condition won't improve, they may expect few benefits from health promotion. Any conversation about health promotion activities must take such expectations into account."[5] Health care providers must provide information to remove potential barriers that limit participation in health promotion, demonstrate the benefits to those with chronic illness, and embrace the challenges of providing health, fitness, and wellness options to all populations in need of preventive care (primary, secondary, or tertiary care). If qualified professionals cannot adequately market their skills and knowledge, less qualified individuals may corner the market on preventive practice and comprehensive health care.

A basic knowledge of key marketing concepts can help the entrepreneurial health care provider develop a strong business that serves the health needs of targeted populations in the community. Each profession in health care has a responsibility to increase awareness of its specialized services for health promotion and link with other health care providers collaboratively to create an effective network to screen and refer for optimal outcomes.

Marketing Mix: The Four Ps

Product, pricing, placement, and *promotion*, the four Ps, are the essential domains of the classic marketing model.[9,10] Marketing plans are developed and implemented within each of these 4 domains to foster the business-to-client relationship.

Product

Product in health promotion and prevention practice may include the programs and resources offered to meet the needs and expectations of targeted clients.[10] The product includes the entire spectrum from tangible goods (eg, a therapy ball for a home exercise program to supplement a group exercise session) to intangible services available to meet consumers' needs (eg, screening for fall risk or yoga classes for older adults). When a product is first introduced, early adopters will rush to use the new product because the mainstream has not yet been enticed to purchase the product. As the mainstream begins to use the product, a growth phase occurs in which the number of sales increases along with the number of clients making purchases. Eventually, the cycle will see a maturation in which the product becomes stable in terms of sales and new clients. Once a product has matured, it can continue unchanged for many years or can slide into a decline. Industry sales and profits notably decrease in this final phase of the product life cycle.[10]

Many strategies can be used to manage the product during its life cycle:

- *Increase frequency of use*: Increasing the client's frequency of using a service or product is a common strategy. For example, encouraging existing customers to participate in additional programming that meets their needs can extend the life cycle of that service.
- *Increase the number of clients*: Health care professionals can increase the number of new clients by educating and converting them to customers of existing programs. Marketing existing programs by using stories of success can help lure potential customers to services, especially when those stories are authenticated by word of mouth.
- *Find a new or alternative use for existing products*: Some health promotion programs are integrated into preexisting medical facilities or community centers. These facilities can extend their programming to individuals with special needs during off-peak hours. For example, one health promotion program features aerobic exercises within an existing rehabilitation gym and offers open gym hours for previous clients and patients.
- When all other strategies fail, repackaging the same product with a new appearance and new marketing campaign is another option.

Pricing

Pricing is the exchange value for a good or service.[10] Determining pricing in the health and wellness sector is sometimes based on competitors' practice and sometimes based on predeterminates, such as insurance company payments or government regulations.

Pricing can be difficult to establish and is often a dynamic entity. The primary issue to consider when establishing a price is that it helps to determine profitability for the organization. In the simplest of terms, collected revenues from the goods and services must exceed the cost of selling those goods and services. Other considerations include the perception of the product or service with the attached price tag. Products with higher-than-average price tags impart an image of prestige and greater quality. Conversely, products with lower-than-average prices may reflect a value purchase or, at times, a below-quality offering. In general, the price of the product should be comparable with local competition without being significantly higher or lower. A method of increasing pricing and profitability is to package or bundle product offerings, giving the appearance of great value but also increasing revenue.[10]

Placement

Placement, or distribution, is the aspect of the marketing mix that is concerned with how, when, and where the product is placed before the target market.[10] Inherent within the domain of distribution and placement are the key factors of the distribution channels and the logistics to make the plan a reality. The distribution channels or supply chain consist of the entire spectrum of events and activities that take the finished good or service from production to the end user. These distribution processes and the inherent efficiencies within the chain can include factors like inventory, materials handling, packaging, ordering, shipping, and warehousing. The logistics of the placement include activities for the coordination and flow of information.

Promotion

The final formal aspect of the marketing mix, *promotion*, accounts for the "...informing, persuading and influencing of the consumer's purchase decision."[11] Its elements include the strategies and plans that are enacted to create an environment in which the consumer will purchase the product or service. The key element of promotion is the marketing communication that appears to the potential buyer through a variety of media (eg, television, print, Internet).[11] For a promotional strategy to be effective, consumers must be made aware of the product or service and how it can meet their needs. If a client is not aware of the product or service, the chances of making a purchase are low.

Packaging

Packaging, although not exclusive enough to warrant its own domain apart from the classic 4 Ps, is something to consider and respect as part of an established or developing marketing campaign (ie, the fifth P).[9] Product packaging is an important part of the perception of the goods and services. Packaging can mean the simple appearance of the insert sleeve in the latest computer program, but it is also the state and condition of the location in which services are provided. A fitness center that has old and antiquated equipment may not be an appealing sell to a potential client.

Another element to consider in the health and wellness sector is the visual discrepancy between healthy people and people with various afflictions or even varying age groups or sexes. Many health clubs establish sex-specific hours in their exercise rooms. Likewise, if the target population is a healthy young adult market, overlapping hours in a swimming pool with an arthritic exercise group or with elementary age children on a field trip may not provide the best packaging of the service.

Health Care Marketing: The SCAP Model

Marketing in the health care world has taken the shape of public relations campaigns, organizational awareness, staff recruitment and retention, direct insurance marketing, and patient satisfaction efforts.[10] In recent years, health care organizations have worked more aggressively to get health and wellness products directly in front of the client. The classic 4 Ps have been redesigned into this model to more appropriately reflect the marketing mix of goods and services within the health care field: service, consideration, access, and promotion (SCAP).[12]

- *Services* that are designed to meet the health and wellness needs of the target market are identified and promoted.
- *Consideration* is the value for the service. In the health care world, direct, cash-based reimbursements are not directed to the organization from the consumer of the service. Deductibles, copayments, and coinsurances are the language of payments, coupled with allowables and preferred networks from the insurance company perspective. Frequently, the consumer does not consider the cost to the provider in the payment of services rendered.
- *Access* is the ease of obtaining the service from the provider. When and how often a service can be accessed is a consideration in the marketing mix and is partly responsible for a client's decision to use a particular service.
- *Promotion* of the health and wellness service is the component that makes the target market aware of the existence of the service. The promotion should gain awareness, impart knowledge, and suggest goods and services to use.

Integrated Marketing

Integrated marketing is an expansion of the classic model of marketing founded on the premise that the individual consumer has unique wants and needs, coupled with a driving effort to produce a consistent marketing message for the consumer. In today's communication generation, the marketer possesses a wide variety of media with which to reach potential consumers (eg, television, Internet, newsprint, radio, e-mail, social media). With such varied opportunities to advertise to the public, great potential exists for the delivery of disjointed and inconsistent messages. Integrated marketing is the push to present a consistent message to the individual consumer. Its 4 foundational elements include the following:

1. Nurturing personal relationships with the customer
2. Using current information technology to encourage interactivity and rapid communication
3. Fostering mission marketing or a shared organizational vision
4. Distributing a consistent message

Nurturing personal relationships was mentioned in the opening of this chapter as one of the most important things for an organization to pursue. Integrated marketing relies on the ability of the organization to connect and make the individual customer feel special. Today's generation of consumers is accustomed to personalization, customization, and immediate gratification. Attempts at personalization are necessary to master if success is the ultimate goal. Information is now global and nearly instantaneous. Understanding the target market and how consumers access information is critical to where, how, and when an organization will use its marketing budget. The best use of funds may be directed at print ads or radio spots; Internet banner ads and e-mail newsletters may provide greater access. Print ads can mention a web link to a wealth of information about fitness, health, wellness, hours of operation, biographies of employees, costs, and even the potential to register or pay fees online.

Fostering mission marketing and supporting a shared organizational vision are valuable elements of the integrated marketing approach. The mission of the organization should be easily understood by the consumer through the marketing and actions of the organization.

Distributing message consistency is the final piece of the integrated marketing. After personalization efforts have been fostered through rapid communication exchange technologies and the mission of the organizations is set and shared through all levels, the message that is distributed should be consistent and to the point. A feeling of familiarity is a major selling point for consumers. When a consumer recognizes a trusted logo or trade name, even if the product is unfamiliar, the consumer is likely to purchase from the familiar company as opposed to an unfamiliar company. The consistency of the message should be easily recognized through uniform themes, color schemes, and logos.

Marketing Strategies for Health and Wellness Centers and Organizations

Before marketing strategies are presented, budget should be discussed. A budget should be developed that matches the goals and objectives of both the marketing plan and the mission of the organization. Many health care organizations develop their marketing budget through a process of what is left over after all other bills have been paid. Although this may be the reality, it is not good business sense. Some experts believe that an organization should spend as much on a marketing plan as its chief competitors. Others disagree. The health care industry, hospitals, insurance companies, and drug corporations have implemented enterprising marketing campaigns directed to the individual consumer.

For adequate budgeting, an annual percentage of gross revenues should be allocated to marketing. Setting the percentage may be a process of trial and error and may range drastically depending on business objectives. A business-to-business organization may allot as little as 1% of revenues. A company looking to introduce a new product on the market may dedicate as much as 50% of initial target revenues to penetrate the market. For instance, a wellness center has projected annual revenues of $200,000 and allocated 10% annually for marketing. If resources are not dedicated to marketing, it is difficult to attract new customers and keep existing customers. If the wellness organization does not work to keep the target audience aware of its services and products, a competing organization will work to make its goods and services readily available to the other organization's customers.

Goodwill

Goodwill is a term used in marketing and corporate valuation that reflects the positive attitude and feelings in the community about the product.[12] Perception of a product or corporate goodwill by the public and potential target market centers on the status, participation, and earned respect within the community. Some organizations establish goodwill by contributing and donating goods and services to sectors of need within the community. Others establish goodwill by providing valued quality products; still others establish goodwill by being long-standing members of and contributors to the community. Establishing goodwill can become an invaluable asset in developing a marketing plan. Products, companies, and wellness causes can build marketing plans on established goodwill by providing special services to underserved populations and sharing their pro bono efforts through public relations.

Logos

Logo and slogan products provide many great opportunities for a consistent message and image.[13] An organization can develop an attractive logo that supports the mission and promotes the organizational objectives as part of an integrated marketing plan. Color themes, logos, and slogans should be used consistently across all marketing venues. Logos and color schemes can be developed internally through the use of various graphic imaging software programs or can be outsourced to local graphic design or Internet-based companies. Logos can be added to polo shirts worn by staff members to present a professional and consistent appearance. Promotional supply companies provide a wide array of creative and professional marketing items. With all of the possible promotional product opportunities to deplete a marketing budget, wise and careful analysis of the anticipated product distribution and expected conversion rate should be considered.

Newsletters

Newsletters, either in print form mailed to current or prospective consumers, or in electronic form circulated via the Internet or e-mail, can provide marketing and consumer information elements about the wellness organizations.[13] This communication tool can be published weekly, monthly, quarterly, semiannually, or annually. Newsletters can contain public health information or specific company information. Biographies about employees or healthy eating tips could be regularly included. Updates on product information and services could supplement a regular newsletter installment. At the minimum, to adhere to an integrated marketing approach, the newsletter should contain familiar product or trade names, logos, coloring, and company contact information. Retail businesses can solicit e-mail addresses from consumers to compile a distribution list for the periodic newsletter.

Websites

Websites have become a staple of information about organizations that provide goods and services to the public. Website design and hosting can be done internally or can be outsourced to companies that provide a professional service. Internet-based websites should adhere to the following simple principles:

- Have an easily identifiable URL
- Have all information accessible in less than 3 mouse clicks
- Have complete company contact information for those potential customers or current clients who wish to reach the company[14]

The URL (uniform resource locator) is more commonly known as the web address for the website. It is the string of characters that appears in the navigation bar of the web browser. Typically, the URL begins with "http://" or "ftp://" and may end in a variety of combinations, including .com, .org, .biz, .net, .tv, or .gov. This domain name should be easily recognizable and remembered but should not take a great deal of effort to key into a web browser. Note that organizations with similar domain names make identification with any company difficult. Also, *cybersquatters* (people who buy domain names corresponding to a famous brand name or trademark in hopes of reselling the domain for a significant profit) may complicate selection of domains. Domain names are secured by paying an annual registration fee to a domain registration company (eg, http://www.networksolutions.com).[13]

Navigation of a website should be easy, with information available with only a few clicks. A navigation bar should contain at least corporate and contact information. A web page that includes frequently asked questions (FAQs) can be of great assistance to the web surfer. Complex website technology can make a website that is slow to download or does not easily run on all web browsers. Although broadband use is growing, many people still access the Internet via more traditional dial-up connections that do not load complicated or graphic-laden websites as easily. It is tempting to use many of the creative tools and software that are at the disposal of website designers, but a site that is too complex for the average user may serve as a source of frustration and reflect negatively on the organization. While developing content for the website, note the key criteria listed in Table 19-1 that evaluates the effectiveness of a health-related website.[13]

Search Engines

Search engines are Internet-based tools that are designed to produce responses or "hits" to keyword queries entered by the computer user.[15] If the wellness organization has a web presence and relies on access to the web from search engines, it is beneficial to work with the major search engine providers to ensure that their products and services appear at or near the top of the list with associated keywords. Few companies dedicate marketing funds to take full advantage of the potential revenue streams from *search engine marketing* (SEM).[15] Detailed strategies to take advantage of this ever-growing and ever-changing technology are beyond the scope of this chapter, but interested organizations can find many dedicated reference books and sources on the Internet itself for this strategy.

Banner Advertisements

Banner advertisements are web-based advertisements in which a website sells or hosts space on their page to other companies or organizations in the form of a banner advertisement or a sidebar advertisement.[13] The banner ad appears either on the top or bottom of the web page. Smaller sidebar advertisements are usually embedded along the periphery of the web page. Users are able to click on the ad, which will take them to a second page with more information or to the direct web page of the advertiser. Soliciting banner or sidebar advertisement space on a host web page should

TABLE 19-1. HEALTH-RELATED WEBSITE EVALUATION FORM

Content

- The purpose of the site is clearly stated or may be clearly inferred.
- The information covered does not appear to be an infomercial (ie, an advertisement disguised as health education).
- There is no bias evident.
- If the site is opinionated, the author discusses all sides of the issue, giving each due respect.
- All aspects of the subject are covered adequately.
- External links are provided to fully cover the subject.

Accuracy

- The information is accurate.
- Sources are clearly documented.
- The website states that it subscribes to Health on the Net code principles.

Author

- The site is sponsored by or is associated with an institution or organization.
- For sites created by an individual, author's/editor's credentials (educational background, professional affiliations, certifications, past writings, experience) are clearly stated.
- Contact information (e-mail, address, and/or phone number) for the author/editor or webmaster is included.

Currency

- The date of publication is clearly posted.
- The revision date is recent enough to account for changes in the field.

Audience

- The type of audience the author is addressing is evident (eg, academic, youth, minority, general).
- The level of detail is appropriate for the audience.
- The reading level is appropriate for the audience.
- Technical terms are appropriate for the audience.

Navigation

- Internal links add to the usefulness of the site.
- Information can be retrieved in a timely manner.
- A search mechanism is necessary to make the site useful.
- A search mechanism is provided.
- The site is organized in a logical manner, facilitating the location of information.
- Any software necessary to use the page has links to download software from the Internet.

(continued)

Table 19-1 (continued). Health-Related Website Evaluation Form

External Links

- Links are relevant and appropriate for this site.
- Links are operable.
- Links are current enough to account for changes in the field.
- Links are appropriate for the audience (eg, sites for the general public do not include links to highly technical sites).
- Links connect to reliable information from reliable sources.
- Links are provided to organizations that should be represented.

Structure

- Educational graphics and art add to the usefulness of the site.
- Decorative graphics do not significantly slow downloading.
- Text-only option is available for text-only web browsers.
- Usefulness of site does not suffer when using text-only option.
- Options are available for disabled persons (eg, large-print, audio).
- If audio and video are components of the site and cannot be accessed, the information on the site is still complete.

Adapted from Potts K. *Web Design and Marketing Solutions for Business Websites.* Berkley, CA: Apres; 2007.

be determined by the documented history of hits or number of times the web page is viewed by potential consumers. A critical factor related to the number of hits is the conversion rate; simply put, this is the number of actual consumers that are converted from the number of hits observed. If a website claims to have 10,000 hits per month but only 15 new customers can be attributed to that ad, the monthly conversion rate is 0.15% (15/10,000). Costs of doing this type of advertisement are directly related to the size of the advertisement, the location (top of the page is premium), and the anticipated conversion rate. Some hosting companies will charge per the actual number of hits generated per month.

Spam, Spim, and Pop-up Ads

Spam, spim, and pop-up advertisements are generally undesirable means to support the marketing objectives of a wellness organization. Spam is unsolicited e-mail advertisements and spim is the instant messaging counterpart of spam.[13] Pop-up ads are the immediate presence of unsolicited windows that open when a website is accessed. The key to these marketing elements is that they are *unsolicited* and are frequently viewed in a negative light by the recipient. Many software companies today are selling products that prevent or block these types of direct communication efforts. Either of these avenues has potentially serious repercussions on the image and goodwill of an organization and should therefore be used judiciously.

Table 19-2 provides additional marketing strategies for health promotion that can be used to reach different target markets.

Table 19-2. Marketing Strategies for Health Promotion

The following marketing strategies may be used to increase the awareness of health and wellness programs:

- *Newsprint Advertisement:* Newspapers and magazines with large circulations reaching hundreds of thousands of people will charge premium rates for full page ads near the front. However, a small 2×2″ ad on the final page of the periodical will not cost as much. Circulations will vary depending on the day of the week the newspaper is published. More people are accessing newspapers via dedicated websites, so this option should be taken into account. The key is to make the most effective use of advertising dollars based on anticipated conversion rates.
- *Television and Radio Spots:* It costs money to get an advertising spot on the air, and the cost is dependent on the duration of time that the spot consumes. When considering television and radio spots, a careful target market analysis should be performed knowing which medium the target market frequently listens to or watches. One efficient way to explore these media is to ask existing customers their preferences. It is worthwhile to take advantage of the expertise of the radio and television stations about development and production of the advertising spot.
- *Scholarships:* A wellness organization could sponsor a scholarship, establishing criteria for receipt of the award and then presenting the award at a local ceremony. Publicity would come in terms of recognition at the ceremony and in the associated program and possibly as a public interest story in a local newspapers.
- *Sports Team and Event Sponsorships:* Purchasing banner ads that adorn a community recreation center, school, or college and printing ads in programs for special events provide exposure and goodwill to a wide array of potential customers.
- *Billboards:* Although billboards are limited in the scope of detailed information they can provide, they can attract attention and provide key information about the organization (eg, how to contact the organization through an Internet address, URL, or phone number).
- *Membership Discounts:* Offering periodic discounts, incentives, or appreciation events for valued clients show them that they are appreciated. Personalized communication (eg, handwritten notes) and cash discounts on products or regular services are additional options for demonstrating appreciation of valued clients. It is more cost effective to keep a valued customer than it is to recruit a new one.
- *Public Interest Stories and Services:* Newspaper columns addressing health and wellness issues and products create public interest and are cost-effective. The drawback of this type of marketing is that it cannot be counted on for consistent distribution because these types of news-based stories are often used as space fillers.
- *Word-of-Mouth Advertising:* This type of advertising is closely related to goodwill because people are often more comfortable using goods and services that trusted friends and family also use. One major drawback of word-of-mouth marketing is the potential for negative comments from disgruntled or unsatisfied customers. Conventional wisdom states that it only takes comments from one unhappy customer to offset the positive comments of 10 happy customers. The trends are common that unhappy people will tell more people about their negative experience than happy people will tell of their positive experience. At the very least, a regular

(continued)

TABLE 19-2 (CONTINUED). MARKETING STRATEGIES FOR HEALTH PROMOTION

program of thanking customers and informing them that their positive comments about their experience are much appreciated. Give clients a discount or referral bonus for every customer that they encourage to use the product. This type of strategy is highly effective and does not consume a significant part of the marketing budget.

- *Outreach Services and Health Fairs*: There is a wide array of plausible options for outreach services at schools, shopping centers, grocery stores, etc. Health fairs in particular have the potential of reaching a large audience in a small amount of time at a relatively low cost. If there is no organized health fair in the immediate region of the health and wellness organization, then this is a wonderful opportunity to organize and sponsor such an event.
- *Product Association*: Physical therapists can work to associate their products (health education, prescription for physical activity, and stress management) with healthy living and stress reduction.
- *Free Promotional Items and Free Services:* The term "free" catches the eye of the consumer but will only be effective if the lure of the free item or service converts potential consumers into regular clients. The success of promotional giveaway items (eg, paper cups, pens, etc) and services should be ultimately measured in a cost-effectiveness analysis, taking into consideration the actual conversion rate for new customers.

SUMMARY

Marketing involves making a personal connection and sustaining a meaningful relationship between clients and health care providers, a relationship built on knowledge, trust, and effectiveness that meet clients' needs. Identifying the target market and using rapid communications technologies to build individual relationships with the potential consumer are key attributes to any well-constructed marketing plan. Additionally, constructing a collaborative network of resources to optimize care builds a strong relationship with potential referral sources.

Health and wellness marketing, although similar to conventional marketing, is probably better reflected in the acronym of SCAP: service, consideration, access, and promotion. An integrated marketing approach is one that fosters a consistency of message and focuses on the needs of the individual. Many strategies, ranging from promotional items to logo-based products, websites, print advertisements, and TV/radio spots, can be used to promote health, fitness, and wellness to the specific populations served by health care providers. The value of preventive practice should be emphasized as the key to optimal health.

REFERENCES

1. Definition of marketing. American Marketing Association. http://www.marketingpower.com/AboutAMA/Pages/DefinitionofMarketing.aspx. Accessed May 30, 2013.
2. Oka RK, King AC, Young DR. Sources of social support as predictors of exercise adherence in women and men ages 50 to 65 years. *Womens Health*. 1995;1(2):161-175.

3. Duncan TE, McAuley E. Social support and efficacy cognitions in exercise adherence: a latent growth curve analysis. *J Behav Med.* 1993;16(2):199-218.
4. Aggarwal B, Liao M, Allegrante J, Mosca L. Low social support level is associated with non-adherence to diet at 1-year in the family intervention trial for heart health (FIT Heart). *J Nutr Educ Behav.* 2010;42(6):380-388.
5. Rimmer JH. Health promotion for people with disabilities: the emerging paradigm shift from disability prevention to prevention of secondary conditions. *Phys Ther.* 1999;79:495-502.
6. How to use data 2020. Healthy People 2020. http://www.healthypeople.gov/2020/data/default.aspx. Accessed June 1, 2013.
7. Data and statistics. Centers for Disease Control and Prevention. http://www.cdc.gov/datastatistics/. Accessed June 1, 2013.
8. Health information for individuals and families. US Department of Health and Human Services Office of Disease Prevention and Health Promotion. http://www.health.gov/. Accessed May 20, 2014.
9. Lesh SG. Integrated marketing for the new millennium. *Bus Educ Technol J.* 2000;2(2):35-37.
10. Marketing 101. Small Business Administration. http://www.sba.gov/content/marketing-101-basics. Accessed May 20, 2014.
11. Janal DS. *Online Marketing Handbook: How to Promote, Advertise, and Sell Your Product and Services on the Internet.* New York, NY: Wiley and Sons; 1998.
12. Longest B, Rakich J, Darr K. *Managing Health Services Organizations & Systems.* 4th ed. Baltimore, MD: Health Professionals Press; 2000.
13. Lesh SG, Konin J, DePalma B. Paths to profits. *Training & Conditioning.* 2002;12(8):20-24.
14. Lesh SG. Innovative technological communication trends in allied health: instant messaging now appearing on the radar screen. Paper presented at: ASAHP Annual Conference; October 20-23, 2004; Tampa, FL.
15. Bruemmer PJ. Establishing a search engine marketing budget. MarketingProfs. http://www.marketingprofs.com/2/bruemmer7.asp. Accessed February 2, 2006.

20

Managing a Prevention Practice
A Business Model

Shawn T. Blakeley, PT, CWI, CEES, MBA and
Catherine Rush Thompson, PT, PhD, MS

"America's health care system is in crisis precisely because we systematically neglect wellness and prevention."—Tom Harkin, Annual Conference: Preventative Medicine 2006, February 2005

PLANNING AND DESIGNING A HEALTH PROMOTION PROGRAM

Vision

Starting a prevention practice may be daunting, but management with an eye toward success can guide and inspire its development. Health care professionals should begin with a vision that embodies the purpose and passion that will sustain efforts during challenges encountered when starting a new business. This vision statement cohesively motivates all engaged in the business to move the program toward the desired goals of improved community health and wellness.

A *vision statement* is a statement or phrase describing long-term desired change resulting from the health organization's or program's work. Ideally, statements are clear, inspirational, memorable, and concise—expressed in as few as 10 words. For example, Healthy People 2020's vision for the nation is a "society in which all people live long, healthy lives."[1]

In formulating a vision statement, fundamental questions include the following[2]:

- What type of prevention practice and health promotion would best serve the community?
- Would the prevention practice complement a preexisting program or would it be created anew?
- What are the populations with unmet health care needs?

Thompson CR.
Prevention Practice and Health Promotion: A Health Care Professional's Guide to Health, Fitness, and Wellness, Second Edition (pp 323-338).

- What areas of expertise can the health care professional offer in the areas of primary, secondary, and tertiary prevention?

One model for fashioning health promotion programs that meet identified needs is the PRECEDE-PROCEED model of health promotion planning.[3] This model, developed over the last quarter century, is based on the following 2 propositions:

1. "Health and health risks are caused by multiple factors.
2. Because health and health risks are determined by multiple factors, efforts to effect behavioral, environmental, and social change must be multidimensional and multisectoral."[3]

The PRECEDE-PROCEED model broadly envisions health promotion encompassing quality of life, health, environment, and lifestyle, with influences from health education, media, advocacy, policy, regulation, resources, and organization. This model has been used to develop cancer prevention and control interventions and smoking cessation programs that encompass medical, educational, and governmental entities. "The goals of the model are to explain health-related behaviors and to design and evaluate the interventions designed to influence both the behaviors and the living conditions that influence them and their sequelae."[3] Using this model, health care professionals can more comprehensively (1) diagnose and evaluate environmental, genetic, and lifestyle factors affecting health; (2) advocate for policies, regulations, and resources for health, fitness, and wellness; and (3) participate in the development of effective strategies to affect the environment, lifestyle behaviors, and society as a whole. This complex process requires professionals with sophisticated skills, evidence-based techniques, and current data to collaborate with organizations and communities for program planning and implementation. Table 20-1 illustrates the stages of comprehensive evaluation, implementation, and evaluation of health promotion programs using the PRECEDE-PROCEED model.

Many programs featuring prevention practice are contained within medically based facilities (eg, hospitals, outpatient clinics, rehabilitation centers), educationally based facilities (eg, preschools, elementary schools, middle schools, high schools, universities), community-based recreational programs (eg, YMCA, Special Olympics), and businesses (eg, corporate wellness and ergonomic programs). Where is the optimal location for prevention practice? The key is to match the community need with the expertise and passion of health care professionals, making the program both convenient and accessible. For example, a physical therapist with expertise working with exercise-related injuries might envision setting up a partnership in a well-established fitness club, enabling a steady flow of clients referred for musculoskeletal injuries. Finally, health care professionals should research available health promotion programs and community resources before reinventing the wheel.

A Promising Business Plan

A promising business plan provides clear objectives, details desired services or products to meet unmet demand, explores prospective funding sources, outlines effective marketing strategies, and lays out a realistic timeline with financial milestones. The business plan provides a blueprint for the intended program, anticipating needs for equipment (purchase and maintenance), supplies, marketing costs, facilities, and qualified personnel. A good resource for developing a business plan is the US Small Business Administration (SBA) (www.sba.gov).[4] According to the SBA, the following 4 rudimentary questions need to be answered before composing a plan[4]:

1. What service or product does your business provide and what needs does it fill?
2. Who are the potential customers for your product or service and why will they purchase it from you?
3. How will you reach your potential customers?
4. Where will you get the financial resources to start your business?

TABLE 20-1. PRECEDE-PROCEED MODEL				
PHASE	**ASSESSMENT**	**IMPLEMENTATION**	**EVALUATION**	**FACTORS**
1	Social			Quality of life
2	Epidemiologic			Health
3	Behavioral & environmental			Behavior, lifestyle, environment
4	Educational & ecological			Predisposing factors, reinforcing factors, enabling factors
5	Administrative policy			Health services, health education, health promotion, policy, regulations
6		Program implementation		Predisposing factors, reinforcing factors, enabling factors
7			Process involved in programming	Behavior, lifestyle, environment
8			Effect of programming	Health
9			Outcome of programming	Quality of life

Adapted from Tolma EL, Cheney MK, Troup P, Hann N. Designing the process evaluation for the collaborative planning of a local turning point partnership. *Health Promot Practice.* 2009;10(4):537-548; and Crosby R, Noar SM. What is a planning model? An introduction to PRECEDE-PROCEED. *J Public Health Dent.* 2011;71 Suppl 1:S7-S15.

Table 20-2 outlines business plan components that should be considered when starting a small business, such as a prevention practice or health promotion program.

Services or Products That Fill an Unmet Need

Before approaching any source of funding, the health care professional must do a *needs assessment* to determine whether the proposed program meets a community need. Health care professionals should thoroughly explore other programs in the area, asking about provided services and needs unmet by competitors. Finding a unique niche eliminates competition and provides the community with desirable options. Some programs have had great success partnering with preexisting mental health and hospital-based programs, opening exercise and educational facilities during after-work hours for those interested in preventive care and health promotion.

Potential Clients

Currently, there is a paucity of specialized programs to meet the needs of individuals with disabilities. For example, although approximately 500,000 children younger than 18 have cerebral palsy,[5] few communities have recreational and leisure-time activities that are designed to be inclusive of this population. Current studies are showing positive findings that support the effectiveness

TABLE 20-2. BUSINESS PLAN COMPONENTS
• *Business Concept*: Describes the business, its product, and the market it will serve. It should point out exactly what will be sold to whom and why the business will hold a competitive advantage.
• *Financial Features*: Highlights the important financial points of the business, including sales, profits, cash flows, and return on investment.
• *Financial Requirements*: Clearly states the capital needed to start the business and to expand. It should detail how the capital will be used and the equity, if any, that will be provided for funding. If the loan for initial capital will be based on security instead of equity, you should also specify the source of collateral.
• *Current Business Position*: Furnishes relevant information about the company, its legal form of operation, when it was formed, the principal owners and key personnel.
• *Major Achievements*: Details any developments within the company that are essential to the success of the business. Major achievements include items like patents, prototypes, location of a facility, any crucial contracts that need to be in place for product development, or results from any test marketing that has been conducted.

of dance combined with other rehabilitation methods to promote movement coordination and motor learning.[6] Dance is also a wonderful opportunity for socialization and creative expression. A specialized dance program serving large populations of children, including those with cerebral palsy and other developmental disabilities, would fill a niche and be both therapeutic and desirable.

Another example is offering programs that accommodate both physical and psychological needs of clients. One of the many barriers to exercise adherence is accessibility and privacy in changing rooms and during activities, especially for individuals with weight management issues. Offering a weight management program that ensures privacy, safety, and effectiveness would likely draw adults who are overweight or obese, estimated to be more than 35% of the population.[7]

Finally, creating a plan that incorporates mechanisms for clients' feedback helps managers hone the program to meet the clients' needs and expectations. Anticipating the need for adjustments over time to meet clients' expectations, the manager should offer alternative plans (plans B and C) in case plan A might fail to yield anticipated results.

Reaching Customers

Chapter 19 discusses the various creative ways that prevention practice can be marketed to the public. If marketed successfully, the practice will develop a steady stream of clients who are supported by the unique services offered by the program. For example, an aquatics program for individuals with arthritis can be provided at a low cost to groups of clients with degenerative arthritis.

To ensure program success, it is important to track participants' progress so that each individual has a sense of personalization and accomplishment toward reaching personal health, fitness, or wellness goals. Finally, incentives for program adherence, such as t-shirts, can provide extrinsic feedback to clients while providing ongoing marketing.

Financial Resources

When planning and designing a prevention practice, managers should carefully examine its feasibility. Can the prevention practice support itself? Are there grant monies that can be used to develop and sustain the envisioned type of health promotion business? Would these services be provided pro bono or offered as part of a corporate program?

Funding may be a stumbling block if the prevention program must be self-sustaining. Few insurance policies cover programs for sustained primary, secondary, and tertiary preventive care needed by many to establish lifelong healthy lifestyles, requiring clients to pay out of pocket for services rendered. One alternative is to seek financial support from existing businesses with a vested business interest, such as vendors of health-related or fitness products. Another alternative is to explore grants and loans supporting societal health and wellness.

Healthy People 2020 is funded through federal dollars and offers grants for health promotion.[1] If the mission of a proposed program meets key objectives of this national initiative, it is possible to obtain government funding. Local and state health agencies receive funding for ongoing prevention programs in their jurisdictions and may award grants to local programs that meet the health care needs of their communities.

Another potential source of funding is the Affordable Health care Act (ACA), detailing prevention resources for each state, providing recommendations for preventive care, and citing initiatives for "building healthier communities by investing in prevention" at its website (http://www.hhs.gov/aca/).[8] The ACA includes the Prevention and Public Health Fund (PPHF), an account developed to support workplace wellness initiative, representing the largest national commitment to investing in wellness and prevention in history. This fund is aimed at waiving cost sharing for preventive services, providing new funding for community preventive services, and creating workplace wellness programs.[9]

A financial accounting of the business investments, ongoing income, and expenses may require the expertise of a bookkeeper or an accountant. The SBA notes: "While poor management is cited most frequently as the reason businesses fail, inadequate or ill-timed financing is a close second."[4] The SBA offers resources that can guide the entrepreneur in determining the appropriate financing for a new business, including a prevention practice.

Legal Considerations

Another major reason why many small businesses fail is because they fail to seek legal help at critical development stages.[4] Company filings and regulations are critical to starting a health promotion practice and managing finances. Budgeting for legal services and following an attorney's guidance helps to safeguard the business from complex legal problems. One helpful government site itemizes legal requirements for businesses and their employees (http://www.business.gov/).[10] Table 20-3 summarizes essential steps for addressing legal compliance for new businesses.

Corporate Wellness

In recent years, health care professionals have been hired by industry to prevent injuries and disease. Many companies are realizing the benefits of corporate wellness and afford health care professionals an opportunity to meet community needs without personal financial risks. Employee wellness programs are uniquely positioned to meet health issues facing a multigenerational workforce.[11] "In companies with a strong culture of health, employees are 3 times as likely as others to report taking action to improve their health."[12] In addition, the strong health culture promotes better performance, as reported by employees. In Meyer and Maltin's[13] review of research on employee commitment and well-being, they conclude that there is "a large body of research demonstrating the benefits of commitment for employers," benefiting both the employees and the employers for a "win-win situation."

Ensuring a Healthy and Productive Workforce

The US Task Force on Disease Prevention and Health Promotion reports that the most effective interventions available to clinicians for reducing the incidence of disease and disability in the United States are those that address the personal health practices of patients.[14] In an effort to

Table 20-3. Legal Aspects of Setting Up a Health Promotion Practice

- *Pick a Name Legally*: A company name cannot infringe on existing businesses, which are typically registered with the Secretary of State in the state where the health promotion practice is located. A free trademark search is an additional measure to ensure no conflicts with existing businesses and can be explored at the US Patent Trademark Office.
- *Incorporate the Business*: A limited liability corporation (LLC), S corporation, and C corporation are popular options for incorporating a business. Each structure has its own advantages and disadvantages, depending on specific circumstances. For example, an LLC provides protection from liability for a small business. Each option should be discussed with a legal advisor.
- *Register the Business Name/DBA*: A DBA (doing business as) must be filed at the state and/or county when that the business name is different from the legal name of the corporation as shown in its articles of incorporation. Consult with legal counsel to determine the need to file a DBA.
- *Get a Federal Tax Identification Number*: Issued by the Internal Revenue Service, the tax ID allows them to track a company's transactions.
- *Become Familiar With Employee Laws*: Management must be mindful of employee rights and legal obligations, including federal and state payroll and withholding taxes, self-employment taxes, antidiscrimination laws, Occupational Safety and Health Administration regulations, unemployment insurance, workers' compensation rules, and wage and hour requirements.
- *Obtain the Necessary Business Permits and Licenses*: Check for the need for business permits and licenses, including, but not limited to, a general business operation license, zoning and land use permits, sales tax license, health department permits, and occupational or professional licenses.
- *File for Trademark Protection*: Although not required by law, registering a trademark allows legal protection and facilitates recovery of properties if the trademark is infringed upon.
- *Open a Bank Account to Start Building Business Credit*: Using business credit separates personal funds from business funds and builds business credit because cash flow provides evidence for taking on a business loan.

Adapted from Akalp N. 8 legal steps for starting your business. Mashable.com. http://mashable.com/2012/02/08/legal-steps-start-business/. Accessed June 1, 2013.

manage the costs incurred with disease and disability of their workforce, corporations are hiring clinicians to address the personal health practices of their employees.

Employee Wellness Profile/Health Risk Appraisal

Employers seek information about their employees' health to determine health-related risks and needed programs for corporate wellness. The wellness profile aggregates individual wellness baselines and measures group health improvements through collective employee reporting.[15] There are several steps the health care professional would follow to administer an employee wellness profile program.

Upon hire, and periodically thereafter, employees complete a personal, confidential written health assessment, usually at the time of their medical physical. Individuals answer questions about their health, physical activity, eating practices, substance use, stress, social health, safety, medical care, and views on health and wellness.

A confidential objective assessment of the individual's current health status is then sent directly to his or her home address. This assessment addresses health needs and lifestyle practices that determine personal well-being.

Their personal score is benchmarked against national averages and used to provide positive reinforcement of good health practices while making recommendations to improve poor ones.

The change of an individual's score over time is assessed and reflects the modifications that employee made in health practices.

The aggregate data from all employee wellness profiles are confidentially reported to the company in an executive summary report. First the demographics of the company are summarized and the major health risks are identified. Health risks such as cardiovascular disease, cancer, lung disease, diabetes, liver dysfunction, and even suicide or depression can be ranked according to prevalence.[7] Furthermore, the exact factors that are contributing to each health risk are identified. In addition to health risks, lifestyle risks such as stress and sleeplessness can also be recognized. Finally, current disease states are identified and quantified.

Actuarial charts can then be used to provide the company with a projected average cost per claim for the upcoming year. This figure can be compared with what similar companies with similar workforces expect to pay when they have had an ongoing comprehensive wellness program in place for a number of years. The difference in expected costs between these 2 companies estimates the economic effect of preventable risk factors. The difference in cost per claim represents a realistic savings that could be used to fund the wellness program. More importantly, the executive summary report identifies which health risks to focus on. For example, a company would be disappointed in attempting to manage the weight of their obese workforce by focusing on diabetes education, when only 3% have contributing risk factors for diabetes. The company would better invest their resources in nutrition education and/or fitness improvement if those areas were defined as the key contributing risk factors to obesity.

When done regularly, health care professionals can use the employee wellness profile as a useful assessment tool to help a company identify health risks, establish wellness goals, assess program effectiveness, and establish the thrust and direction of upcoming health and wellness needs. In a nutshell, employee wellness profiles allow for health surveillance.

Implementing a Corporate Wellness Program

The health care professional's goal when implementing a corporate wellness program is to assist employees in adopting positive behaviors to lead healthier lives and integrating social, mental, emotional, spiritual, and physical aspects of wellness. High-quality corporate wellness programs are congruent with the company's values, have a well-stated mission or primary objective, and have secondary objectives that are fluid and change periodically, depending on the needs of the workforce.

Several different methods are used to educate a workforce regarding health hazards, to reinforce good health practices, and to encourage change in undesirable health habits. Wellness programming must be customized to the needs and culture of each organization. What works well in one industry may be ineffective for another. Table 20-4 lists the range of strategies that can be incorporated throughout a given year. Table 20-5 lists common topics and screenings offered in corporate wellness programs.

Benefits of a successful corporate wellness program are abundant. Sometimes immediate improvement can be attained in employee productivity and morale, enhanced recruitment and retention, and improved overall corporate image. Other advantages can be realized shortly after

Table 20-4. Strategies for Corporate Wellness

Assessments	• Routine health screenings (eg, blood pressure, glucose) • Health risk assessments • Fitness assessments • Biomedical screenings • Wellness assessments • Quality of life assessments
Programs	• Lunch-n-learn programs • Incentive programs • One-on-one disease management programs • Annual employee health fairs • Group activities offering group support • Individualized counseling • Lectures tailored to employee needs • Competitions
Resources and media	• Newsletters • Targeted mailings • 800 number access for health information and advice • Self-care books • Interactive website • Company's intranet (Q&A, wellness chat rooms) • Apps for health and wellness • On-site health clinic • Vouchers for a clinical office visit • Exercise facilities • Healthy meal offerings onsite

implementation, such as decreased short- and long-term disability costs, workers' compensation costs, employee absenteeism, and overall health care costs. In one case study, the major return on investment came from a reduction in the rate of increased medical costs.[16]

The major challenge with corporate health promotion programs is that the benefits are most often in the form of costs *avoided* rather than in cost *savings*. Because it is difficult to calculate or see costs avoided, estimating the financial benefits of a program is complex and may be difficult to sell within an organization. Additionally, the costs that are avoided can vary greatly due to differing workforce populations, different sites, dissimilar industries, and variations between health promotion programs. However, because the most effective interventions for reducing the incidence of disease and disability involve addressing personal health practices, a comprehensive corporate wellness program guided by an employee wellness profile is an excellent place for clinicians to start.

Table 20-5. Workplace Health Promotion

• Smoking cessation	• Body fat profiles
• Stress management	• Blood pressure checks
• Life balance	• Pulmonary function testing
• Weight measurement and management	• Diabetes risk assessment
• Personal training	• Blood glucose levels
• Onsite chair massages	• Depression screening
• Flu shots	• Bone density screening
• CPR/first aid training	• Spiritual wellness
• Back care	• Vision and hearing screenings
• Cumulative trauma risk reduction/prevention	• Stroke assessment
• Carpal tunnel prevention	• AED (automated electronic defibrillator) training
• Nutrition	• Women's health
• Blood-borne pathogen training	• Time management
• Proper lifting techniques	• Anger management
• Posture and body alignment	• Financial management
• Cholesterol screening	

Essential Functions Testing and Post-Offer Screening

The Americans With Disabilities Act of 1990 (ADA) outlaws discrimination against individuals with disabilities in state and local government services, public accommodations, transportation, and telecommunications.[17] Individuals with disabilities must be assessed to determine whether they are capable of performing required job duties or receive accommodations. Also, individuals at risk for illness or injury need to be similarly assessed to determine their work capabilities and appropriate job skills. One way a company can promote a healthy workforce is by testing employees to ensure that they are physically capable of performing the functions that are deemed essential for their specific position. Hundreds of thousands of worker are either injured or killed in workplace accidents.[18] Essential functions testing allows a company to identify target groups at risk for injury and implement controls that keep the environment safe for all workers.

Most post-offers screens include the following parts:

- *Informed consent.* The individual signs a standard release from liability and answers general questions designed to uncover any physical restrictions or limitations that the individual may have. The goal is to find out if the test is contraindicated, such as in the case of a pregnancy.
- *General global screen.* Heart rate and blood pressure are taken and compared against the American Heart Association standards. Range of motion is charted from head to toe, and a strength grade for major muscle groups is documented. Postural malalignment is charted, and screens for common musculoskeletal disorders are performed. These pre-employment baseline measurements are compared with the employee's medical history questionnaire to identify inconsistencies. Additionally, a physician or therapist may use this baseline data to compare postinjury impairments to pre-employment status.

- *Postinjury intervention.* Objective measurements are used to develop a specific postinjury medical or legal intervention. For example, after a work-related hand injury, the employee's pre-employment grip strength may be used by the treating physician or therapist to establish his or her goals. The company may only be responsible for rehabilitating the employee to preinjury status vs normal limits. If a baseline strength measurement is not available, then frequently the company may be expected to rehabilitate the individual to a level that is close to the standard for a person the same age and sex, even if the individual is weaker than that standard. Although all of these pre-employment baselines are useful and important, most states will not allow a company to deny employment based on their results.
- *Essential functions testing.* This component of employment screening involves testing an individual to see whether he or she is capable of safely performing the essential functions of a designated job. The employee either passes or fails, and failure constitutes legal grounds to deny employment.

It is best if the vendor who administers the essential functions test is the same who developed the essential functions for the job. Positional tolerances, lifting, carrying, pushing, pulling, reaching, fine motor skills, bending, stooping, kneeling, crawling, walking, driving, twisting, squatting, stairs, ladders, ramps, curbs, poles, reading, color discrimination, depth perception, hearing sensitivity, tactile discrimination, and temperature discrimination are frequently tested. The law varies, but some states may require that the essential functions be defined in a written job description for testing to commence.

Additionally, most states require that all individuals applying for a position be tested in an attempt to prevent discrimination. Frequently, an employer will expect the vendor who is administering the test to provide information regarding the employability of the individual. It is important that the vendor simply administer the test and deliver the results. The employer should make all judgment and decisions regarding employment of the individual.

Essential functions testing is most commonly done pre-employment, as a contingency for employment (ie, a job offer is conditional on its successful completion). However, more companies are doing periodic testing of their workforce to help identify the population that cannot safely perform their jobs.

The essential functions test can also be a useful tool when a physician is determining an injured worker's fitness for duty. In other words, if the patient has not achieved strength or mobility levels to successfully complete the test, then the physician will frequently assign a restricted or modified work status to keep the patient safe while justifying the need for more rehabilitation. Testing allows the health care professional to observe an unsafe work practice, such as improper lifting, and document that proper training was provided. An essential functions test empowers a company to appropriately match employees to safe and appropriate jobs.

Ensuring a Healthy and Benign Work Environment

In addition to screening individuals for their capabilities and matching them to appropriate job tasks, health care professionals can analyze each job task to determine whether it is as safe as possible to perform. In this sense, health care professionals are experts in ergonomics, or the science of fitting jobs to people.

Comprehensive Company-Wide Ergonomics Program

The goal of a corporate ergonomics program is to reduce risk factors known to be associated with the development of musculoskeletal and cumulative trauma disorders. Physical, environmental, organizational, and psychosocial risk factors should be considered. Much like a corporate wellness program, an ergonomics program should be congruent with the company's values, have a well-stated mission or primary objective, and, at times, have a changing secondary focus depending on the thrust and needs of the company at the time. This serves as an action plan or road map, keeping the program on a straight and narrow path.

The initial step is to locate the problem in particular departments or jobs:

- *Document analysis*: By reviewing the company's injury history, one can identify trends. For example, there might be a disproportionate number of injuries in one department or an increase in a specific diagnosis noticed in a particular job. Analyzing the injury history often points the ergonomist in an appropriate direction.
- *Symptom surveys*: Symptom surveys or comfort-level surveys assign ratings of discomfort by body part and can be used to identify jobs or departments where the workers experience sub-reportable levels of discomfort. Symptom surveys target symptoms of pain, numbness, tingling, burning, or swelling that (1) occurred in the previous 12 months, (2) last for at least one week, (3) occur at least once per month, and (4) are not caused by an acute injury. The results of these surveys help identify departments where symptoms of discomfort exist but where these symptoms are masked by a low incidence of documented injuries.
- *Departmental Checklist*: Some ergonomists will blanket whole departments with a risk factor checklist. Some checklists will assign a combined risk factor score with an established threshold, indicating the need for a more in-depth analysis. Many online resources provide ergonomics checklists for both physically demanding and sedentary jobs.
- *Identification of Offending Risk Factors*: Both physical and psychological risk factors need to be appraised and identified. Psychosocial risk factors include machine-paced tasks, incentive pay, routine overtime, electronic monitoring of employees, limited ability to influence daily decisions, and monotonous tasks. Other risk factors include extreme posture, velocity of motion, repetition of tasks, total task duration, nerve compression, vibration, cold temperatures, and force required to accomplish the task.
- *Final Assessment*: The final assessment regarding the degree of total risk is a fine balance of all of the above conditions. For example, a task may require an extreme posture with high velocity and vibration, but if the task duration is negligible, then the task may be benign.

Ergonomics Task Force

An ergonomics task force is frequently formed to identify and evaluate possible solutions. This task force can comprise several members, including representatives from employee health, a safety office employee, a medical office employee, company engineers, employee representatives, the ergonomist, and a union representative, if applicable. This committee examines design specifications, analyzes similar operations/industries, reviews the literature for solutions, talks to vendors/trade association/organizations/specialists, and generally brainstorms to determine a solution to presenting problems.

Solutions fall into 1 of 3 categories. First, administrative controls reduce the frequency, duration, and severity of exposures to the risk factors. Job rotation, mandatory rest periods, job enhancement, stretching programs, conditioning programs, light/modified work duties, and supervision are all examples of administrative controls. Second, engineering controls are one-time changes that protect all employees. Engineering controls are permanent and involve physical changes to workstations, equipment, the production facility, or any other relevant aspect of the work environment to reduce or eliminate the presence of risk factors. Third, work practice controls are procedures for safe and proper work and specific for each task or workplace. Personal protective equipment, appropriate training, job simulation/practice, correct lifting techniques, proper tool maintenance, and correct use of workstations are all examples of work practice controls. The solutions selected should address the particular risk factors involved.

The ergonomics committee should meet periodically to ensure solution implementation and follow-up. A status report should be maintained to track ergonomics issues, solution implementation, and current status. The committee should conduct continuous ergonomics monitoring to identify potential problems. Rarely are all existing risk factors identified, and as jobs are added or changed, new risk factors are continually being created. A yearly review of the ergonomics program should be conducted to assess its effectiveness, track the status of ergonomics goals, and establish the direction of upcoming health and safety needs.

Ensuring Healthy and Appropriate Work Practices

Healthy individuals working in a healthy environment can still incur injury if they are performing tasks in an unhealthy way. The body mechanics involved in performing a specific task can be evaluated by a health care professional, and health education can be personalized to the needs of an individual client.

Defining Essential Job Functions

One role of a health care professional, typically a physical therapist or occupational therapist, has always been to help people function as independently as possible in performing the motor tasks required to fulfill important roles in their lives. These motor tasks are sometimes self-evident. For example, the motor task of transferring sit-to-stand is essential to getting out of a chair and fulfilling certain life roles.

Work is one important life role for most people. However, in work settings the motor tasks are not self-evident and must be defined. For example, an assembly plant may need to specify the amount required to lift, push, or pull to function in a particular job. These work-related motor tasks are called the essential functions for a job. Positional tolerances, lifting, carrying, pushing, pulling, reaching, fine motor skills, bending, stooping, kneeling, crawling, walking, driving, twisting, squatting, stairs, ladders, ramps, curbs, poles, reading, color discrimination, depth perception, hearing sensitivity, tactile discrimination, and temperature discrimination are examples of essential functions.

The duration of each essential function should be identified in accordance with the US Department of Labor *Dictionary of Occupational Titles* as follows[19]:

- Occasional = 1% to 33% of the shift
- Frequent = 34% to 66% of the shift
- Constant = 67% to 100% of the shift

Well-defined essential functions are useful to companies for several reasons.

Essential functions are legally required for companies that choose to physically test their employees against them. For example, a company cannot deny employment to an individual who is unable to lift 50 pounds if that motor task is not deemed essential to function in that job.

Essential functions are useful when suggesting job rotation. For example, rotating from one fine motor task to another may not reduce exposure to similar risk factors; however, rotation from a fine motor task to a gross motor task may.

If harmful risk factors are uncovered during the job analysis, this can serve as a trigger to the ergonomic committee for follow-up before it leads to injury. Preventive work station stretches are often created from the essential functions. Otherwise, the prevention-based stretches may miss their target.

Essential functions give physicians important information with which they can make decisions regarding an individual's work status. Restricted or light duty can keep an injured worker safe yet productive on the job.

Essential functions give health care professionals and occupational therapists job-related rehabilitation goals. If a patient is required to carry 25 pounds at work and he or she is currently unable to do so, then the therapist has a sound, objective, and valid goal.

Essential functions allow for companies to either place injured workers or assess whether they can make reasonable accommodations to the worksite. The ADA contains specific guidelines that define the rights and obligations for companies and employees.[20] As jobs experience change and modification, so do the essential functions. Therefore, the essential functions should be updated on a regular schedule and modified when job modifications occur. Essential functions are the cornerstone from which many other worksite prevention measures are developed (Table 20-6).

Preventive Job-Specific Work Station Stretches

Health care professionals have always provided injured workers with useful information during their rehabilitation about how to prevent another injury. However, companies are starting to recognize the value this information can have to noninjured workers. Preventive work station stretching and strengthening routines are another way clinicians help companies manage their workers' compensation costs.

Developing a preventive job-specific program begins with a jobsite analysis. Observation of different workers performing the same job helps to establish the essential functions for a particular position. From these essential functions, the clinician can identify the structures in one's body that absorb and generate forces. A stretching and strengthening program can then be recommended that is customized for that particular position.

Providing this routine empowers the employee to be proactive about his or her health and wellness at work. Companies will frequently have a health care professional train a shift leader to lead his or her group through the program when arriving to work or returning from break. Some corporations even take roll or document participation in the stretching program. This record can sometimes be used to demonstrate a company's proactive approach or illustrate an employee's noncompliance.

Summary

Starting a prevention practice begins with a passionate vision, followed by a clearly articulated business plan outlining the need, the target niche filled by the business, and resources to ensure success. With backgrounds in health, fitness, and wellness, as well as knowledge about business practices, legal considerations, and financial resources, health care professionals can build their companies in multiple directions providing primary, secondary, and/or tertiary preventive care and health promotion to those with disabilities or chronic illness. Additionally, health care providers can collaborate with communities and businesses to provide screenings, evaluate workplace ergonomics, develop adaptations to enhance participation, and offer interventions to prevent and treat illness and injury. Screening individuals' fitness, health, and wellness for their job responsibilities, leisure-time activities, and activities of daily living, as well as promoting health, fitness, and wellness across the lifespan, are all aspects of prevention practice where health care professionals can excel.

References

1. Healthy People 2020 framework. US Department of Health and Human Services. http://healthypeople.gov/2020/consortium/HP2020Framework.pdf. Accessed May 20, 2014.
2. Green LW, Kreuter MW. *Health Promotion Planning: An Educational and Ecological Approach*. 3rd ed. Mountain View, CA: Mayfield Publishing; 1999.

TABLE 20-6. ESSENTIAL FUNCTION ANALYSIS: QUESTIONS

PRELIMINARY QUESTIONS

- Does the position exist to perform this job function?
- What is the employer's judgment regarding which functions or job requirements are essential?
- Would the position be fundamentally different if this function or job requirement was altered?
- Is the number of employees to whom this function or job requirement could be given limited?
- Is this a highly specialized function or job requirement?
- What would be the consequences if this function or job requirement was not included?
- Is there a current incumbent in this position who performs this function or meets the job requirements?
- Did the incumbent of this position perform this function or meet the job requirements?
- Are the essential functions of this job linked to a specific location?
- What type of supervision is required over this position while performing job duties?

PHYSICAL REQUIREMENTS

What are the physical requirements in an 8-hour workday for the following activities?

Activity duration: Occasional=1% to 33% Frequent=34% to 66% Constant=67% to 100%

Sitting	Standing	Walking	Crawling	Climbing	Pushing or pulling	
Bending	Crouching	Kneeling	Balancing	Talking	Reaching overhead	
Lifting (in lb)	10 or less	11 to 25	26 to 50	51 to 75	76 to 100	Over 100
Carrying (in lb)	10 or less	11 to 25	26 to 50	51 to 75	76 to 100	Over 100
Repetitive use of hands/arms			Repetitive use of legs		Grasping	
Eye/hand coordination			Fine manipulation			

MENTAL REQUIREMENTS

What are the mental requirements in an 8-hour workday for the following activities?

Activity duration: Occasional=1% to 33% Frequent=34% to 66% Constant=67% to 100%

Handling stress	Adjusting to changes	Thinking analytically
Concentrating on tasks	Discriminating colors	Remembering names
Using effective verbal communication	Remembering details	Making decisions
Research & data analysis	Examining/observing emotions details	

ADDITIONAL INFORMATION

List other information helpful in understanding the physical, mental, and performance requirements of the position.

(continued)

Table 20-6 (continued). Essential Function Analysis: Questions

HEALTH & SAFETY

What health and safety standards are required of an incumbent in this job category?

ENVIRONMENTAL FACTORS

What are the environmental factors encountered at this job?

Exposure:	*Occasional = 1% to 33%*		*Frequent = 34% to 66%*		*Constant = 67% to 100%*		
Inside	Dirty	Outside	Dusty	Humid	Wet	Hot	Cold
Odors	Hazards		Fumes, gases		Chemical	Biological	
Radiation	High places		Temperature		Working with others		
Walking on uneven ground			Working around others		Working alone		
Being around equipment & machinery							
Driving cars, trucks, forklifts & other equipment							

PERFORMANCE REQUIREMENTS

What are the performance requirements for the job?

- Maintain stamina during workday
- Working at various temperatures
- Staying organized
- Operates equipment
- Meeting deadlines
- Directing others
- Attendance
- Writing
- Attending work
- Using math/calculations
- Working effectively with coworkers

TOOLS & EQUIPMENT

List machines, tools, equipment, and motor vehicles used in the performance of the duties (eg, "Computer," "Operate forklift up to 4000 pounds capacity," "Respirator equipment requirement").

REQUIREMENTS OF THE POSITION

List certificates, licenses, or education required (eg, "Requires valid license as a registered nurse in the State of Washington").

List additional knowledge, skills, and abilities required for this position and tell why required.

Adapted from Essential and marginal job function analysis. Pennsylvania State University. http://www.psu.edu/dept/aaoffice/pdf/emjfa_current1.pdf. Accessed May 20, 2014.

3. Crosby R, Noar SM. What is a planning model? An introduction to PRECEDE-PROCEED. *J Public Health Dent.* 2011;71 Suppl 1:S7-S15.
4. Create your business plan: executive summary. US Small Business Administration. http://www.sba.gov/content/executive-summary. Accessed May 20, 2014.
5. Prevalence and incidence of cerebral palsy. CerebralPalsy.org. http://cerebralpalsy.org/about-cerebral-palsy/prevalence-of-cerebral-palsy/. Accessed May 20, 2013.
6. Cerebral palsy and dance. National Center on Health, Physical Activity, and Disability. http://www.ncpad.org/895/5018/Cerebral~Palsy~and~Ballet#sthash.SeFFzQAP.dpuf. Accessed May 20, 2013.
7. Adult obesity facts. Centers for Disease Control and Prevention. http://www.cdc.gov/obesity/data/adult.html. Accessed May 20, 2013.
8. Affordable Healthcare Act: basics and background. American Public Health Association. http://www.apha.org/advocacy/Health+Reform/ACAbasics/. Accessed May 20, 2014.
9. Haberkorn J. The Prevention and Public Health Fund. Health Affairs. http://www.healthaffairs.org/healthpolicybriefs/brief.php?brief_id=63. Accessed October 22, 2013.
10. Learn about business law & regulations. US Small Business Administration. http://www.sba.gov/category/navigation-structure/starting-managing-business/starting-business/understand-business-law-r. Accessed May 20, 2014.
11. Blumenthal D. Employer-sponsored health insurance in the United States: origins and implications. *N Engl J Med.* 2006;355(1):82-88.
12. Isaac FW. Sustaining a culture of health and well-being at Johnson & Johnson. DFW Business Group of Health. http://dfwbgh.org/wellness2010/Culture_of_Health.pdf. Accessed November 1, 2011.
13. Meyer J, Maltin E. Employee commitment and well-being: a critical review, theoretical framework and research agenda. *J Vocat Behav.* 2010;77:323-337.
14. Steps to a Healthier US. US Public Health Department Office of Disease Prevention and Health Promotion. http://odphp.osophs.dhhs.gov/. Accessed May 20, 2013.
15. Employer program. Wellness Management Systems. http://www.wellnessmanagementsystems.com/%28S%28cakbpb55eoaohj45ovmyf255%29%29/clients/wms/detail.aspx?iid=225&AspxAutoDetectCookieSupport=1. Accessed May 20, 2013.
16. The business case for a corporate wellness program: a case study of General Motors and the United Auto Workers Union. The Commonwealth Fund. http://www.commonwealthfund.org/Search.aspx?search=Corporate+Wellness&filefilter=1. Accessed June 1, 2013.
17. The ADA: your responsibilities as an employer. US Equal Employment Opportunity Commission. http://www.eeoc.gov/facts/ada17.html. Accessed June 1, 2013.
18. Injuries, illnesses, and fatalities. US Department of Labor Bureau of Labor Statistics. http://www.bls.gov/iif/. Accessed June 1, 2013.
19. Standard occupational classification. US Department of Labor Bureau of Labor Statistics. http://www.bls.gov/soc/home.htm. Accessed May 30, 2013.
20. Title III highlights. US Department of Justice. Civil Rights Division. Disability Rights Section. http://www.ada.gov/t3hilght.htm. Accessed June 10, 2014.

Appendix A
Brief Health Information

Adapted from the WHO's International Classification of Functioning, Disability and Health

Name of client: ______________________ Date of birth: ______________ Age: ______

Examiner: ______________________________ Date of screen: ______________

Location of screening: ____

GENERAL HEALTH SCREEN:

Rate your physical health in the past month? Very good [ ] Good [ ] Moderate [ ] Bad [ ] Very bad [ ]

Rate your mental and emotional health in the past month? Very good [ ] Good [ ] Moderate [ ] Bad [ ] Very bad [ ]

Do you currently have any disease(s) or disorder(s)? [ ] NO [ ] YES

If YES, please specify:

____

Did you ever have any significant injuries that had an effect on your level of functioning? [ ] NO [ ] YES

If YES, please specify:

____

Have you been hospitalized in the last year? [ ] NO [ ] YES

If YES, please specify reason(s) and for how long:

______________________________; _____ days

______________________________; _____ days

______________________________; _____ days

Thompson CR.
Prevention Practice and Health Promotion: A Health Care Professional's Guide to Health, Fitness, and Wellness, Second Edition (pp 339-345).

Are you taking any medications, over-the-counter drugs, or supplements (either prescribed or over the counter)? [ ] NO [ ] YES

If YES, please specify major medications; note allergies or poor reactions:

____

Are you receiving any kind of treatment for your health? [ ] NO [ ] YES

If YES, please specify:

____

ACTIVITIES:

Do you have any person assisting you with your self-care, shopping, or other daily activities? [ ] NO [ ] YES

If YES, please specify person and assistance they provide:

____

IN THE PAST MONTH, have you cut back (ie, reduced) your usual activities or work because of your *health condition*? (a disease, injury, emotional reasons or alcohol or drug use) [ ] NO [ ] YES

If yes, how many days? ________

IN THE PAST MONTH, have you been totally unable to carry out your usual activities or work because of your *health condition*? (a disease, injury, emotional reasons or alcohol or drug use) [ ] NO [ ] YES

If yes, how many days? ________

Daily activities:

Sedentary activities (hr): ________________ Mild physical activity (hr) ________________

Moderate physical activity (hr) ________________ Vigorous physical activity (hr) ________________

Leisure activities: How would you describe the type, intensity, and duration of your physical activity (on a weekly basis)?

Type: ______________________________

Duration: ______________________________

Frequency: ______________________________

Intensity: ______________________________

BODY STRUCTURE/BODY FUNCTION:

Anthropometrics: Height (in): ________ Weight (lb): ________

Hips (in): ________ Waist (in): ________

Hips-to-waist ratio: ________

Male: Excellent: < 0.85 Good: 0.85 to 0.90

Female: Excellent: < 0.75 Good: 0.75 to 0.80

Body mass index: Healthy range: Male: 19.1 to 25.8 Female: 20.7 to 26.4

Vital signs: Normal ranges for the average healthy adult at rest:

Blood pressure: ______ 90/60 to 120/80 mm Hg

Breathing: ______ 12 to 18 breaths per minute

Pulse: ______ 60 to 100 beats per minute

Temperature: ______ 97.8°F to 99.1°F/average 98.6°F

Family history:

___ Allergies ___ Arthritis ___ Alcoholism

___ Cancer ___ Diabetes ___ High blood pressure

___ Kidney disease ___ Mental illness ___ Seizure disorders

___ Stroke ___ Other (*list:* ______)

General health: Weight (lb): ______

___ Fatigue ___ Weakness ___ Malaise

___ Fever ___ Illness (*describe:* ______)

Immunizations: Are immunizations current? Yes ___ No ___

What is your travel history? ______

______

Birth history: Vaginal ______ C-section ______ Full-term? Yes ___ No ___

Any complications ______

Medical history (prior to the past year):

Serious accidents (date, injury, length of care) ______

Hospitalizations (date, injury, length of care) ______

Surgeries (date, injury, length of care) ______

Serious illness (date, injury, length of care) ______

Skin: ___ Skin problems ___ Sun exposure ___ Sun protection

___ Any special needs for personal care for skin and hair

Vision: ___ Glasses or contacts ___ Any problems with vision ___ Vision screen

Ears: ___ Earaches ___ Infections

___ Discharge from ear ___ Ringing (tinnitis) ___ Dizziness (vertigo)

Nose and sinuses:

___ Discharge from the nose ___ Discharge from the sinuses ___ Sinus pain

___ Unusual/frequent cold ___ Change in sense of smell

Mouth and throat:

_____ Pain _____ Toothache _____ Lesions/sores on mouth

_____ Lesions/sores on throat _____ Changes in the mouth or throat

_____ Altered taste _____ Jaw pain

Neck: _____ Neck pain _____ Limitations in neck movement

_____ Lumps, swelling, tenderness, or other discomfort

Respiratory system:

_____ History of asthma _____ Chest pain _____ Shortness of breath

_____ Cough _____ Wheezing

Cardiovascular system:

_____ Pain near heart with exertion _____ Pain near heart without exertion

_____ Dizziness when standing up _____ Personal history of any heart problems

_____ Problems breathing when sleeping

Peripheral vascular system:

_____ Coldness _____ Numbness _____ Tingling

_____ Swelling of legs or hands _____ Pain in legs _____ Varicose veins

_____ Discolored hands or feet _____ History of vascular problems

Gastrointestinal system: Frequency of bowel movement _______

_____ Changes in appetite _____ Food intolerance _____ Heartburn

_____ Abdominal pain _____ Rectal bleeding _____ Flatulence (gas)

_____ Nausea and vomiting _____ Recent changes in stool

_____ Constipation or diarrhea _____ Rectal conditions _____ High fiber in diet

_____ Use of antacids/laxatives

Urinary system: Frequency of urination _______

_____ Problems with urgency _____ Pain with urination _____ Unusual color

_____ Other problems

Reproductive system:

Male genital system:

_____ Penis or testicular pain _____ Sores or lesions _____ Discharge

_____ Lumps _____ Hernia

Female genital system:

Menstrual history (last period, duration, cycle): ____________________

Pregnancy history: ____________________

_____ Vaginal itching
_____ Discharge
_____ Age of menopause
_____ Menopausal signs or symptoms
_____ Postmenopausal bleeding

Male and female sexual history:

_____ In relationship with intercourse
_____ Aspects of sex satisfaction
_____ Contraception is satisfactory
_____ Awareness of family planning
_____ Familiar with sex education
_____ Awareness of sexually transmitted diseases
_____ Presence of sexually transmitted diseases

Musculoskeletal system:

_____ History of arthritis; gout; joint pain, swelling, or stiffness; deformity
_____ Range of motion limitations
_____ Muscular pain
_____ Muscle cramps
_____ Muscle weakness
_____ Gait problems
_____ Problems with coordination
_____ Back pain
_____ Joint stiffness
_____ Limitations in movement
_____ History of back problems or disk disease

Neurological system:

_____ History of seizures, blackouts, strokes, fainting, headaches
_____ Motor problems: tics, tremors, paralysis, or coordination problems
_____ Sensory: numbness, tingling
_____ Memory: loss, disorientation
_____ Mood change
_____ Depression
_____ History of mental health dysfunction

Hematologic system:

_____ Bleeding problems
_____ Excessive bruising
_____ Lymph node swelling
_____ Exposure to toxins and radiation
_____ Blood transfusions and reactions ____________________

Endocrine system:

_____ History of diabetes
_____ Thyroid disease
_____ Intolerance to heat and cold
_____ Change in skin pigmentation/texture
_____ Excessive sweating

_____ Abnormal relationship between appetite and weight (*describe*: ____________________

____)

_____ Abnormal hair distribution _____ Nervousness

_____ Tremors _____ Need for hormone therapy

ENVIRONMENTAL FACTORS: (*Note physical and/or social barriers and facilitators*)

Do you use any assistive device such as glasses, hearing aid, wheelchair, etc? [ ] NO [ ] YES

If YES, please specify:

____

Do you wear any orthotics, shoe inserts, splints, or other devices? [ ] NO [ ] YES

If YES, please specify:

____

Home: Social relationships: _____ Positive _____ Negative _____ Neutral

Physical: _____ Number of stories _____ Steps to enter

_____ Fire alarms (updated batteries)

Work: Social relationships: _____ Positive _____ Negative _____ Neutral

Physical: _____ Ergonomic workstation

____

PERSONAL FACTORS:

Race: ____________________________

Ethnicity: ____________________________

Do you smoke? [ ] NO [ ] YES

Do you consume alcohol or drugs? [ ] NO [ ] YES

_____ Tobacco _____ Alcohol _____ Drugs

If YES, please specify average daily quantity ____________________________

Education (highest level):

____

Sleep and rest: How would you describe your sleep behavior?

Sleep schedule ____

Typical duration of sleep ____________________________________

Typical sleep posture ______________________________________

Does your partner interfere with your sleep? If so, how: ____________________

Other comments: ____

Nutrition: How would you describe your eating behavior?

_____ Healthy _____ Unhealthy

Overall diet: ____

_____ Caffeine (tea, coffee, cola drinks) intake

_____ Use of vitamins _____ Food allergies or intolerance

Mealtime habits: ____

PARTICIPATION:

Role in a relationship with significant other:

_____ Spouse _____Committed relationship

Roles as a parent:

Children (ages and sexes): ____

Roles in the community: ____

WELLNESS: Positive stressors: ____

Negative stressors: ____

Stress management/coping strategies: ______________________________

Spirituality: ____

Signs of stress:

Behavioral: ____

Emotional: ____

Cognitive: ____

Physical: ____

Appendix B
Developmental History

Child's name: ______________ Parent's name: ___________ Occupation: ___________

Child's birthdate: ___________ Parent's name: ___________ Occupation: ___________

Child's age: ______________ Today's date: ___________

PART I: Prenatal history—Questions related to mother's pregnancies and this delivery

1. Have you been pregnant before?
2. If you have been pregnant before, how many times?
3. Were there problems during other pregnancies? If so, please specify:

4. What was the length of this pregnancy?
   Number of weeks' gestation: _____ Duration of labor for this child: _____
5. Type of delivery: vaginal? _____ C-section? _____ Any complications?

PART II: Child's early history—Questions about this child's early development

1. What was the condition of your child at birth (eg, healthy, at risk, requiring neonatal intensive care)?
2. What problems were evident at birth?
3. Were you aware of any problems before your child's birth?
4. What was your child's APGAR score at 1 minute?
5. What was your child's APGAR score at 5 minutes?
6. What was your child's birth weight?
7. What was your child's height at birth?
8. What were your child's sleep patterns after birth?

Thompson CR.
Prevention Practice and Health Promotion: A Health Care Professional's Guide to Health, Fitness, and Wellness, Second Edition (pp 347-349).

9. Has your child had any problems with sleep since birth?
10. What is your child's favorite activity?
11. How does your child react to movement?
12. Is your child toilet trained?
13. Are there any problems related to your child's toileting?
14. Has your child been hospitalized since birth? (specify):
15. Does your child have allergies? (specify):
16. Does your child have a history of ear infections? (specify):
17. Is your child teething now?
18. Does your child have any other medical problems or had medical tests to rule out possible medical problems?
19. Note the age of each of the following developmental milestones:

    Sitting alone _____ Crawling on all fours _____ Walking alone _____
    Running _____ Creeping upstairs _____ Creeping down stairs _____
    Catching a large ball _____ Using words _____ 2-word sentences _____
    3- to 4-word sentences _____ Asking questions _____ Drinking from a cup _____
    Dressing self _____ Using a spoon _____ Using a knife _____
    Using markers or crayons _____
20. Describe your child's general coordination and balance:
21. Describe your child's ability to communicate:

PART III: Present status—Current care, concerns, and managment

1. Parent(s) concerns:
2. Current medications:
3. Current illnesses:
4. Current medical diagnosis(es):

5. Current sleeping patterns and related problems:

6. Current eating habits and related problems:

7. Interaction with other children:

8. Attendance at day care, play groups, other (specify):

9. Current coordination in movement—both small and large movements:

10. Current coordination in movement—using hands:

11. Describe language at present:

12. Physician's name:
13. Physician's address:
14. Physician's phone:
15. Names of other specialists working with your child:

16. What is the family's history since the birth of this child (eg, moves, changes, significant traumas, or other problems)?:

17. Names and ages of siblings:

18. Are the other siblings in good general health? If not, please describe:

19. Other comments:

Appendix C
Resources for Health, Fitness, and Wellness

Apps

A wide range of applications (apps) for health, fitness, and wellness are currently available for use, some at no charge. These apps range from body mass index (BMI) calculators, recipes, and tracking of lifestyle behaviors to user-friendly anatomy, first aid, and disease-specific applications. A simple search of the Internet using the term "app" and the desired topic yields helpful results. Their use depends on the needs of the clinician, client, and program. In "Smartphone Technology and Apps: Rapidly Changing Health Promotion," Kratzke and Cox[1] state: "It is recommended that development of new health promotion programs using smartphones and apps include evidence-based guidelines for chronic disease management, improved physician-patient interaction, and improved access to services from a distance." This study challenges health care providers to share their outcomes using the various apps available in the marketplace to provide the best resources for their clients.

Websites

The following sites provide extensive information and are linked to updated information related to health, fitness, and wellness.

American Association of Retired Persons
http://www.aarp.org/health/fitness/info-06-2010/prevention_and_wellness_resources.html

The Prevention and Wellness Resources for Leaders features a Workplace Health Promotion Tool Kit as well as online health tools for the following topics:

- AARP health record tool
- BMI calculator

Thompson CR.
Prevention Practice and Health Promotion: A Health Care Professional's Guide to Health, Fitness, and Wellness, Second Edition (pp 351-357).

- Care provider locator
- Drug interaction checker
- Doughnut hole calculator
- Drug compare
- Drug savings tool
- Health encyclopedia
- Health law guide: Affordable Care Act
- Health savings account calculator
- Health learning tool
- Learning centers: lists over 1000 of the most common diseases and conditions
- Long-term care calculator
- Many Strong: manage care for a loved one by building an online community
- Medicare summary notice decoder
- Pill identifier
- Symptom checker
- Visual MD

American Congress of Obstetricians and Gynecologists (ACOG)
http://www.acog.org

Topics include breast cancer; breastfeeding; abuse; abnormal bleeding; endometrial cancer; gynecologic cancers; health care policy; labor and delivery; lesbian, bisexual, and transgender women; menopause; neonatal or infant; ovarian cancer; pelvic support problems or incontinence.

American College of Sports Medicine
http://www.acsm.org/

This site features resources (books, DVDs, wearables, and posters) on business and management, fitness/personal training, nutrition and weight control, special populations, sports medicine, stress management, special populations, wall charts, and tools.

American Medical Association
http://www.ama-assn.org/ama

The Public Health site offers the following health topics: improving health outcomes, AMA Healthier Life Steps, alcohol and other drug abuse, smoking and tobacco control, eliminating health disparities, educating physicians on controversies and challenges in health, vaccination resources, roadmaps for clinical practice, veterans' health, public health preparedness and disaster response, aging and community health, adolescent health, and Building a Healthier Chicago (BHC).

Addition links provide more detailed information about the following:

- Childhood obesity
- Healthy eating resources
- Patient assistance program directory
- Resources for older drivers
- Atlas of the body

- Adolescent health handouts
- Caregiver self-assessment
- Smoking and tobacco control

American Physical Therapy Association
http://www.apta.org

This professional organization offers a broad spectrum of health, fitness, and wellness educational materials, including the following:

- American Physical Therapy Association Public Relations Manual: A How-To
- Why It Feels Right to Put Your Health in the Hands of a Physical Therapist
- Fit Kids
- FUNfitness: A Screening Kit to Assess Children's Flexibility, Strength & Balance
- Fit Teens
- Fit for the Fairway: A Posture Assessment for Golfers
- Golfers: Take Care of Your Back
- Balance and Falls Awareness Event Kit
- What You Need to Know About Balance and Falls
- What You Need to Know About Arthritis
- Fitness: A Way of Life
- Taking Care of Your Back
- What You Need to Know About Neck Pain
- What You Need to Know About Carpal Tunnel Syndrome
- Taking Care of Your Hand, Wrist, and Elbow
- Taking Care of Your Shoulder
- Taking Care of Your Foot and Ankle
- Taking Care of Your Knees
- Taking Care of Your Hips
- What You Need to Know About Osteoporosis
- You Can Do Something About Incontinence
- For Women of All Ages
- For the Young at Heart
- Secret of Good Posture
- Scoliosis: What Young People and Their Parents Need to Know

American Psychological Association
http://www.apa.org/

This organization has a wealth of information for mental health issues, including attention deficit hyperactivity disorder, aging, anger, anxiety, autism, bipolar disorder, bullying, children, death and dying, eating disorders, emotional health, ethics, hate crimes, natural disasters, parenting, trauma, violence, and workplace issues.

American Public Health Association
http://www.apha.org/

This site offers a wide range of information for public health and health promotion for the nation. The link to Advocacy & Policy includes information related to the following:

- Advocacy tips
- Advocacy activities
- Health reform
- Priorities (creating health equity, ensuring the right to health care, and building a public health infrastructure)
- Reports, issue briefs, fact sheets, and webinars

American Occupational Therapy Association
http://www.aota.org/

This organization has some unique resources for health protection, advocacy, and caregivers, including the following:

- Emergency preparedness and disaster response
- Caregiver toolkit
- Advocacy

Centers for Disease Control and Prevention
http://www.cdc.gov/

The Centers for Disease Control and Prevention (CDC) has a vast array of resources for disease control and prevention. Information for the following topics are linked to this site:

- Diseases and conditions
- Healthy living
- Emergency preparedness response
- Injury, violence, and safety
- Environmental health
- Workplace safety and health
- Data and statistics
- Global health
- Travelers' health
- Life stages and populations

Gateway to Health Communication and Social Marketing Practice
http://www.cdc.gov/healthcommunication/

This site offers a range of resources for enhancing health communication and social marketing campaigns and programs, including "tips for analyzing and segmenting an audience, choosing appropriate channels and tools, or evaluating the success of your messages or campaigns."

- Audience
- Campaigns
- Research/evaluation

- Channels
- Tools and templates
- Risk communication

Chronic Disease Prevention and Health Promotion
http://www.cdc.gov/chronicdisease/index.htm

This CDC site outlines program for the following issues and conditions:

- Cancer
- Community health
- Diabetes
- Heart disease and stroke
- Nutrition, physical activity, and obesity
- Oral health
- Population health
- Preventing chronic disease
- Reproductive health
- Smoking and tobacco use

National Institute of Occupational Safety and Health
http://www.cdc.gov/niosh/

This CDC site offers resources for the following topics: workplace safety, industries and occupations, diseases and injuries, safety and prevention, hazards and exposures, chemicals, emergency preparedness and response.

US Department of Health & Human Services: Prevention
http://www.hhs.gov/safety/index.html

This site focuses on preventive care with resources regarding the following:

- Exercise and fitness
- Diet, nutrition, and eating right
- Healthy lifestyle
- Vaccination/immunizations
- The environment and your health

National Center for Complementary and Alternative Medicine
http://nccam.nih.gov/

For evidence-based information regarding complementary and alternative medicine, this site provides the following links:

- Topics A-Z: Research-based info from acupuncture to zinc
- Safety: Safety info for a variety of products and practices
- Herbs at a glance: Uses and side effects of herbs and botanicals.
- How to find a practitioner: Information on seeking complementary and alternative medicine treatment.

President's Council on Fitness, Sports, and Recreation
http://www.fitness.gov/

This site has abundant resources for fitness, including physical activity guidelines for Americans, exercise and physical activity for older adults, Go4Life (an exercise and physical activity campaign from the National Institute on Aging, designed to help older adults fit exercise and physical activity into their daily life), HealthFinder (wide range of health topics selected from more than 1600 government and nonprofit organizations to bring you reliable health information), Let's Move! (tips for families, community leaders, schools, mayors and local leaders, chefs, and health care providers on what they can do to end childhood obesity), state-based physical activity program directory, and We Can! (Ways to Enhance Children's Activity & Nutrition).

Senior Net
http://www.seniornet.org/php/default.php

This site lists helpful health tips and links to health promotion and prevention practice for older adults, including the following:

- Exercise for older adults: information from the National Institutes of Health (http://nihseniorhealth.gov/exercise/toc.html)
- Info on Aging (http://www.infoaging.org/expert.html)
- Elder Page (http://www.aoa.dhhs.gov/elderpage.html)
- The National Senior Citizens' Law Center (http://www.nsclc.org/)
- American Association of Retired Persons (http://www.aarp.org)
- Secrets of Aging (http://www.secretsofaging.org/)
- Stealing Time (http://www.pbs.org/stealingtime/)
- The Administration on Aging (http://www.aoa.dhhs.gov/)
- National Osteoporosis Foundation (http://www.nof.org/)

US Centers for Medicare & Medicaid Services
https://www.healthcare.gov/

This site provides information related to the Affordable Health Care Act for all constituencies and a Health insurance marketplace for comparing various options for health care.

U.S. Consumer Product Safety Commission
http://www.cpsc.gov/en/Safety-Education/

This site focuses on safety with updated product safety information, educational modules, and safety guides for the public.

- Safety education: all-terrain vehicles, carbon monoxide, cribs, magnets, pool safety, window pull cords
- Safety guides: kids and babies, toys, homes, sports/fitness/recreation, outdoor and garden

US Department of Health and Human Services
http://www.hhs.gov/aca/

This site offers resources regarding the Affordable Health Care Act resources, health insurance, Medicare and Medicaid, families, diseases, preparedness, and prevention.

Reference

1. Kratzke C, Cox C. Smartphone technology and apps: rapidly changing health promotion. *International Electronic Journal of Health Education*. 2012;15:72-82.

Financial Disclosures

Shawn T. Blakeley has no financial or proprietary interest in the materials presented herein.

Ann Marie Decker has no financial or proprietary interest in the materials presented herein.

Shannon DeSalvo has no financial or proprietary interest in the materials presented herein.

Dr. Amy Foley has no financial or proprietary interest in the materials presented herein.

Dr. Martha Highfield has no financial or proprietary interest in the materials presented herein.

Dr. Steven G. Lesh has no financial or proprietary interest in the materials presented herein.

Dr. Gail Regan has no financial or proprietary interest in the materials presented herein.

Dr. Ellen F. Spake has no financial or proprietary interest in the materials presented herein.

Mike Studer has no financial or proprietary interest in the materials presented herein.

Dr. Catherine Rush Thompson has no financial or proprietary interest in the materials presented herein.